Guide to the
Dissection of the Dog

Guide to the
Dissection of the Dog

Eighth Edition

Howard E. Evans, PhD, AVMA (Hon.)
Professor Emeritus of Veterinary and Comparative Anatomy
Department of Biomedical Sciences
College of Veterinary Medicine
Cornell University
Ithaca, New York

Alexander de Lahunta, DVM, PhD, DACVIM-Neurology, DACVP (Hon.)
James Law Professor of Veterinary Anatomy, Emeritus
College of Veterinary Medicine
Cornell University
Ithaca, New York

ELSEVIER

ELSEVIER

3251 Riverport Lane
St. Louis, Missouri 63043

GUIDE TO THE DISSECTION OF THE DOG, EIGHTH EDITION   ISBN: 978-0-323-39165-8

Notices

Knowledge and best practice in this field are constantly changing. As new research and experience broaden our understanding, changes in research methods, professional practices, or medical treatment may become necessary.

Practitioners and researchers must always rely on their own experience and knowledge in evaluating and using any information, methods, compounds, or experiments described herein. In using such information or methods they should be mindful of their own safety and the safety of others, including parties for whom they have a professional responsibility.

With respect to any drug or pharmaceutical products identified, readers are advised to check the most current information provided (i) on procedures featured or (ii) by the manufacturer of each product to be administered, to verify the recommended dose or formula, the method and duration of administration, and contraindications. It is the responsibility of practitioners, relying on their own experience and knowledge of their patients, to make diagnoses, to determine dosages and the best treatment for each individual patient, and to take all appropriate safety precautions.

To the fullest extent of the law, neither the Publisher nor the authors, contributors, or editors, assume any liability for any injury and/or damage to persons or property as a matter of products liability, negligence or otherwise, or from any use or operation of any methods, products, instructions, or ideas contained in the material herein.

Previous editions copyright © 2010, 2004, 2000, 1996, 1988, 1980, 1971.

Library of Congress Cataloging-in-Publication Data
Names: Evans, Howard E., author. | DeLahunta, Alexander, 1932- author.
Title: Guide to the dissection of the dog / Howard E. Evans, PhD, Professor
   Emeritus of Veterinary and Comparative Anatomy, Department of Biomedical
   Sciences, New York State College of Veterinary Medicine, Cornell
   University, Ithaca, New York; Alexander de Lahunta, DVM, PhD, DACVIM,
   DACVP, James Law Professor of Veterinary Anatomy, Emeritus Rye, New
   Hampshire.
Description: Eighth Edition. | St. Louis, Missouri : Elsevier, [2017] |
   Includes bibliographical references and index.
Identifiers: LCCN 2015038543 | ISBN 9780323391658 (hardcover : alk. paper)
Subjects: LCSH: Dogs--Anatomy. | Dogs--Dissection.
Classification: LCC QL813.D64 M54 2017 | DDC 636.7--dc23 LC record available at http://lccn.loc.
gov/2015038543

Director, Content Strategy: Penny Rudolph
Content Development Manager: Jolynn Gower
Senior Content Development Specialist: Brian Loehr
Publishing Services Manager: Jeff Patterson
Book Production Specialist: Carol O'Connell
Design Direction: Brian Salisbury

Printed in China

Last digit is the print number: 9   8   7

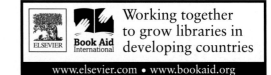

Preface

This edition of *Guide to the Dissection of the Dog* has changed considerably since it was first published as a paperback in 1947 by Malcolm Miller, DVM, PhD, previously Professor and Head of the Department of Anatomy in the New York State Veterinary College at Cornell University. In 1971, *Miller's Guide to the Dissection of the Dog* by Evans and de Lahunta was published in a new format with additional illustrations. Subsequent editions altered the procedures for dissection, added illustrations, and gave instructions for palpation of the live dog. Several editions have been translated into Japanese, Spanish, Portuguese, Korean, and Chinese. This eighth edition includes changes in many figures and the addition of new ones. There is a short atlas of transverse sections of the dog brain selected from the *Brain of the Dog in Section*, by Marcus Singer, and relabeled in accordance with present nomenclature. All terms used are from the latest, free electronic version of the fifth edition of *Nomina Anatomica Veterinaria*.

The purpose of this guide is to facilitate a thorough dissection so as to learn basic mammalian structure and specific features of the dog. We have attempted to emphasize what we believe is essential anatomical knowledge for a veterinary curriculum. The descriptions are based on the dissection of embalmed, arterially injected adult dogs of mixed breeds.

A more detailed consideration of the structures dissected can be found in the fourth edition of *Miller's Anatomy of the Dog* by Evans and de Lahunta published in 2013 by Elsevier.

Howard E. Evans
Alexander de Lahunta

Acknowledgments

We are grateful to many students and colleagues throughout the world for their corrections and helpful suggestions for improvement. Of particular help were Professors Wally Cash of Kansas State, Anton Hoffman of Texas A&M, Elaine Coleman and Mahmoud Mansour of Auburn University, and Gheorghe Constantinescu at the University of Missouri in Columbia, Missouri. We have tried to strike a balance in detail so that teachers can choose what suits their courses best. Our teaching colleagues at Cornell—Marne Fitzmaurice, Abraham Bezuidenhout, Cornelia Farnum, Linda Mizer, John Hermanson, and Paul Maza—have been very helpful. All of our former Deans—George Poppensiek, Robert Phemister, Edward Melby, Franklin Loew, and Donald Smith—have supported our efforts. Our former Dean, Michael Kotlikoff, now Provost of Cornell University, continues to encourage us. Technical and clerical support was cheerfully provided by Pamela Schenck and Jen Patterson. Our veterinary college librarians were very helpful, particularly Susanne Whitaker.

Most of the illustrations were prepared by the late Marion Newson, RN, medical illustrator in the Department of Anatomy. Other drawings were made by former illustrators Pat Barrow, Louis Sadler, and William Hamilton. We especially thank Michael Simmons, the past College Illustrator, for his illustrations and skillful corrections.

Contents

Illustrations

Tables

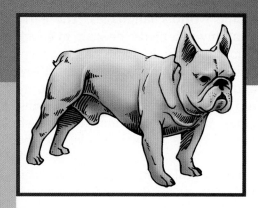

Anatomical Terminology

CHAPTER OUTLINE

Anatomy is the study of structure. Physiology is the study of function. Structure and function are inseparable as the foundation of the science and art of medicine. One must know the parts before one can appreciate how they work. **Gross anatomy,** the study of structures that can be dissected and observed with the unaided eye or with a hand lens, forms the subject matter of this guide.

The anatomy of one part in relation to other parts of the body is **topographical anatomy.** The practical application of such knowledge in the diagnosis and treatment of pathological conditions is **applied anatomy.** The study of structures too small to be seen without a light microscope is **microscopic anatomy.** Examination of structure in even greater detail is possible with an electron microscope and constitutes **ultrastructural anatomy.** When an animal becomes diseased or its organs function improperly, its deviation from the normal is studied as **pathological anatomy.** The study of the development of the individual from the fertilized oocyte to birth is **embryology,** and from the zygote to the adult it is known as **developmental anatomy.** The study of abnormal development is **teratology.**

MEDICAL ETYMOLOGY AND ANATOMICAL NOMENCLATURE

The student of anatomy is confronted with an array of unfamiliar terms and names of anatomical structures. A better understanding of the language of anatomy helps make its study more intelligible and interesting. For the publication of scientific papers and communication with colleagues, the mastery of anatomical terminology is a necessity. To ensure knowledge of basic anatomical terms, a medical dictionary should be kept readily accessible and consulted frequently. It is very important to learn the spelling, pronunciation, and meaning of all new terms encountered. Vertebrate structures are numerous, and in many instances common names are not available or are so vague as to be meaningless. One soon realizes why it is desirable to have an international glossary of terms that can be understood by scientists in all countries. Acquisition of a medical vocabulary can be aided by the mastery of Greek and Latin roots and affixes.

Our present medical vocabulary has a history dating back more than 2000 years and reflects the influences of the world's languages. The early writings in anatomy and medicine were in Greek and later almost entirely in Latin. As a consequence, most anatomical terms stem from these classical languages. Latin terms are commonly translated into the vernacular of the person using them. Thus the Latin *hepar* becomes the English *liver,* the French *foie,* the Spanish *higado,* and the German *Leber.*

Although anatomical terminology has been rather uniform, differences in terms have arisen between the different fields and different countries. In 1895 a group of anatomists proposed a standard list of terms derived from those in use throughout the world. This list, known as the *Basle Nomina Anatomica* (BNA), formed the basis for the present sixth edition of *Nomina Anatomica* (NA) 1989, which was prepared by the International Anatomical Nomenclature Committee (IANC) and adopted by the International Congress of Anatomists in Paris in 1955. Of the 5640 standard terms, more than 80% are continued from the BNA. In response to dissatisfaction with the work of the last committee (IANC), the International Federation of Associations of Anatomists created a new committee in 1989, the Federative Committee on Anatomical Terminology (FCAT), to write *Terminologia Anatomica* (TA), which was published in 1998. This new list of terms gives each term in Latin accompanied by the current usage in English-speaking countries. There is an index to Latin and English terms as well as to eponyms (Thieme Publishers, Stuttgart and New York). Both the NA and TA lists are for human anatomy.

The International Committee on Veterinary Anatomical Nomenclature (ICVAN), appointed by the World Association of Veterinary Anatomists in 1957, published *Nomina Anatomica Veterinaria* (NAV) for domestic mammals in 1968. These terms, as revised in the fifth edition in 2005 (published on the World Wide Web), serve as the basis for the nomenclature used in this guide.

DIRECTIONAL TERMS

An understanding of the following planes, positions, and directions relative to the animal body or its parts is necessary to follow the procedures for dissection (Fig. 1-1).

PLANE: A surface, real or imaginary, along which any two points can be connected by a straight line.

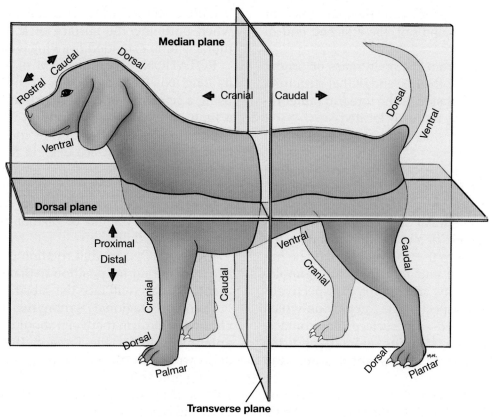

Fig. 1-1 Directional terms.

Median Plane: Divides the head, body, or limb longitudinally into equal right and left halves. Sagittal Plane: Passes through the head, body, or limb parallel to the median plane. Transverse Plane: Cuts across the head, body, or limb at a right angle to its long axis or across the long axis of an organ or a part. Dorsal Plane: Runs at right angles to the median and transverse planes and thus divides the body or head into dorsal and ventral portions.

DORSAL: Toward or relatively near the upper surface (as opposed to the supporting surface) of the head, body, and tail. This surface is opposite to the supporting surface in the standing animal. On the limbs it applies to the upper or front surface of the carpus, tarsus, metapodium, and digits (opposite to the side with the pads).

VENTRAL: Toward or relatively near the supporting surface and the corresponding surface of the head, neck, thorax, and tail. This term is never used for the limbs.

MEDIAL: Toward or relatively near the median plane.

LATERAL: Away from or relatively farther from the median plane.

CRANIAL: Toward or relatively near the head; on the limbs it applies proximal to the carpus and tarsus. In reference to the head, it is replaced by the term *rostral.*

ROSTRAL: Toward or relatively near the nose; applies to the head only.

CAUDAL: Toward or relatively near the tail; on the limbs it applies proximal to the carpus and tarsus. Also used in reference to the head.

The adjectives for directional terms may be modified to serve as adverbs by replacing the ending *al* with the ending *ally,* as in *dorsally.*

Certain terms whose meanings are more restricted are used in the description of organs and appendages.

INTERNAL or INNER: Close to, or in the direction of, the center of an organ, body cavity, or structure.

EXTERNAL or OUTER: Away from the center of an organ or structure.

SUPERFICIAL: Relatively near the surface of the body or the surface of a solid organ.

DEEP: Relatively near the center of the body or the center of a solid organ.

PROXIMAL: Relatively near the main mass or origin; in the limbs and tail, the attached end of that structure.

DISTAL: Away from the main mass or origin; in the limbs and tail, the free end of that structure.

RADIAL: On that side of the forearm (antebrachium) in which the radius is located.

ULNAR: On that side of the forearm in which the ulna is located.

TIBIAL and FIBULAR: On the corresponding sides of the leg (crus), the tibial side being medial and the fibular side being lateral.

In the dog and similar species, the paw is that part of the thoracic or pelvic limb distal to the radius and ulna or to the tibia and fibula. The human hand (manus) and foot (pes) are homologous with the forepaw and hindpaw, respectively.

PALMAR: The aspect of the forepaw on which the pads are located—the surface that contacts the ground in the standing animal—and the corresponding surface of the metacarpus and carpus.

PLANTAR: The aspect of the hindpaw on which the pads are located—the surface that contacts the ground in the standing animal—and the corresponding surface of the metatarsus and tarsus. The opposite surface of both forepaw and hindpaw is known as the *dorsal surface.*

AXIS: The central line of the body or any of its parts.

AXIAL, ABAXIAL: Of, pertaining to, or relative to the axis. In reference to the digits, the functional axis of the limb passes between the third and fourth digits. The axial surface of the digit faces the axis, and the abaxial surface faces away from the axis.

The following terms apply to the various basic movements of the parts of the body.

FLEXION: The movement of one bone in relation to another in such a manner that the angle formed at their joint is reduced. The limb is retracted or folded; the digit is bent; the back is arched dorsally.

EXTENSION: The movement of one bone upon another such that the angle formed at their joint increases. The limb reaches out or is extended; the digit is straightened; the back is straightened. Extension beyond 180 degrees is overextension.

ABDUCTION: The movement of a part away from the median plane.

ADDUCTION: The movement of a part toward the median plane.

CIRCUMDUCTION: The movement of a part when outlining the surface of a cone (e.g., the thoracic limb extended drawing a circle).

ROTATION: The movement of a part around its long axis (e.g., the action of the radius when using a screwdriver). The direction of rotation of a limb or segment of a limb on its long axis is designated by the direction of movement of its cranial or dorsal surface (e.g., in medial rotation of the arm, the crest of the greater tubercle is turned medially).

SUPINATION: Lateral rotation of the appendage so that the palmar or plantar surface of the paw faces medially.

PRONATION: Medial rotation of the appendage from the supine position so that the palmar or plantar surface will face the substrate.

Common regional synonyms include **brachium** for the arm (between shoulder and elbow), **antebrachium** for the forearm (between elbow and carpus), **thigh** for the pelvic limb (between the hip and stifle), and **crus** for the leg (between stifle and tarsus). The pelvic limb is not the leg. Only the crus is the leg.

On radiographs the view is described in relation to the direction of penetration by the x-ray: from point of entrance to point of exit of the body part before striking the film. Oblique views are described with combined terms. A view of the carpus with the x-ray tube perpendicular to the dorsal surface and the film on the palmar surface would be a dorsopalmar view. If the x-ray tube is turned so that it points toward the dorsomedial surface of the carpus and the film is on the palmarolateral surface, the view would be dorsomedial-palmarolateral oblique. If the animal is lying on its right side, adjacent to the radiographic film, the radiograph is a left-to-right lateral view.

DISSECTION

The dog provided for dissection has been humanely prepared by injection of pentobarbital for anesthesia through the cephalic vein and by exsanguination through a cannula inserted in the common carotid artery. This procedure allows the pumping action of the heart to empty the blood vessels before the injection of embalming fluid consisting of 5% formalin, 2% phenol, and 30% ethanol in aqueous solution. It is injected under 5 lb of pressure over a period of approximately 30 minutes. After embalming, the arteries are injected with red latex, also through the common carotid artery, from a 50-mL hand syringe. A well-kept specimen facilitates dissection and study throughout the course. Gauze moistened with 2% phenoxyethanol, 1% phenol, or other antifungal agents helps to prevent spoilage. Plastic bags can be used to wrap the paws and head and plastic sheeting to cover the entire specimen to prevent desiccation between dissection periods. Refrigeration is helpful for storage but is not essential.

There are certain principles and procedures that are generally accepted as aids in the learning of anatomy. The purpose of the dissection is to gain a clear understanding of the normal structures of the body and their relationships, and an appreciation for individual variation. Radiography and the more recent development of imaging procedures such as computed tomography (CT), magnetic resonance imaging (MRI), and ultrasonography (US) require a clear understanding of these relationships and the ability to interpret three-dimensional anatomy from two-dimensional views. (For a presentation of canine gross anatomy in planar section correlated with US and CT, see Feeney et al. in the Bibliography.)

2 CHAPTER

The Skeletal and Muscular Systems

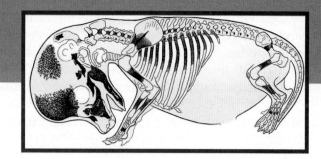

CHAPTER OUTLINE

Before dissection of muscles is explained, the bones of that region (Fig. 2-1) are described. A thorough understanding of the relationships of muscles and bones facilitates learning the muscular attachments and functions.

The **appendicular skeleton** includes the bones of the thoracic girdle and forelimbs and the pelvic girdle and hindlimbs (Table 2-1, Fig. 2-2).

The **axial skeleton** consists of the bones of the skull; hyoid apparatus; cartilages of the larynx; and bones of the vertebral column, ribs, and sternum.

BONES OF THE THORACIC LIMB

The **thoracic girdle** consists of paired scapulae and clavicles (see Fig. 2-10). The scapula is large, whereas the **clavicle** is reduced. The dog's clavicle (see Fig. 2-10) is a small oval plate located cranial to the shoulder within the clavicular tendon in the brachiocephalicus muscle (see Fig. 2-12). The clavicle is one of the first bones to show a center of ossification in the fetal dog, but in the adult it is partly or completely cartilaginous. It is frequently visible in dorsoventral radiographs of the trunk, medial to the shoulder joint.

Scapula

The scapula (Figs. 2-3 and 2-4), a flat, approximately triangular bone, possesses two surfaces, three borders, and three angles. The ventral angle is the distal or articular end that forms the **glenoid cavity**, and the constricted part that unites with the expanded blade is referred to as the **neck**.

Table **2-1**	Bones of the Appendicular Skeleton
Thoracic Limb (Forelimb)	**Pelvic Limb (Hindlimb)**
Thoracic Girdle	**Pelvic Girdle**
Scapula	Ilium
Clavicle	Ischium
	Pubis
Arm or Brachium	**Thigh**
Humerus	Femur
	Patella
Forearm or Antebrachium	**Leg or Crus**
Radius	Tibia
Ulna	Fibula
Forepaw or Manus	**Hindpaw or Pes**
Carpal bones	Tarsal bones
Metacarpal bones	Metatarsal bones
Phalanges	Phalanges

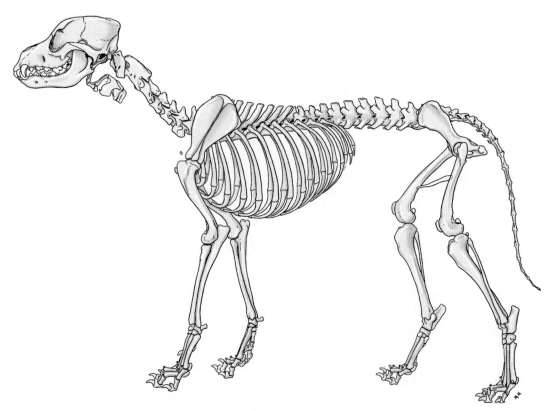

Fig. 2-1   Skeleton of male dog. A, Lateral view of skeleton.

Continued

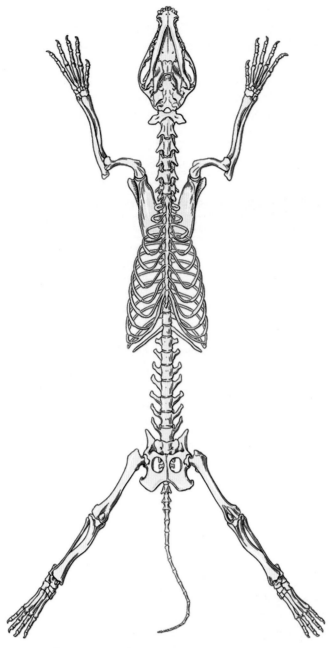

Fig. 2-1—cont'd B, Ventral view of skeleton. (Part B from Evans HE, de Lahunta A: *Miller's anatomy of the dog*, ed 4, St Louis, 2013, Saunders.)

The lateral surface (see Fig. 2-3, *A*) of the scapula is divided into two nearly equal fossae by a shelf of bone, the **spine** of the scapula. The spine is the most prominent feature of the bone. It begins at the dorsal border as a thick, low ridge and becomes thinner and wider toward the neck. In all breeds the free border is slightly thickened, and in some it is everted caudally. The distal end is a truncated process, the **acromion**, where part of the deltoideus muscle arises. On a continuation of the spine proximally, the omotransversarius attaches. The remaining part of the spine provides a place for insertion of the trapezius and for origin of that part of the deltoideus that does not arise from the acromion.

The **supraspinous fossa** is the entire lateral surface cranial to the spine of the scapula. The supraspinatus arises from all but the distal part of this fossa.

The **infraspinous fossa**, caudal to the spine, is triangular, with the apex at the neck. The infraspinatus arises from the infraspinous fossa.

The medial or costal surface has two areas (see Fig. 2-3, *B*). A small proximal and cranial rectangular area, the **serrated face**, serves as insertion for the serratus ventralis muscle. The large remaining part of the costal surface is the **subscapular fossa**, which is nearly flat and usually presents three straight muscular lines that converge distally. The subscapularis arises from the whole subscapular fossa.

The **cranial border** of the scapula is thin. Near the ventral angle the border is concave as it enters into the formation of the neck. The notch thus formed is the **scapular notch**. The dorsal end of the cranial border thickens and, without definite demarcation at the **cranial angle**, is continuous with the dorsal border.

The **dorsal border** extends from the **cranial** to the **caudal angles**. In life it is capped by a narrow band of cartilage, but in the dried specimen the cartilage is destroyed by ordinary preparation methods. The rhomboideus attaches to this border.

Just proximal to the ventral angle, the thick **caudal border** bears the **infraglenoid tubercle**, from which arise the teres minor and the long head of the triceps. The middle third of the caudal border of the scapula is broad and smooth; part of the subscapularis and the long head of the triceps arise from it. Somewhat less than a third of the dorsal segment of the caudal border is thick and gives rise to the teres major.

The **ventral angle** forms the expanded distal end of the scapula. The adjacent constricted part, the **neck**, is the segment of the scapula distal to the spine and proximal to the expanded part of the bone that forms the glenoid cavity. Clinically, the ventral angle is by far the most important part of the scapula, because it enters into the formation of the shoulder joint. The **glenoid cavity** articulates with the head of the humerus. Observe the shallowness of the cavity.

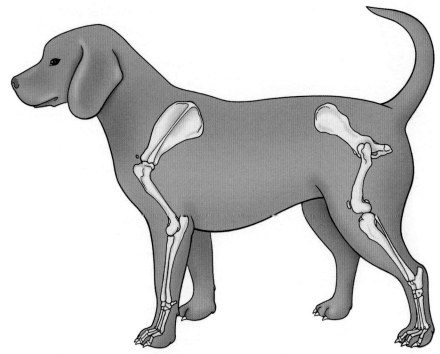

Fig. 2-2 Topography of appendicular skeleton.

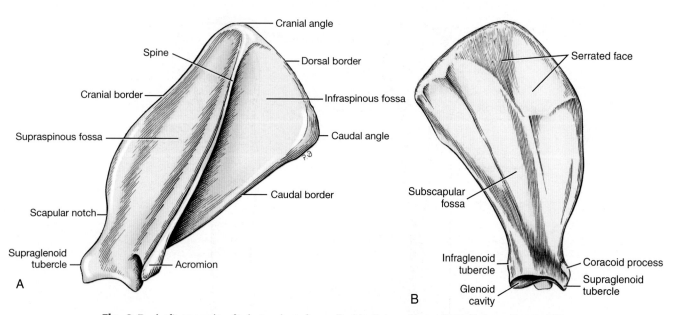

Fig. 2-3 Left scapula. **A,** Lateral surface. **B,** Medial surface. (Part B from Evans HE, de Lahunta A: *Miller's anatomy of the dog,* ed 4, St Louis, 2013, Saunders.)

The **supraglenoid tubercle** is an eminence at the cranial part of the glenoid cavity. The tubercle shows a slight medial inclination on which a small tubercle, the **coracoid process**, can be distinguished. The coracobrachialis arises from the coracoid process, whereas the biceps brachii arises from the supraglenoid tubercle.

LIVE DOG

Palpate the borders of the scapula, spine, acromion, and supraglenoid tubercle.

Humerus

The humerus (Fig. 2-5) is located in the arm, or brachium. This bone enters into the formation of

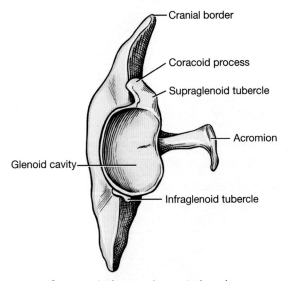

Fig. 2-4   Left scapula, ventral angle.

both the shoulder joint and the elbow joint. The shoulder joint is formed by the articulation of the scapula and humerus; the elbow joint is formed by the articulation of the radius and ulna with each other and with the humerus. The proximal extremity of the humerus includes the head, neck, and the greater and lesser tubercles. The distal extremity, the condyle, includes the trochlea, capitulum, and the radial and olecranon fossae, which communicate proximal to the trochlea through the supratrochlear foramen. The medial and lateral epicondyles are situated on the sides of the condyle. The body of the humerus lies between the two extremities.

The **head** of the humerus is the part that articulates with the glenoid cavity of the scapula. It presents more than twice the area of the glenoid cavity and is elongated sagittally. Although the shoulder joint is a typical ball-and-socket joint, it normally undergoes only flexion and extension. The **intertubercular groove** begins at the cranial

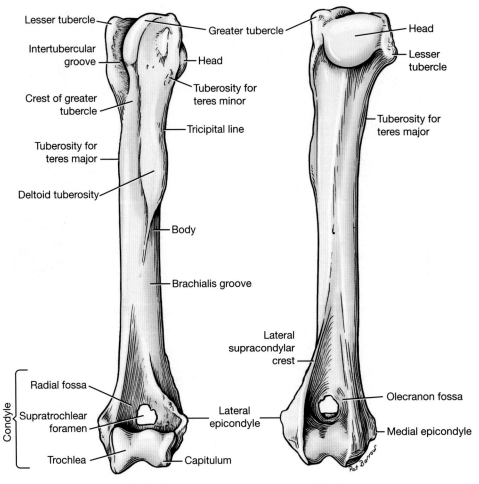

Fig. 2-5   Left humerus, cranial and caudal views.

end of the articular area. It lodges the tendon of origin of the biceps brachii and is deflected toward the median plane by the **greater tubercle**, which forms the craniolateral part of the proximal extremity. The greater tubercle is convex at its summit and, in most breeds, higher than the head. It is continued distally in the body of the humerus by the crest of the greater tubercle. The greater tubercle receives the insertions of the supraspinatus and the infraspinatus and part of the deep pectoral. Between the head of the humerus and the greater tubercle are several foramina for the transmission of vessels. The infraspinatus is inserted on the smooth facet on the lateral side of the greater tubercle. The **lesser tubercle** lies on the medial side of the proximal extremity of the humerus, caudal to the intertubercular groove. It is not as high or as large as the greater tubercle. The subscapularis attaches to its proximal border. The **neck** of the humerus is not distinct except caudally. It is the line along which the head and parts of the tubercles have fused with the body.

The **cranial surface** of the humerus is distinct in the middle third of the body, where it furnishes attachment for the brachiocephalicus and part of the pectorals. Distally it fades but may be considered to continue to the medial lip of the trochlea. On the proximal third of the cranial border are two ridges. They continue to the cranial and caudal parts of the greater tubercle. The ridge that extends proximally in a craniomedial direction is the **crest of the greater tubercle** and is also the cranial border of the bone. This forms part of the area of insertion of the pectorals and the cleidobrachialis.

The ridge extending to the caudal part of the greater tubercle is on the **lateral surface** of the humerus. Distally it is thickened to form the **deltoid tuberosity**. The deltoideus inserts here. From this tuberosity to the caudal part of the greater tubercle, the ridge forms the prominent **tricipital line**. The lateral head of the triceps arises from this line. The teres minor inserts on the **tuberosity of the teres minor** adjacent to the proximal extremity of the tricipital line. The smooth **brachialis groove** is on the lateral surface of the body. The brachialis, which originates in the proximal part of the groove, spirals around the bone in the groove so that distally it lies on the craniolateral surface. Distal to this groove is the thick **lateral supracondylar crest**. The extensor carpi radialis

and part of the anconeus attach here. The crest extends distally to the lateral epicondyle.

The **caudal surface** is smooth and rounded transversely and ends in the deep olecranon fossa.

The **crest of the lesser tubercle** crosses the proximal end of the **medial surface** and ends distally at the **teres major tuberosity**. The teres major and latissimus dorsi are inserted on this tuberosity. Caudal and proximal to this, the medial head of the triceps arises and the coracobrachialis is inserted. Approximately the middle third of the medial surface is free of muscular attachment and is smooth.

The distal end of the humerus, including its articular areas and the adjacent fossae, is the **humeral condyle**. The articular surface is divided unevenly by a low ridge. The large area medial to the ridge is the **trochlea**, which articulates with both the radius and the ulna and extends proximally into the adjacent fossae. The articulation with the trochlear notch of the ulna is one of the most stable hinge joints (ginglymus) in the body. The small articular area lateral to the ridge is the **capitulum**, which articulates only with the head of the radius.

The **lateral epicondyle** is smaller than the medial one and occupies the enlarged distolateral end of the humerus proximal to the capitulum. It gives origin to the common digital extensor, lateral digital extensor, ulnaris lateralis, and supinator. The lateral collateral ligament of the elbow also attaches here. The lateral supracondylar crest extends proximally from this epicondyle and is the origin for the extensor carpi radialis.

The **medial epicondyle** is the enlarged distomedial end of the humerus proximal to the trochlea. Its caudal projection deepens the olecranon fossa. The anconeus arises from this projection. The elevated portion of the medial epicondyle serves as origin for flexor carpi radialis, flexor carpi ulnaris, pronator teres, and the superficial and deep digital flexor muscles. The medial collateral ligament of the elbow also attaches here.

The **olecranon fossa** is a deep excavation of the caudal part of the humeral condyle. It receives the anconeal process of the ulna during extension of the elbow. On the cranial surface of the humeral condyle is the **radial fossa**, which communicates with the olecranon fossa by an opening, the **supratrochlear foramen**. No soft structures pass through this foramen.

Radius

The radius and ulna are the bones of the antebrachium, or forearm. It is important to know that they cross each other obliquely so that the proximal end of the ulna is medial and the distal end is lateral to the radius. The radius (Fig. 2-6), the shorter of the two bones of the forearm, articulates proximally with the humerus and distally with the carpus. It also articulates with the ulna, proximally by its caudal surface and distally near its lateral border.

The proximal extremity consists of head, neck, and tuberosity. The **head** of the radius, like the whole bone, is widest medial to lateral. It forms proximally an oval, depressed articular surface, the **fovea capitis**, which articulates with the capitulum of the humerus. The smooth caudal border of the head is the **articular circumference** for articulation with the radial notch of the ulna. The small **radial tuberosity** lies distal to the neck on the medial border of the bone. The biceps brachii and brachialis insert in part on this tubercle.

The **body** of the radius is compressed so that it possesses cranial and caudal surfaces and medial and lateral borders. It is slightly convex cranially. At the carpal end, the body blends without sharp demarcation with the enlarged distal extremity. The caudal surface of the radius is roughened and slightly concave. It has a ligamentous attachment to the ulna. Distally it broadens and becomes the expanded caudal surface of the distal extremity. The cranial surface of the radius, convex transversely, is relatively smooth throughout.

The distal extremity of the radius is the **trochlea**. Its carpal articular surface is concave. On the lateral surface of the distal extremity is the **ulnar notch**, a slightly concave area with a facet for articulation with the ulna. The medial surface of the distal extremity ends in a rounded projection, the **styloid process**. The medial collateral ligament of the carpus attaches proximal to the styloid process. The cranial surface of the distal extremity presents three distinct grooves. The most medial groove, which is small, short, and oblique, contains the tendon of the abductor digiti I longus. The middle and longest groove, extending proximally on the shaft of the radius, is for the extensor carpi radialis. The most lateral of the grooves on this surface is

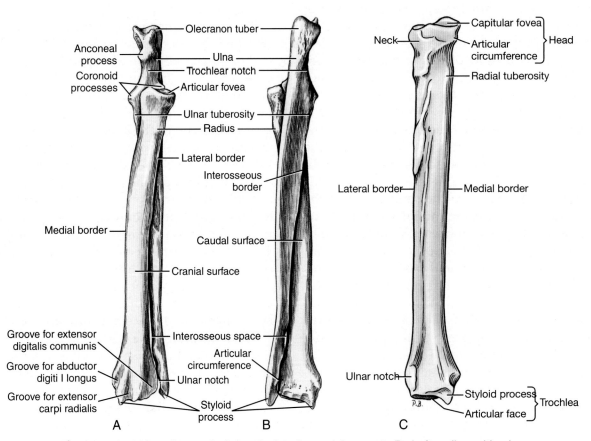

Fig. 2-6 A, Left radius and ulna articulated, cranial aspect. **B,** Left radius with ulna articulated, caudal aspect. **C,** Left radius, caudal view. (Parts A and B from Evans HE, de Lahunta A: *Miller's anatomy of the dog*, ed 4, St Louis, 2013, Saunders.)

wide and of variable distinctness. It contains the tendon of the common digital extensor.

Ulna

The ulna (Figs. 2-6, 2-7) is located in the caudal part of the forearm. It exceeds the radius in length and is irregular in shape and generally tapers from its proximal to its distal end. Proximally the ulna is medial to the radius and articulates with the trochlea of the humerus by the **trochlear notch** and with the articular circumference of the radius by the **radial notch**. This forms the elbow. Distally the ulna is lateral and articulates with the radius medially and with the ulnar and accessory carpal bones distally.

The proximal extremity is the **olecranon**, which includes the olecranon tuber and the anconeal process. It serves as a lever arm for the extensor muscles of the elbow. It is four-sided, laterally compressed, and medially inclined. Its proximal

end, the **olecranon tuber**, is grooved cranially and enlarged and rounded caudally. The triceps brachii, anconeus, and tensor fasciae antebrachii attach to the caudal part of the olecranon. The ulnar portions of the flexor carpi ulnaris and deep digital flexor arise from its medial surface.

The **trochlear notch** is a smooth, vertical, half-moon–shaped concavity facing cranially. The whole trochlear notch articulates with the trochlea of the humerus. At its proximal end a sharp-edged, slightly hooked **anconeal process** fits into the olecranon fossa of the humerus when the elbow joint is extended. At the distal end of the notch are the **medial** and **lateral coronoid processes**, which articulate with the humerus and radius. The medial coronoid process is larger. Between these processes is the radial notch for articulation with the articular circumference of the radius.

The **body** of the ulna is three-sided in its middle third; proximal to this the bone is compressed laterally, whereas the distal third gradually loses its borders, becomes irregular, and is continued by the pointed distal extremity. The **ulnar tuberosity** is a small, elongated eminence on the medial surface of the bone at its proximal end, just distal to the medial coronoid process. The biceps brachii and the brachialis insert on this eminence. The **interosseous border** is distinct, rough, and irregular, especially at the junction of the proximal and middle thirds of the bone, where a large, expansive, but low eminence is found. This eminence indicates the place of articulation with the radius by means of a heavy ligament. Frequently, a vascular groove medial to the crest marks the position of the caudal interosseous artery. This groove is most conspicuous in the middle third of the ulna. The body shows a distinct caudal concavity.

The distal extremity of the ulna is the head with its prominent **styloid process**. A part of this process articulates with the ulnar and accessory carpal bones. The head articulates medially with the radius.

Carpal Bones

The term **carpus** (Figs. 2-8 through 2-10) is used to designate that part of the extremity between the antebrachium and metacarpus that includes all the soft structures as well as the bones. The carpus includes seven small, irregular bones arranged into two rows. These are most conveniently studied on radiographs. The proximal row contains three bones. The largest of these, the **intermedioradial**

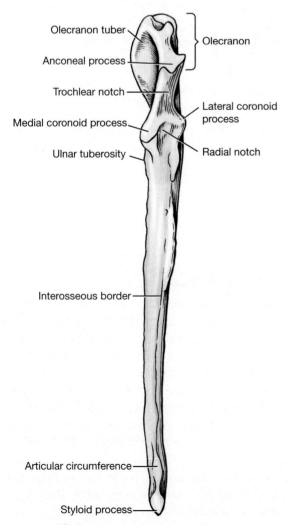

Olecranon tuber

Anconeal process

Olecranon

Trochlear notch

Medial coronoid process

Lateral coronoid process

Ulnar tuberosity

Radial notch

Interosseous border

Articular circumference

Styloid process

Fig. 2-7 Left ulna, cranial view.

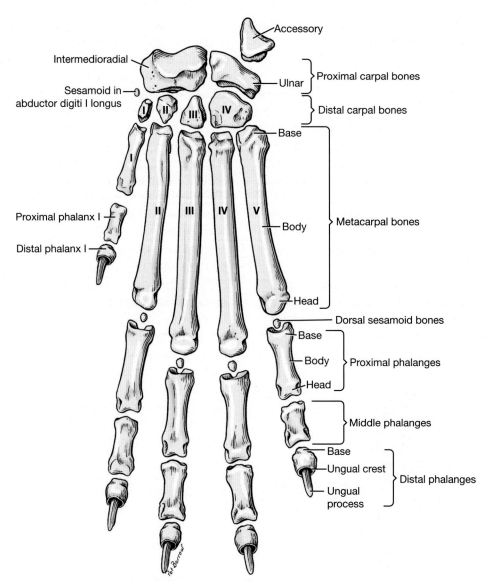

Fig. 2-8 Bones of left forepaw, dorsal view.

carpal, is on the medial side and articulates proximally with the radius. The **ulnar carpal** is the lateral member of the proximal row. Its palmar portion projects distally palmar and lateral to the fourth carpal bone. The **accessory carpal**, the palmar member, is a short rod of bone that articulates with the styloid process of the ulna and the ulnar carpal bone and serves as a lever arm for some of the flexor muscles of the carpus. The distal row consists of four bones numbered from the medial to the lateral side. From the smallest on the medial side, these are the **first, second, third,** and **fourth carpal bones.** The fourth carpal bone is the largest and articulates with the base of the fourth and fifth metacarpals.

Metacarpal Bones

The **metacarpus** (see Figs. 2-8 and 2-9) contains five bones. The metacarpal bones are long bones in miniature, possessing a slender **body**, or shaft, and large extremities. The proximal extremity is the **base**, and the distal one is the **head**. The metacarpals, like the carpals and digits, are numbered from medial to lateral. Proximally all articulate principally with the corresponding carpal bones, except the fifth, which articulates with the fourth carpal. Distally all articulate with the corresponding proximal phalanges. Note the sagittal ridge on the head for articulation with the sagittal groove in the base of the corresponding proximal phalanx. The interosseous muscles largely fill the

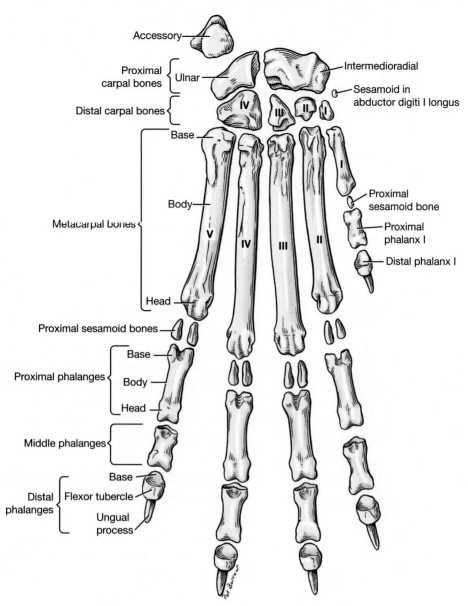

Fig. 2-9   Bones of left forepaw, palmar view.

intermetacarpal spaces palmar to the metacarpal bones.

The first metacarpal bone is atypical. It is a vestigial structure, but unlike the first metatarsal bone in the hindpaw, it is constantly present.

Phalanges

In the forepaw there are three phalanges for each of the four main digits (see Figs. 2-8 and 2-9); the first digit, or pollex, a dewclaw, has two phalanges. Each proximal and middle phalanx has a proximal **base**, a **body**, and a distal **head**.

On the distal phalanx, a thin shelf of bone, the **ungual crest**, overlaps the claw and forms a band of bone around the proximal portion of the claw.

The **ungual process** is a curved conical extension of the distal phalanx into the claw. The rounded dorsal part of the base is the **extensor process** on which the common digital extensor tendon is inserted. A small process on the palmar surface is the **flexor tubercle** for insertion of the deep digital flexor tendon.

Two **proximal sesamoid bones** are located in the interosseous tendons on the palmar surface of each metacarpophalangeal joint (digits II–V). Four small **dorsal sesamoid bones** (none for the first digit) are embedded in the common digital extensor tendons as they pass over the metacarpophalangeal joints (see Figs. 2-8 and 2-9).

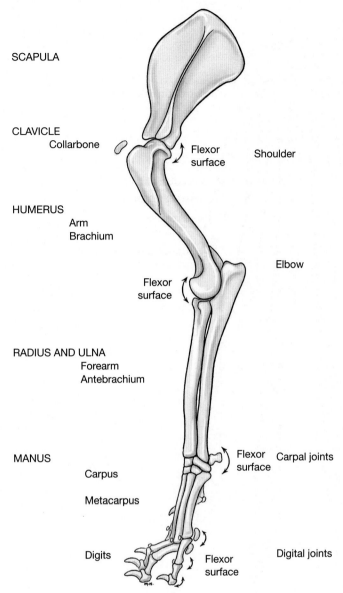

SCAPULA

CLAVICLE
Collarbone

Flexor surface

Shoulder

HUMERUS
Arm
Brachium

Flexor surface

Elbow

RADIUS AND ULNA
Forearm
Antebrachium

MANUS
Carpus
Metacarpus

Flexor surface

Carpal joints

Digits

Flexor surface

Digital joints

Fig. 2-10 Left forelimb skeleton and flexor surfaces of the joints.

LIVE DOG

Flex and extend the shoulder joint. Palpate the greater tubercle of the humerus. Follow its cranial part to the crest of the greater tubercle and cranial border of the humerus. Palpate the groove medial to the greater tubercle and its crest. Palpate the deltoid tuberosity on the lateral surface of the body and the epicondyles on the condyle of the humerus. Note the width of the condyle at the elbow and the more prominent medial epicondyle.

Because of the size of the medial epicondyle, most elbow joint separations (luxations) caused by injury result in the humerus being displaced medial to the ulna. Note that replacement would require flexion of the elbow to allow the anconeal process of the ulna to pass over the crest of the lateral epicondyle.

Flex and extend the elbow. Palpate the olecranon tubercle proximally, the head of the radius laterally, and the medial coronoid process of the ulna medially deep to the muscles. Note that the combined radius and ulna at the elbow are not as wide as the humeral condyle. Flex and extend the antebrachiocarpal joint and palpate the styloid process of the radius medially and ulna laterally.

Flex and extend the carpus. Note that the major motion is at the antebrachiocarpal joint. Palpate the accessory carpal. Palpate the metacarpals and phalanges and flex and extend the metacarpophalangeal and interphalangeal joints. Note that the flexor surface of the metacarpophalangeal joint is the palmar surface despite being the wider angle while bearing weight. Note the relationship of the metacarpal pad to the metacarpophalangeal joints and the digital pads to the distal interphalangeal joints.

MUSCLES OF THE THORACIC LIMB
Superficial Structures of the Thorax

General study of the ventral surface of the trunk should be made before the dissection of the thoracic region is begun. Find the **umbilicus**. This is represented by a scar that may be either flat or slightly raised and is located on the midventral line, one third to one fourth of the distance from the xiphoid cartilage to the scrotum or vulva. In most dogs it is hidden by hair. The umbilicus is irregularly oval and may be from a few millimeters to a centimeter in length. The umbilicus serves as a landmark in abdominal surgery. Notice that the hair over a large area around the umbilicus slants toward it, thus forming a **vortex**.

Pick up a fold of skin, or **common integument**, which consists of an outer thin epithelium, the **epidermis**, and an underlying thicker layer of connective tissue, the **dermis**. Skin thickness varies on different parts of the body, depending on the extent of the dermis. Notice that the skin is thickest in the neck region, thinner over the sternum, and thinnest on the ventral surface of the abdomen; also notice that the skin of the dorsum of the neck and thorax is loosely attached.

The mammae vary in number from 8 to 12, but 10 is average. They are situated in two rows, usually opposite each other. The number is usually reduced in the smaller breeds.

When 10 glands are present, the cranial 4 are the **thoracic mammae**, the following 4 are the **abdominal mammae**, and the caudal 2 are the **inguinal mammae**. When the abdominal and inguinal mammae are maximally developed, the glandular tissue in each row appears to form a continuous mass. The mammae lie in areolar connective tissue and are not fused to the body wall. The cranial pair of thoracic mammae are smaller than the other pair. Each mamma has a papilla, or nipple, that is partly hairless and contains about 12 openings, but these vary and are difficult to see if the animal is not lactating.

The costal cartilages of the tenth, eleventh, and twelfth ribs unite with each other to form the **costal arch**. Palpate this arch and the caudal border and free end of the last or thirteenth rib. This rib does not attach to the costal arch and is therefore called a "floating rib."

Make a midventral incision *through the skin only* from the cranial end of the neck to the umbilicus (Fig. 2-11). From the umbilicus extend a transverse incision to the mid-dorsal line on the **left side**. From a point on the midventral incision directly opposite the arm, extend a transverse incision to the left elbow. Make a complete circular incision through the skin around the elbow. Extend a third transverse incision from the cranial end of the midventral incision to the mid-dorsal line on the left side. This should pass just caudal to the ear. Carefully reflect the skin of the thorax and neck to the mid-dorsal line. The skin will be intimately fused with the thin underlying **cutaneous** muscle over the neck, thorax, and abdomen. The muscle should be left on the specimen as far as is possible.

The subcutaneous tissue that now confronts the dissector is composed of areolar tissue and fascia. **Areolar tissue** appears as a thin layer of loose, irregularly arranged connective tissue that often contains fat. **Fascia** is a denser, more regularly arranged thin layer of connective tissue. It is more fibrous, and it envelops the body beneath the skin and encloses individual muscles or groups of muscles. The **superficial fascia** is deep to the areolar tissue, forming the deep portion of the subcutaneous tissue that covers the entire body. It blends with the **deep fascia**, which is more firmly attached to the muscle that it encloses. These are not always easily distinguished from each other. The areolar tissue is often distended with embalming fluid. (Clinical subcutaneous injections are made into this tissue.) When the fatty areolar tissue and fascia with vessels and nerves are removed from a muscle, the muscle is said to be "cleaned."

All muscles have attachments. In most instances the more proximal attachment, the part that moves the least, is considered the **origin**. The **insertion** is the more distal attachment, or the part that moves the most. The origin is usually a direct attachment of the muscle cells to the bone. The insertion often is by a tendon or aponeurosis extending from the muscle cells to the bone. A **tendon** consists of dense, regularly arranged fibrous connective tissue organized into a small, well-defined bundle. An **aponeurosis** has the same consistency as a tendon, but the fibrous tissue is arranged as a thin sheet of tissue. A **ligament** is dense fibrous connective tissue between bones, although the term is also used for a variety of thin fibrous connections between organs or between an organ and the body wall.

Read before you dissect! In many instances, during the study of muscles, a description of a specific muscle will be given before the instructions for dissection. At no time should muscles be removed or even transected without instructions. In each instance clean the exposed surface of the muscle being described, isolate its borders, and verify its origin and insertion. If the muscle is to be "transected," free it from underlying structures first. As each muscle is defined, visualize its attachments and position on the skeleton and understand its function.

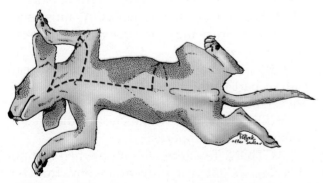

Fig. 2-11 Dissection position and first skin incisions.

The **cutaneous trunci** (see Figs. 2-15 and 2-17) is a thin sheet of muscle that covers most of the dorsal, lateral, and ventral walls of the thorax and abdomen. It has no direct bony attachments. It is more closely applied to the skin than to underlying structures and is often reflected with the skin before being observed. Like all cutaneous muscles, it is developed in the superficial fascia of the thorax and abdomen. Caudal to the shoulder the fibers sweep obliquely toward the axilla; farther caudally they are principally longitudinal and arise from the superficial fascia over the pelvic region.

The attachments of the cutaneous trunci are the superficial fascia of the trunk and the skin. The muscle sends a fasciculus to the medial side of the forelimb; caudal and ventral to this the fibers fray out over the deep pectoral muscle. The cutaneous trunci twitches the skin. It is innervated by the lateral thoracic nerve. In the male dog there is a distinct development of this muscle adjacent to the ventral midline caudal to the xiphoid. This is the **preputial muscle**, which passes caudally and radiates into the prepuce, forming an arch with the muscle of the opposite side. It functions to support the cranial end of the prepuce during the nonerect state and to pull the prepuce back over the glans penis after erection and protrusion.

Sever the axillary and ventral attachments of the cutaneous trunci and reflect it dorsally. *Caution:* Beneath the thin cutaneous trunci is the thicker latissimus dorsi muscle, which should be left in place on the lateral side of the trunk.

LIVE DOG

Grasp the skin in several areas and note the variation in thickness. Note where it is especially loose and suitable for subcutaneous injections of fluids. Pinch the skin over the side of the thorax and observe the skin wrinkling that occurs because of reflex activity of the cutaneous trunci muscle. Palpate the costal arch to locate the last floating rib. Feel for the umbilicus.

Extrinsic Muscles of the Thoracic Limb and Related Structures

The extrinsic muscles of the thoracic limb are those that attach the limb to the axial skeleton; the intrinsic muscles extend between the bones that compose the limb itself. Extrinsic muscles of the thoracic limb are as follows:
- Superficial pectoral
- Deep pectoral
- Brachiocephalicus
- Omotransversarius
- Trapezius
- Rhomboideus
- Latissimus dorsi
- Serratus ventralis

In the ventral thoracic region are the superficial and deep pectoral muscles, which extend between the sternum and the humerus. Thoroughly clean these muscles. In thin specimens this will require little dissecting. In pregnant or lactating bitches, it will require reflecting the two thoracic mammae caudally, and in fat specimens the forelimb will probably have to be manipulated so that the borders of the muscles are clearly discernible before cleaning. Always clean the extremities of a muscle as well as the middle part. Actually see and feel the attachments. Visualize the muscle's position and action on the skeleton and attempt to palpate it on a live dog.

1. The two **superficial pectoral muscles** (see Figs. 2-12, 2-14, 2-18) lie on each side under the skin between the cranial part of the sternum and the humerus. Their caudal border is thin; their cranial border is thick and rounded and forms the caudal border of a triangle at the base of the neck. The smaller **descending pectoral** is superficial to the transverse pectoral, which it obliquely crosses from its origin on the first sternebra to its insertion on the crest of the greater tubercle of the humerus. The **transverse pectoral** arises from the first two or three sternebrae and inserts over a longer distance on the crest of the greater tubercle of the humerus. It is related on its deep surface to the deep pectoral muscle (ascending pectoral). At their insertions these muscles lie between the brachiocephalicus in front and the biceps brachii and humerus behind. Clean both of these superficial pectoral muscles. Transect them 1 cm from the sternum, and reflect them toward the humerus. As muscle attachments are being cleaned, examine the skeletal parts involved.

   ORIGIN: The first two sternebrae and usually a part of the third; the fibrous raphe between adjacent muscles.

   INSERTION: The whole crest of the greater tubercle of the humerus.

   ACTION: To adduct the limb when it is not bearing weight or to prevent the limb from being abducted when bearing weight.

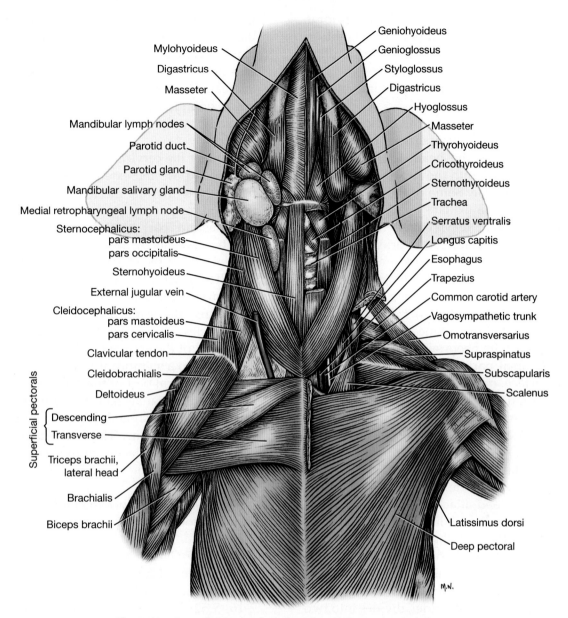

Fig. 2-12 Superficial muscles of neck and thorax, ventral view.

INNERVATION: Ventral branch of spinal nerves C7 and C8.

2. The **deep pectoral muscle** (see Figs. 2-12, 2-14, 2-15, 2-16, 2-18) extends from the sternum to the humerus and is larger and longer than the superficial pectoral muscles. It lies largely under the skin, the thoracic mammae, and the ventral portion of the **cutaneous trunci**. The papilla of the caudal thoracic mamma usually lies at the caudal border of the muscle. Only the cranial part is covered by the superficial pectoral muscles. An abdominal slip of this muscle is often present on the caudolateral border. Transect the deep pectoral muscle 2 cm

from, and parallel to, the sternum, and clean the distal part to its insertion.

ORIGIN: The ventral part of the sternum and the fibrous raphe between fellow muscles; the deep abdominal fascia in the region of the xiphoid cartilage (the caudal end of the sternum).

INSERTION: The major portion partly muscular, partly tendinous on the lesser tubercle of the humerus; an aponeurosis to the greater tubercle and its crest; the caudal part to the medial brachial fascia.

ACTION: When the limb is advanced and fixed in a supporting position: to pull the trunk cranially and to extend the shoulder joint. When the limb is not supporting weight: to draw the limb caudally and flex the shoulder joint. To adduct the limb.

INNERVATION: Caudal pectoral nerves (C8, T1).

The **superficial fascia of the neck** is continued on the head as the superficial fascia of the various regions of the head. Caudally it becomes continuous with the superficial brachial and pectoral fasciae. Some of the fascia is also continued into the axillary space. Notice that the external jugular vein is completely wrapped by it. Save this vein for future orientation. The cutaneous muscles of the neck are completely enveloped by the fascia. Only the platysma will be dissected.

The **platysma** (see Figs. 3-2, 5-21, *A*) is the best developed of the cutaneous muscles of the neck and head. Its fibers sweep cranioventrally over the dorsal part of the neck and over the lateral surface of the face. The muscle may have been reflected with the skin. Its insertion will be seen when the head is dissected.

3. The **brachiocephalicus** (see Figs. 2-12 through 2-15, 2-18, 3-1) of the dog is a compound muscle developmentally, although it appears as one muscle that extends from the arm to the head and neck. One end attaches on the distal third of the humerus, where it lies between the biceps brachii medially and the brachialis laterally. Proximally on the humerus it partly covers the pectoral muscles at their insertions and lies craniomedial to the deltoid muscle. It crosses the cranial surface of the shoulder, divides into two parts, and obliquely traverses the neck. At the shoulder a faint line crosses the muscle. This is the edge of a fibrous plate, the **clavicular intersection**, on the deep surface of which the vestigial **clavicle** (collarbone) is connected. A band of connective tissue can be felt extending from this vestigial clavicle to the manubrium of the sternum and to the scapula. Although the clavicle has lost its functional significance in the dog, it is still considered the origin of the components of the brachiocephalicus muscle. Thus the muscle distal to the clavicular intersection that attaches to the humerus is the **cleidobrachialis**. The muscle that extends from the clavicular tendon to the neck and head is the **cleidocephalicus**. The cleidocephalicus has two parts: a thin **pars cervicalis**, which attaches to

the dorsal midline of the neck (formerly called the *cleidocervicalis*), and beneath it a thicker **pars mastoidea**, which attaches to the mastoid process of the skull (formerly called the *cleidomastoideus*). The cervical part of the cleidocephalicus is bounded caudally by the trapezius and cranially by the occipital part of the sternocephalicus.

Transect the cervical part of the cleidocephalicus to expose the extent of the mastoid part below. Note that the mastoid part runs toward the head deep to the sternocephalicus. Transect the mastoid part of the muscle and search for the clavicle by inserting a finger on the medial side of the clavicular intersection.

ATTACHMENTS: All attachments are movable, but the clavicle or clavicular intersection is considered the origin for purposes of naming the muscles. The cleidobrachialis attaches to the distal end of the cranial border of the humerus. There is also a significant fascial tie into the axilla. The cervical part of the cleidocephalicus attaches to the cranial half of the mid-dorsal fibrous raphe and sometimes to the nuchal crest of the occipital bone. The mastoid part of the cleidocephalicus attaches to the mastoid part of the temporal bone with the sternomastoideus muscle.

ACTION: To advance the limb; to extend the shoulder joint and draw the neck and head to the side.

INNERVATION: Accessory nerve and ventral branches of cervical spinal nerves.

4. The **sternocephalicus** (see Figs. 2-12, 2-15, 2-16, 5-52) arises on the sternum and inserts on the head. At the cranial end of the sternum the muscle is thick, rounded, and closely united with its fellow of the opposite side. Even after the main parts of the paired muscle diverge, there may be considerable crossing of fibers between the two on the ventral surface of the neck. The dorsal border of the sternocephalicus is adjacent to the ventral border of the cleidocephalicus. The external jugular vein crosses its lateral surface obliquely (see Fig. 3-2). Notice that the cranial part of the muscle divides into two parts and that the thicker ventral portion is closely related to the mastoid part of the cleidocephalicus. The ventral or **mastoid part** of the sternocephalicus (formerly the sternomastoideus) is similar to the mastoid part of the

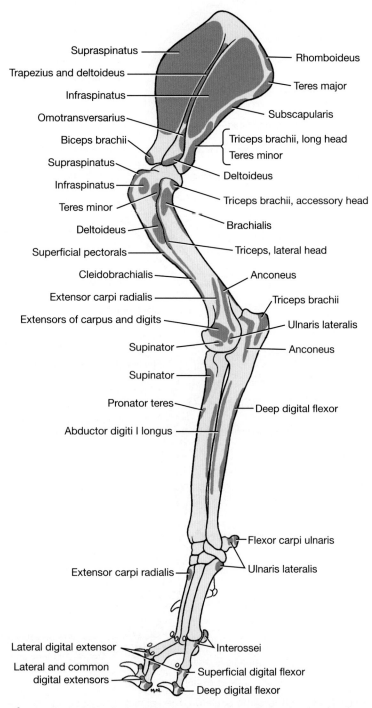

Supraspinatus

Trapezius and deltoideus

Infraspinatus

Omotransversarius

Biceps brachii

Supraspinatus

Infraspinatus

Teres minor

Deltoideus

Superficial pectorals

Cleidobrachialis

Extensor carpi radialis

Extensors of carpus and digits

Supinator

Supinator

Pronator teres

Abductor digiti I longus

Extensor carpi radialis

Lateral digital extensor

Lateral and common
digital extensors

Rhomboideus

Teres major

Subscapularis

Triceps brachii, long head

Teres minor

Deltoideus

Triceps brachii, accessory head

Brachialis

Triceps, lateral head

Anconeus

Triceps brachii

Ulnaris lateralis

Anconeus

Deep digital flexor

Flexor carpi ulnaris

Ulnaris lateralis

Interossei

Superficial digital flexor

Deep digital flexor

Fig. 2-13 Left forelimb skeleton, lateral view of muscle attachments.

cleidocephalicus in shape and insertion. It represents the chief continuation of the sternocephalicus to the head. The thin but wide dorsal portion of the sternocephalicus is the **occipital part** (formerly the sternooccipitalis).

ORIGIN: The first sternebra or manubrium.

INSERTION: The mastoid part of the temporal bone and the nuchal crest of the occipital bone.

ACTION: To draw the head and neck to the side.

INNERVATION: Accessory nerve and ventral branches of cervical spinal nerves.

Transect the left sternocephalicus close to the manubrium and reflect it. The sternohyoid and sternothyroid muscles are both covered by the deep fascia of the neck and lie dorsal to the sternocephalicus at their origin.

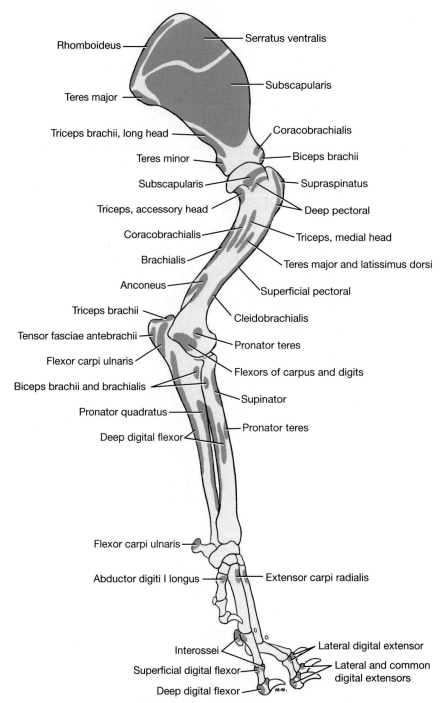

Fig. 2-14   Left forelimb skeleton, medial view of muscle attachments.

The **sternohyoideus** (see Figs. 2-12 and 5-33) lies on the trachea, covered by the sternocephalicus caudally. A midventral groove indicates the separation of right and left muscles.

ORIGIN: The first sternebra and the first costal cartilage.

INSERTION: The basihyoid bone.

ACTION: To pull the tongue and larynx caudally.

INNERVATION: Ventral branches of cervical spinal nerves.

The **sternothyroideus** (see Figs. 2-12 and 5-33) is covered at its origin by the sternohyoideus. The sternothyroideus inserts on the lateral surface of the thyroid cartilage. The left muscle is bounded dorsally by the esophagus and medially by the trachea. Notice that a tendinous intersection runs across the muscle 3 or 4 cm cranial to its origin. It

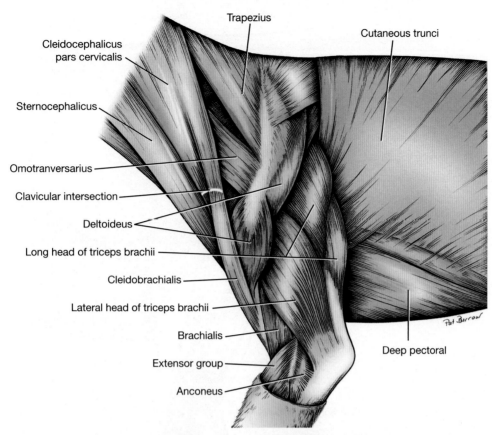

Fig. 2-15 Superficial muscles of left scapula and brachium.

is at this level that the sternohyoideus separates from the sternothyroideus.

ORIGIN: The first costal cartilage.

INSERTION: The caudolateral surface of the thyroid cartilage.

ACTION: Same as the sternohyoideus—to draw the larynx and tongue caudally.

INNERVATION: Ventral branches of cervical spinal nerves and hypoglossal nerve.

5. The **omotransversarius** (see Figs. 2-12, 2-13, 2-15, 2-17, 3-1, 3-2) is in a deeper plane than the cleidocephalicus. It is straplike and extends from the distal end of the spine of the scapula to the atlas. It is related to the deep cervical fascia medially. Its caudal part is subcutaneous, but cranially it is covered by the cervical part of the cleidocephalicus. Transect the omotransversarius through its middle and reflect each half toward its attachment. This will expose the **superficial cervical lymph nodes** located cranial to the scapula (see Fig. 3-26).

ATTACHMENTS: The distal end of the spine of the scapula; cranially, the transverse process (wing) of the atlas.

ACTION: To advance the limb or flex the neck laterally.

INNERVATION: Accessory nerve.

The **deep fascia of the neck** is a strong wrapping that extends under the sternocephalicus, omotransversarius, and cleidocephalicus muscles. It covers the sternohyoideus and sternothyroideus ventrally and surrounds the trachea, thyroid gland, larynx, and esophagus. The deep fascia that covers the common carotid artery, vagosympathetic nerve trunk, internal jugular vein, and tracheal lymphatic trunk is the **carotid sheath**. Locate these structures in the carotid sheath between the omotransversarius dorsally and the sternothyroideus ventrally. The deep fascia of the neck continues dorsally and laterally to invest the deep cervical muscles.

The **supraspinous ligament** (see Fig. 2-84) connects the dorsal aspects of all vertebral spines except the cervical vertebrae (do not dissect at this time). The **nuchal ligament**, composed predominantly of yellow elastic fibrous tissue, extends from the spine of the first thoracic vertebra to the spine of the axis. The **median raphe** of the neck is a longitudinal fibrous septum between right and left epaxial muscles dorsal to the nuchal ligament. It serves as the attachment for many of the cervical muscles.

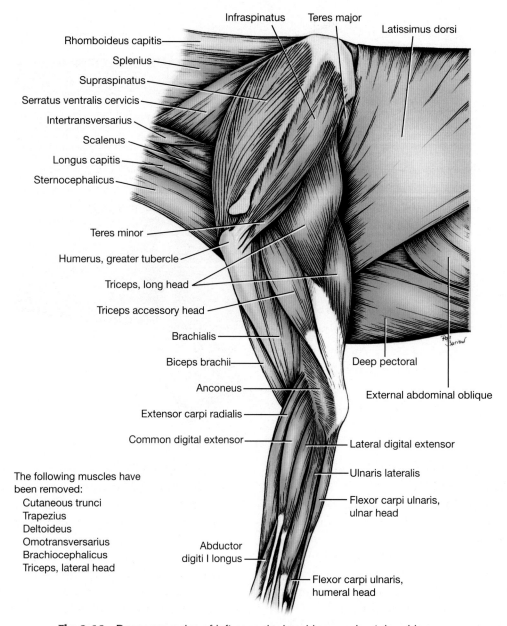

Infraspinatus   Teres major

Latissimus dorsi

Rhomboideus capitis

Splenius

Supraspinatus

Serratus ventralis cervicis

Intertransversarius

Scalenus

Longus capitis

Sternocephalicus

Teres minor

Humerus, greater tubercle

Triceps, long head

Triceps accessory head

Brachialis

Biceps brachii

Anconeus

Extensor carpi radialis

Common digital extensor

Deep pectoral

External abdominal oblique

Lateral digital extensor

Ulnaris lateralis

Flexor carpi ulnaris,
ulnar head

The following muscles have
been removed:
  Cutaneous trunci
  Trapezius
  Deltoideus
  Omotransversarius
  Brachiocephalicus
  Triceps, lateral head

Abductor
digiti I longus

Flexor carpi ulnaris,
humeral head

Fig. 2-16   Deeper muscles of left scapula, brachium, and antebrachium.

Observe these during the dissection of the following muscles.

6. The **trapezius** (see Figs. 2-13, 2-15) is thin and triangular. It is divided into **cervical** and **thoracic** parts, separated by an aponeurosis. The muscle as a whole extends from the median raphe of the neck and the supraspinous ligament to the spine of the scapula. The cervical part is overlapped by the cervical part of the cleidocephalicus whereas the thoracic part overlaps the latissimus dorsi. Transect the trapezius by making an arching cut through the muscle, beginning at the middle of the cranial border. Extend it over the dorsal border of the scapula and continue through the

aponeurotic area to the middle of the caudal border. Reflect the muscle to its attachments.

ORIGIN: The median raphe of the neck and the supraspinous ligament from the level of the third cervical vertebra to the level of the ninth thoracic vertebra.

INSERTION: The spine of the scapula.

ACTION: To elevate and abduct the forelimb.

INNERVATION: Accessory nerve.

7. The **rhomboideus** (see Figs. 2-13, 2-14, 2-16, 2-76, *A*) lies beneath the trapezius and holds the dorsal border of the scapula close to the body. It has capital, cervical, and thoracic parts. The narrow **rhomboideus capitis** attaches the

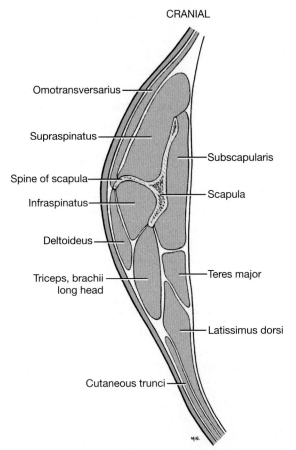

CRANIAL

Omotransversarius

Supraspinatus

Spine of scapula

Infraspinatus

Deltoideus

Triceps, brachii
long head

Cutaneous trunci

Subscapularis

Scapula

Teres major

Latissimus dorsi

Fig. 2-17   Transverse section through middle of left scapula.

cranial dorsal border of the scapula to the nuchal crest of the occipital bone. The **rhomboideus cervicis** runs from the median raphe of the neck to the dorsal border of the scapula. The **rhomboideus thoracis** is short and thick, connecting the spines of the first seven thoracic

vertebrae to the dorsal border of the scapula. Its caudal border is deep to the latissimus dorsi. The cervical and thoracic parts of the rhomboideus are contiguous on the dorsal border of the scapula. Transect the entire muscle a few centimeters from the scapula.

ORIGIN: The nuchal crest of the occipital bone; the median fibrous raphe of the neck; the spinous processes of the first seven thoracic vertebrae.

INSERTION: The dorsal border and adjacent surfaces of the scapula.

ACTION: To elevate the forelimb and draw the scapula against the trunk.

INNERVATION: Ventral branches of cervical and thoracic spinal nerves.

8. The **latissimus dorsi** (see Figs. 2-14, 2-16 through 2-18) is large and roughly triangular. It lies caudal to the scapula, where it covers most of the dorsal and some of the lateral thoracic wall. Clean its ventrocaudal border. Directly caudal to the forelimb, transect the latissimus dorsi at a right angle to its fibers.

ORIGIN: The thoracolumbar fascia from the spinous processes of the lumbar and the last seven or eight thoracic vertebrae; a muscular attachment to the last two or three ribs.

INSERTION: The teres major tuberosity of the humerus and the teres major tendon.

ACTION: To draw the free limb caudally as in digging; to flex the shoulder joint.

INNERVATION: Thoracodorsal nerve (C7, C8, T1).

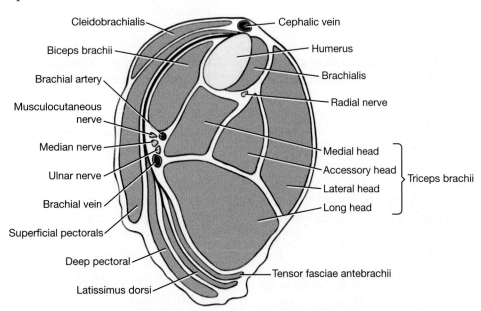

Cleidobrachialis

Biceps brachii

Brachial artery

Musculocutaneous
nerve

Median nerve

Ulnar nerve

Brachial vein

Superficial pectorals

Deep pectoral

Latissimus dorsi

Cephalic vein

Humerus

Brachialis

Radial nerve

Medial head

Accessory head

Lateral head

Long head

Triceps brachii

Tensor fasciae antebrachii

Fig. 2-18   Transverse section through middle of right brachium.

The **thoracolumbar fascia** is deep fascia of the trunk. It arises from the supraspinous ligament and spines of the thoracic and lumbar vertebrae; covers the muscles of the vertebrae, ribs, and abdomen; and fuses with the opposite fascia on the ventral midline along a median fibrous raphe, the **linea alba**. The thoracolumbar fascia serves as an attachment for numerous muscles. It will be dissected with the abdominal muscles.

9. The **serratus ventralis cervicis** and **serratus ventralis thoracis** (Figs. 2-14, 2-16, 2-76, 2-82) form a continuous large fan-shaped muscle that passes from the cervical vertebrae and ribs to the dorsomedial aspect of the scapula and acts as a sling to support the body between the limbs. Visualize the attachments in a standing dog to appreciate how the trunk is suspended between the limbs. Abduct the forelimb. This will require severing the axillary artery and vein, the nerves contributing to the brachial plexus, and the axillary fascia. As the forelimb is progressively abducted, the attachment of the serratus ventralis will detach from the serrated face of the scapula. Because the forelimb is removed at this stage of the dissection, the detachment of the serratus ventralis may be completed. It is the only extrinsic muscle of the forelimb that has not been transected.

ORIGIN: The transverse processes of the last five cervical vertebrae and the first seven or eight ribs ventral to their middle.

INSERTION: The dorsomedial third of the scapula (serrated face).

ACTION: To support the trunk and depress the scapula.

INNERVATION: Ventral branches of cervical spinal nerves and the long thoracic nerve (C7).

LIVE DOG

Stand over a dog and palpate on both sides the superficial pectoral muscles from in front of the thoracic limbs and the deep pectoral muscles from behind. Place your fingers on the sternum and grasp the deep pectoral between your fingers medially and your thumb laterally. Extend the neck and palpate the brachiocephalicus, which will be stretched taut by this maneuver. With the neck extended, palpate the sternocephalicus, sternohyoideus, and sternothyroideus muscles at their attachment to the first sternebra. Palpate the trachea and appreciate the muscles that must be separated to expose the trachea to open it (a tracheostomy).

Palpate the spines of the thoracic vertebrae. The cervical spines caudal to the axis are not palpable. Try to separate the dorsal border of the scapula from the thoracic vertebral spines. The trapezius and rhomboideus prevent this. Palpate the sides of the thorax covered by the latissimus dorsi and feel its ventral border.

Visualize the attachments of the serratus ventralis muscles and how they keep the limb attached to the trunk when the dog is supporting weight. Occasionally, their termination on the scapula is torn by injury. This results in an abnormal elevation of the limb when the dog bears weight, and the dorsal border of the scapula will protrude dorsally beside or above the level of the thoracic spines.

Intrinsic Muscles of the Thoracic Limb

Lateral scapula and shoulder
Deltoideus
Infraspinatus
Teres minor
Supraspinatus
Medial scapula and shoulder
Subscapularis
Teres major
Coracobrachialis
Caudal arm
Tensor fasciae antebrachii
Triceps brachii
Anconeus
Cranial arm
Biceps brachii
Brachialis
Cranial and lateral forearm
Extensor carpi radialis
Common digital extensor
Lateral digital extensor
Ulnaris lateralis
Supinator
Abductor digiti I longus
Caudal and medial forearm
Pronator teres
Flexor carpi radialis
Superficial digital flexor
Flexor carpi ulnaris
Deep digital flexor
Pronator quadratus

Lateral Muscles of the Scapula and Shoulder

1. The **deltoideus** (see Figs. 2-13, 2-15, 2-17) is composed of two portions that fuse and act in

common across the shoulder. The scapular part arises as a wide aponeurosis from the length of the scapular spine and covers the infraspinatus. The latter muscle can be seen through this aponeurosis and should not be confused with the deltoideus. Observe the acromial part of the deltoideus, which arises from the acromion and has a fusiform shape. Both portions of the muscle fuse before they insert on the deltoid tuberosity of the humerus. Transect the combined muscle 2 cm distal to the acromion and reflect the stumps. Free the scapular part from the infraspinatus and work under the aponeurosis of origin to verify its attachment to the spine of the scapula.

ORIGIN: The spine and acromial process of the scapula.

INSERTION: The deltoid tuberosity.

ACTION: To flex the shoulder.

INNERVATION: Axillary nerve.

2. The **infraspinatus** (see Figs. 2-13, 2-16, 2-17) is fusiform and lies principally in the infraspinous fossa. Transect the infraspinatus halfway between its extremities. Free and reflect the distal half from the scapula by scraping the fibers away from the spine and fossa with the handle of the scalpel. Reflect the distal half to its insertion on the side of the greater tubercle. This will expose a **subtendinous synovial bursa** between the tendon of insertion and the greater tubercle of the humerus. A bursa is a closed connective tissue sac containing synovial fluid, which reduces friction.

ORIGIN: The infraspinous fossa.

INSERTION: A small, circumscribed area on the lateral side of the greater tubercle of the humerus.

ACTION: To extend or flex the joint, depending on the degree of extension or position of the joint when the muscle contracts. To abduct the shoulder and to rotate the humerus laterally. To prevent medial rotation when weight bearing and provide lateral stability to the shoulder joint.

INNERVATION: Suprascapular nerve.

3. The **teres minor** (see Figs. 2-13, 2-16), a small, wedge-shaped muscle, is now exposed caudal to the shoulder joint. It is covered superficially by the deltoideus.

ORIGIN: The infraglenoid tubercle and distal third of the caudal border of the scapula.

INSERTION: The teres minor tuberosity of the humerus.

ACTION: To flex the shoulder, rotate the shoulder laterally, and prevent medial rotation when bearing weight.

INNERVATION: Axillary nerve.

4. The **supraspinatus** (see Figs. 2-12, 2-13, 2-14, 2-16, 2-17, 2-19, 2-27), which is wider and larger than the infraspinatus, is largely covered by the cervical part of the trapezius and the omotransversarius. It lies in the supraspinous fossa and extends over the cranial border of the scapula so that a part of the muscle is closely united with the subscapularis medially. Clean and observe the insertion on the greater tubercle of the humerus.

ORIGIN: The supraspinous fossa.

INSERTION: The greater tubercle of the humerus, by a thick tendon.

ACTION: To extend and stabilize the shoulder joint.

INNERVATION: Suprascapular nerve.

Medial Muscles of the Scapula and Shoulder

1. The **subscapularis** (see Figs. 2-12, 2-13, 2-14, 2-17, 2-19) occupies the entire subscapular fossa, the boundaries of which it overlaps slightly. The supraspinatus is closely associated with it cranially, whereas the teres major has a similar relation caudally. Clean the insertion but do not transect the muscle.

ORIGIN: The subscapular fossa.

INSERTION: The lesser tubercle of the humerus.

ACTION: To adduct, extend, and medially stabilize the shoulder joint. To rotate the shoulder joint medially and prevent lateral rotation when bearing weight.

INNERVATION: Subscapular nerve. Considerable support is provided to the shoulder joint by the subscapularis muscle medially, the teres minor and infraspinatus muscles laterally, and the supraspinatus cranially. Luxation will not occur without injury to the joint capsule and its glenohumeral ligaments (see Fig. 2-29).

2. The **teres major** (see Figs. 2-13, 2-14, 2-16, 2-17, 2-19, 2-27), directly caudal to the subscapularis, belies its descriptive name because it is not round but has three surfaces. Its proximal end arises from the subscapularis and the proximal caudal border of the scapula. Fibers extend distally to attach to the tendon of insertion of the latissimus dorsi. Work between the distal half of the muscle and the subscapularis.

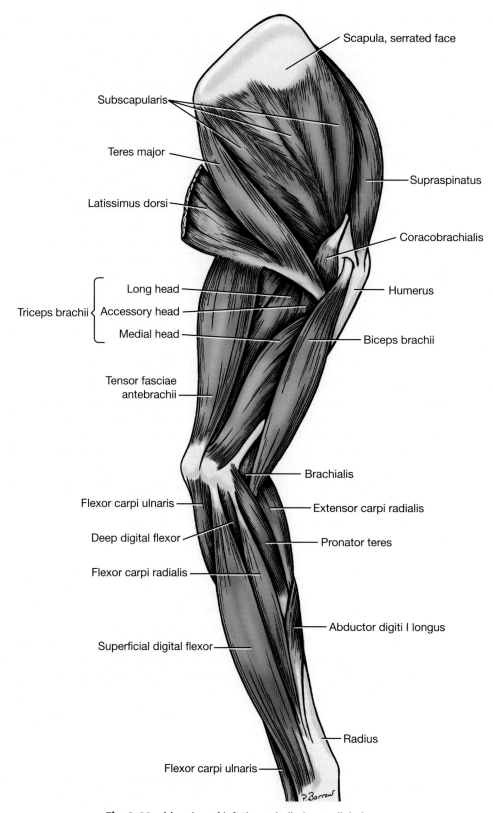

Fig. 2-19 Muscles of left thoracic limb, medial view.

Observe the close relationship between the teres major and the latissimus dorsi as they approach their insertion on the proximal medial surface of the body of the humerus. Transect the teres major and reflect the combined insertion to expose the belly of the coracobrachialis muscle.

ORIGIN: The caudal angle and adjacent caudal border of the scapula; the caudal surface of the subscapularis.

INSERTION: The teres major tuberosity of the humerus.

ACTION: Flex the shoulder joint, rotate the shoulder joint medially, and prevent lateral rotation when weight bearing.

INNERVATION: Axillary nerve.

3. The **coracobrachialis** (see Figs. 2-14, 2-19) crosses the medial surface of the shoulder obliquely. It is a small spindle-shaped muscle that arises from the coracoid process of the scapula by a relatively long tendon that courses caudodistally across the lesser tubercle. There it crosses the tendon of insertion of the subscapularis. The tendon of the coracobrachialis is provided with a synovial sheath as it crosses the lesser tubercle of the humerus. The muscle belly is distal to the lesser tubercle and medial to the origin of the medial head of the triceps. The conjoined tendon of the teres major and latissimus dorsi crosses the insertion of the coracobrachialis. Notice that the coracobrachialis tendon courses cranial to the center of the shoulder. This accounts for its action as an extensor muscle of the shoulder joint. Free the coracobrachialis and isolate the tendon of origin by cutting into its tendon sheath.

ORIGIN: The coracoid process of the scapula.

INSERTION: The crest of the lesser tubercle of the humerus proximal to the teres major tuberosity.

ACTION: To adduct, extend, and stabilize the shoulder joint.

INNERVATION: Musculocutaneous nerve.

LIVE DOG

Locate the spine of the scapula and palpate the supraspinatus cranial to it and the infraspinatus and the scapular part of the deltoideus caudal to it. Find the acromion and palpate the acromial part of the deltoideus and the deltoid tuberosity. Palpate the greater tubercle and the acromion and estimate the middle position on a line between these structures. A needle inserted at this point through the deltoideus, cranial to the infraspinatus, will enter the shoulder joint. Rotate the arm medially and laterally. The restriction to lateral rotation is by the teres major and subscapularis, whereas the restriction to medial rotation is by the teres minor and infraspinatus. Injury that tears the termination of the latter muscles allows excessive medial rotation. In the weight-bearing phase of walking, this causes the elbow to abduct.

Occasionally, injury to the infraspinatus results in shortening of the muscle by contracture when it heals. This results in a constant excessive lateral rotation of the shoulder joint, and the dog stands with the elbow adducted. This persists during the swing phase (protraction), when there is also a compensatory abduction of the paw. On manipulation there is increased restriction to medial rotation of the shoulder joint. This can be corrected by cutting the tendon of the contracted infraspinatus. An overall function of the infraspinatus, supraspinatus, subscapularis, and coracobrachialis is to act as collateral ligaments to stabilize the shoulder joint medially and laterally during normal gait.

Caudal Muscles of the Arm (Brachium)

This group is a large, muscular mass that almost completely fills the space between the caudal border of the scapula and the olecranon. It consists of three muscles: the triceps brachii, the tensor fasciae antebrachii, and the anconeus. By far the largest of these muscles is the triceps brachii. All of the caudal muscles of the arm are extensors of the elbow joint.

1. The **tensor fasciae antebrachii** (see Figs. 2-14, 2-18, 2-19) is a thin strap that extends from the latissimus dorsi to the medial fascia of the forearm and the olecranon. It lies on the long head of the triceps brachii.

ORIGIN: The fascia covering the lateral side of the latissimus dorsi.

INSERTION: The olecranon.

ACTION: To extend the elbow joint.

INNERVATION: Radial nerve.

2. The **triceps brachii** in the dog consists of four heads instead of the usual three, with a common tendon to the olecranon tuber. Only the long head arises from the scapula. The other three arise from the proximal end of the humerus.

The **long head** (see Figs. 2-13 through 2-19, Fig. 2-27) completely bridges the humerus. It arises from the caudal border of the scapula and inserts on the olecranon tuber. It appears to have two bellies. Caudal to the shoulder, palpate a groove between the long and lateral heads of the triceps. Separate these two heads along this groove.

Expose the tendon of the long head and notice the subtendinous bursa between it and the groove of the olecranon. Notice how the tendons of the other heads blend with that of the long head.

ORIGIN: The caudal border of the scapula.

INSERTION: The olecranon tuber.

ACTION: To extend the elbow joint and flex the shoulder joint.

INNERVATION: Radial nerve.

The **lateral head** (see Figs. 2-12, 2-13, 2-15, 2-18, 2-20, 2-27) of the triceps brachii lies distal to the long head, caudal to the acromial part of the deltoideus, and lateral to the accessory head, which it covers. Transect the aponeurotic origin of the lateral head and reflect it to expose the underlying accessory and medial heads. This also exposes the brachialis muscle.

ORIGIN: The tricipital line of the humerus.

INSERTION: The olecranon tuber.

ACTION: To extend the elbow joint.

INNERVATION: Radial nerve.

The **accessory head** (see Figs. 2-13, 2-14, 2-16, 2-18, 2-19, 2-27) lies between the lateral and medial heads.

ORIGIN: The neck of the humerus.

INSERTION: The olecranon tuber.

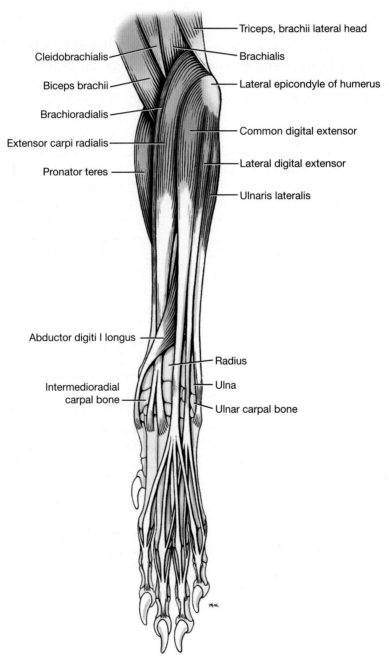

Fig. 2-20   Muscles of left antebrachium, cranial view.

ACTION: To extend the elbow joint.

INNERVATION: Radial nerve.

The **medial head** (Figs. 2-14, 2-18, 2-19, 2-23, 2-27) lies caudally on the humerus lateral and caudal to the biceps brachii. Separate the muscle from the long head caudally and from the accessory head laterally. The long tendon of the accessory head is closely bound to its lateral surface.

ORIGIN: The crest of the lesser tubercle near the teres major tuberosity.

INSERTION: The olecranon.

ACTION: To extend the elbow joint.

INNERVATION: Radial nerve.

3. The **anconeus** (see Figs. 2-13 through 2-16, 2-23) is a small muscle located almost completely in the olecranon fossa. Reflect the insertion of the lateral head of the triceps to uncover the lateral surface of this muscle. Notice that the most distal fibers lie in a transverse plane. On the lateral side, cut the origin of the anconeus from the lateral supracondylar crest and epicondyle. Reflect it to expose the elbow joint capsule. Open the joint capsule to expose the elbow joint at the level of the anconeal process of the ulna.

ORIGIN: The lateral supracondylar crest and the lateral and medial epicondyles of the humerus.

INSERTION: The lateral surface of the proximal end of the ulna (the olecranon).

ACTION: To extend the elbow joint.

INNERVATION: Radial nerve.

LIVE DOG

Palpate the triceps brachii caudal to the arm and its termination on the olecranon. Appreciate the function of this muscle in extension of the elbow joint to support the weight of the animal in standing and during locomotion. Avulsion of its tendon or denervation of this muscle will cause the limb to collapse when weight is placed on it. Lightly striking the triceps tendon at the olecranon tuber will elicit reflex contraction and cause extension of the elbow joint in some dogs.

Cranial Muscles of the Arm

1. The **biceps brachii** (see Figs. 2-12, 2-13, 2-14, 2-16, 2-18 through 2-20, 2-23, 2-27, 2-30) has only one head. It is a long, fusiform muscle that lies on the medial and cranial surfaces of the humerus. It completely bridges this bone as it arises on the supraglenoid tuberosity of the scapula and inserts on the proximal ends of the radius and ulna. It is covered superficially by the pectoral muscles. Clean the muscle and transect it through its middle. Reflect the proximal half to its origin. This will require severing the **transverse humeral retinaculum**, a band of fibrous tissue that joins the greater and lesser tubercles and holds the tendon of origin in the intertubercular groove. An extension of the shoulder joint capsule (the **intertubercular bursa**) acts as a synovial sheath for this tendon. Reflect the distal half of the biceps to the proximal end of the radius and ulna, where it meets the brachialis tendon and bifurcates. The tendons of insertion lie on the elbow joint capsule, covering its medial collateral ligament. Delay cleaning these tendons until after the pronator teres muscle has been dissected.

ORIGIN: The supraglenoid tubercle.

INSERTION: The ulnar and radial tuberosities.

ACTION: To flex the elbow joint and extend the shoulder joint.

INNERVATION: Musculocutaneous nerve.

2. The **brachialis** (see Figs. 2-12 through 2-16, 2-18 through 2-20, 2-30) should be studied from the lateral side. It is a long, thin muscle that lies in the brachialis groove of the humerus. From the proximal third of this groove, the brachialis curves laterally and cranially as it courses distally, crosses the elbow, and inserts by a terminal tendon on the medial side of the proximal end of the ulna. A large part of its lateral surface is covered by the lateral head of the triceps. Distally, it runs medial to the origin of the extensor carpi radialis. Its insertion will be dissected later with the biceps brachii insertion. These are deep to the pronator teres.

ORIGIN: The proximal third of the lateral surface of the humerus.

INSERTION: The ulnar and radial tuberosities.

ACTION: To flex the elbow joint.

INNERVATION: Musculocutaneous nerve.

LIVE DOG

Palpate the crest of the greater tubercle and, medial to it, feel the tendon of the biceps brachii in the intertubercular groove covered by the termination of the pectoral muscles. This part of the tendon is covered by a synovial sheath that is continuous with the shoulder joint capsule. Swelling of the tendon sheath will be felt when there is increased synovial fluid from lesions of the tendon, its sheath, or the shoulder joint. Distally in the arm, feel the terminal portions of the biceps brachii medially and the brachialis laterally on the cranial aspect of the elbow. Both muscles can be palpated here. Lightly striking these muscles at this site with a blunt object will elicit reflex contraction and elbow flexion in some dogs.

Before the rest of the skin is removed from the thoracic limb, examine the foot pads. The small pad that protrudes palmar to the carpus is the **carpal pad**. The largest in the paw, the **metacarpal pad**, is on the palmar side of the metacarpophalangeal joints and is triangular. The **digital pads** are ovoid and flattened. Each is located palmar to the distal interphalangeal joint.

Make a midcaudal incision through the skin from the olecranon through the carpal and metacarpal pads to the interdigital space between digits III and IV. Reflect the skin, dissect it free from the fascia, and remove it from the forelimb. The pads are closely attached to the underlying structures but may be dissected free and removed. Be careful not to cut too deeply and sever the underlying small tendons. Work distally on each of the four main digits and completely remove the skin and digital pads.

The areolar part of the subcutaneous tissue distal to the elbow is scanty. The principal veins and cutaneous nerves lie in large part on the superficial fascia of the antebrachium. For descriptive purposes, the superficial and deep fascia distal to the elbow may be divided into antebrachial, carpal, metacarpal, and digital parts.

The **deep antebrachial fascia** forms a single dense sleeve for the muscles of the forearm on the caudal surface. Make an incision through the deep antebrachial fascia from the olecranon to the accessory carpal bone. Carefully reflect the fascia cranially on the forearm. At first, the fascia is easily reflected because it lies on the epimysium of the muscles beneath. Cranially, it sends delicate septal leaves between muscles, and on reaching the radius, it firmly unites with its periosteum.

Cranial and Lateral Muscles of the Forearm (Antebrachium)

The cranial and lateral antebrachial muscles are, from cranial to caudal, the extensor carpi radialis, supinator, common digital extensor, lateral digital extensor, ulnaris lateralis, and abductor pollicis longus. Most of these muscles arise from the lateral epicondyle of the humerus. A slender, inconstant muscle, the brachioradialis (see Figs. 2-20, 2-21), arises from the lateral supracondylar crest of the humerus, adjacent to the extensor carpi radialis, and passes distally and medially to insert on the distal fourth of the radius. If present, the muscle is frequently removed with the skin.

1. The **extensor carpi radialis** (see Figs. 2-13, 2-14, 2-16, 2-19 through 2-22, 2-27) is the largest of the craniolateral antebrachial muscles. It lies on the cranial surface of the radius throughout most of its course and is easily palpated in the live dog. The tendon looks single but is distinctly double throughout its distal third. These closely associated tendons run first under the tendon of the abductor digiti I longus, then in the middle groove of the radius farther distally, and finally over the carpus. They are held in place on the dorsal surface of the carpus by the **extensor retinaculum** (see Fig. 2-22). This is a transversely oriented condensation of carpal fascia that aids in holding in grooves all the tendons that cross the dorsum of the carpus. Between bundles of tendons the extensor retinaculum dips down to blend with the fibrous dorsal part of the joint capsule. Define by dissection the proximal and distal margins of the extensor retinaculum, but do not sever it along the tendons.

    ORIGIN: The lateral supracondylar crest.

    INSERTION: The small tuberosities on the dorsal surfaces of the base of metacarpals II and III.

    ACTION: To extend the carpal joints.

    INNERVATION: Radial nerve.

2. The **common digital extensor** (see Figs. 2-13, 2-14, 2-16, 2-20 through 2-22, 2-27) is shaped like, and lies caudal to, the extensor carpi radialis on the lateral side of the forearm. The four individual tendons that leave the muscle are closely combined where they cross the cranial surface of the abductor digiti I longus and then the carpus; here they are held in the lateral groove of the radius by the extensor retinaculum. Distal to the ligament the four tendons diverge, and each goes to the distal phalanx of the four main digits. Dissect the tendon of the common extensor that goes to the third or fourth digit. Free the tendon as it crosses each of the joints. It often contains a sesamoid bone at the metacarpophalangeal joint. Insertion is on the extensor process of the distal phalanx.

    ORIGIN: The lateral epicondyle of the humerus.

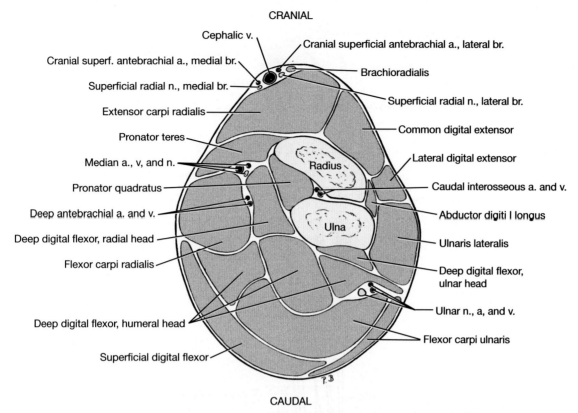

Fig. 2-21 Transverse section of right antebrachium between proximal and middle thirds.

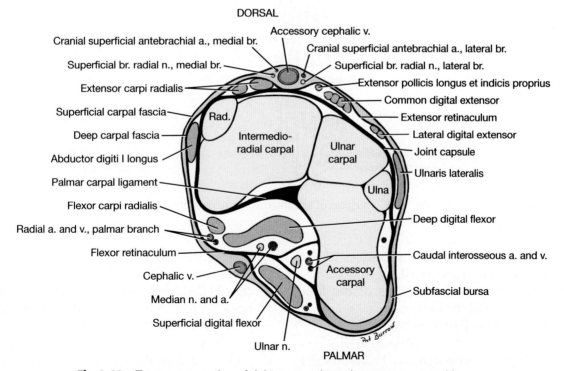

Fig. 2-22 Transverse section of right carpus through accessory carpal bone.

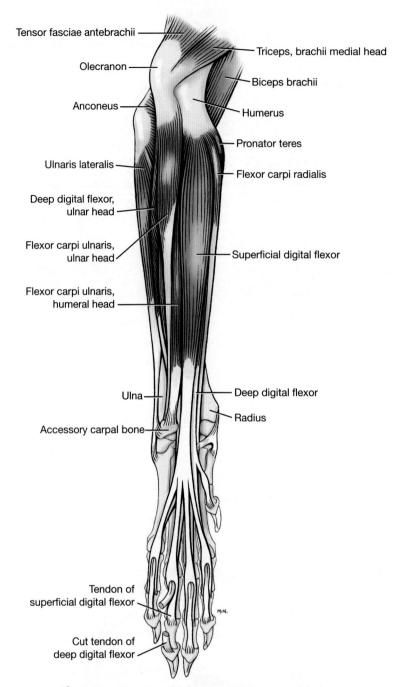

Tensor fasciae antebrachii

Olecranon

Anconeus

Ulnaris lateralis

Deep digital flexor,
ulnar head

Flexor carpi ulnaris,
ulnar head

Flexor carpi ulnaris,
humeral head

Ulna

Accessory carpal bone

Tendon of
superficial digital flexor

Cut tendon of
deep digital flexor

Triceps, brachii medial head

Biceps brachii

Humerus

Pronator teres

Flexor carpi radialis

Superficial digital flexor

Deep digital flexor

Radius

Fig. 2-23   Muscles of left antebrachium, caudal view.

INSERTION: The extensor processes of the distal phalanges of digits II, III, IV, and V.

ACTION: To extend the joints of the four principal digits and the carpus.

INNERVATION: Radial nerve.

Notice that the distal interphalangeal joint is in a marked degree of overextension. This is brought about by the elastic **dorsal ligament**, which lies on each side of the common digital extensor tendon. The ligament attaches proximally to the

sides of the base of the middle phalanx. Distally, it attaches to the dorsal surface of the ungual crest of the distal phalanx (see Fig. 2-26). Its elasticity hyperextends the distal interphalangeal joint and thus retracts the claw.

3. The **lateral digital extensor** (see Figs. 2-13, 2-14, 2-16, 2-20 through 2-22) is about half the size of the common digital extensor. It lies between the common digital extensor and the ulnaris lateralis. Its tendon begins at the middle of

the forearm, passes under the extensor retinaculum in a groove between the radius and ulna, and immediately splits into three branches. The main part of each tendon attaches to the extensor process of the distal phalanx of digits III, IV, and V in common with the common digital extensor tendon.

ORIGIN: The lateral epicondyle of the humerus.

INSERTION: The proximal ends of all the phalanges of digits III, IV, and V, but mainly

the extensor processes of the distal phalanges of these digits.

ACTION: To extend the carpal joints of the carpus and digits III, IV, and V.

INNERVATION: Radial nerve.

4. The **ulnaris lateralis** [extensor carpi ulnaris] (Figs. 2-13, 2-16, 2-20 through 2-24) is larger than the lateral digital extensor and lies caudal to it. It is bounded deeply by the ulna and the large flexor group of muscles, which lie caudal

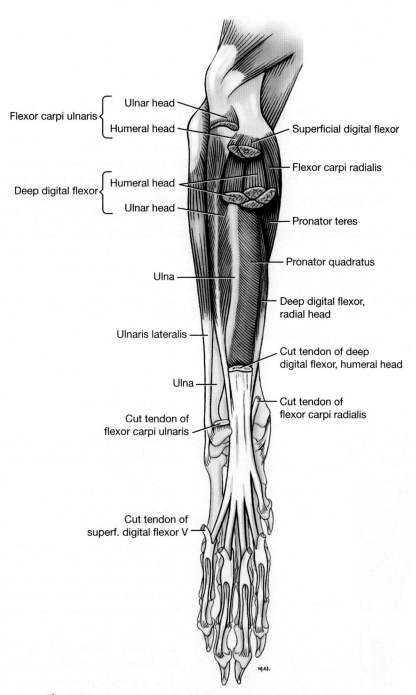

Fig. 2-24 Deep muscles of left antebrachium, caudal view.

and medial to it. It is the only flexor to arise on the lateral epicondyle. Expose the muscle and notice the two tendons of insertion.

ORIGIN: The lateral epicondyle of the humerus.

INSERTION: The lateral aspect of the proximal end of metacarpal V and the accessory carpal bone.

ACTION: To abduct the manus and flex the carpal joints and support the carpus when extended to support weight.

INNERVATION: Radial nerve.

5. The **supinator** (Figs. 2-13, 2-14, 2-25) is short, broad, and flat and obliquely placed across the lateral side of the flexor surface of the elbow joint. It is covered superficially by the extensor carpi radialis and common digital extensors, which should be transected in the middle of their muscle bellies and reflected. The supinator lies principally on the proximal fourth of the radius. There is a sesamoid bone in this muscle where it crosses the head of the radius.

ORIGIN: The lateral epicondyle of the humerus.

INSERTION: The cranial surface of the proximal fourth of the radius.

ACTION: To rotate the forearm laterally so that the palmar side of the paw faces medially (supination); to flex the elbow joint.

INNERVATION: Radial nerve.

6. The **abductor digiti I longus** (see Figs. 2-13, 2-14, 2-16, 2-20 through 2-22) lies primarily in the

groove between the radius and ulna and is triangular. Displace the digital extensors so that the bulk of the muscle is uncovered. Clean the muscle and transect its tendon as it obliquely crosses the extensor carpi radialis. There is a sesamoid bone in its tendon where it crosses the medial surface of the carpus. This muscle is also called the *extensor carpi obliquus* in domestic animals.

ORIGIN: The lateral border and cranial surface of the body of the ulna; the interosseous membrane.

INSERTION: The proximal end of metacarpal I.

ACTION: To abduct the first digit or pollex and extend the carpal joints.

INNERVATION: Radial nerve.

Caudal and Medial Muscles of the Forearm

The deep antebrachial fascia has been removed from this group of muscles. It will be necessary to clean the tendons of insertion when dissecting the individual muscles. The muscles in this group include, from the radius caudally, the pronator teres, the flexor carpi radialis, the deep digital flexor, the superficial digital flexor, and the flexor carpi ulnaris.

1. The **pronator teres** (Figs. 2-13, 2-14, 2-19 through 2-21, 2-23 through 2-25) extends obliquely across the medial surface of the elbow. It is round in transverse section at its origin and flat at its insertion. It lies between the extensor carpi radialis cranially and the flexor carpi radialis caudally. Displace adjacent muscles to see its origin and insertion.

ORIGIN: The medial epicondyle of the humerus.

INSERTION: The medial border of the radius between the proximal and middle thirds.

ACTION: To rotate the forearm medially so that the palmar side of the paw faces the ground (pronation); to flex the elbow.

INNERVATION: Median nerve.

Clean the tendons of insertion of the biceps and brachialis muscles, which are now exposed. The tendon of insertion of the biceps splits into two parts (see Fig. 2-30). The larger of the two inserts on the ulnar tuberosity and the smaller inserts on the radial tuberosity. The terminal tendon of the brachialis inserts between these two tendons of the biceps, primarily on the ulnar tuberosity.

2. The **flexor carpi radialis** (see Figs. 2-14, 2-19, 2-21 through 2-24) lies between the pronator

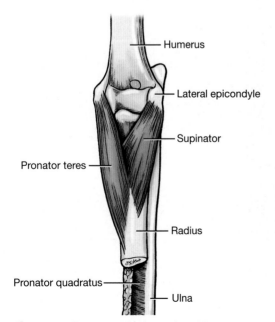

Fig. 2-25 Rotators of left antebrachium.

Humerus

Lateral epicondyle

Supinator

Pronator teres

Radius

Pronator quadratus

Ulna

teres cranially and the superficial digital flexor caudally. It covers the deep digital flexor, part of which can be seen. The flexor carpi radialis has a thick, fusiform belly, which, partly imbedded in the deep flexor, extends only to the middle of the radius. There it gives rise to a flat tendon that is augmented by fibers leaving the medial border of the radius. Clean the tendon to the point where it passes through the carpal canal deep to a thick layer of fibrous tissue on the palmar side of the carpus, the **flexor retinaculum** (see Fig. 2-22). Do not cut through this fibrous tissue now. A synovial sheath extends from the distal end of the radius almost to the insertion of the muscle on the palmar surface of the second and third metacarpal bones. This will be exposed later.

ORIGIN: The medial epicondyle of the humerus and the medial border of the radius.

INSERTION: The palmar side of the base of metacarpals II and III.

ACTION: To flex the carpal joints.

INNERVATION: Median nerve.

3. The **superficial digital flexor** (Figs. 2-13, 2-14, 2-19, 2-21 through 2-24, 2-26, 2-27) lies beneath the skin and antebrachial fascia on the caudomedial side of the forearm. It covers the deep digital flexor and is fleshy almost to the carpus. Its tendon is at first single, then crosses the palmar (flexor) surface of the carpus medial to the accessory carpal bone in the carpal canal, where it is covered by the superficial part of the flexor retinaculum, and finally divides into four tendons of nearly equal size. These insert on the palmar surfaces of the base of the middle phalanges of the four principal digits. At the metacarpophalangeal joint, each forms a collar, the **flexor manica**, around the deep flexor tendon that passes through it. Clean each of the individual tendons as far as the metacarpophalangeal joints. Transect the muscle at the middle of the antebrachium. Transect the superficial part of the flexor retinaculum and turn the distal part of the superficial digital flexor toward the digits. Because all parts of the superficial digital flexor tendon are similar, only that to the third digit will be dissected. The superficial and deep digital flexor tendons are held firmly in place at the metacarpophalangeal joint by the **palmar annular ligament**, which crosses the flexor manica (see Fig. 2-26). If any of the structures mentioned next are not clearly seen on the third digit, they should be verified on one or more of the other main digits. Observe that the tendon of the superficial digital flexor, which forms a flexor manica (see Fig. 2-26), sheathes the deep digital flexor for a distance of more than 1 cm at the metacarpophalangeal joint. The superficial digital flexor tendon lies on the palmar side of the deep flexor tendon at the proximal end of its encircling sheath but on the dorsal side at the distal end. The superficial flexor tendon with its sheath and the deep flexor tendon are in a common synovial membrane, the **digital synovial sheath**.

ORIGIN: The medial epicondyle of the humerus.

INSERTION: The palmar surface of the base (proximal end) of the middle phalanges of digits II, III, IV, and V.

ACTION: To flex the carpal, metacarpophalangeal, and proximal interphalangeal joints of digits II, III, IV, and V.

INNERVATION: Median nerve.

4. The **flexor carpi ulnaris** (see Figs. 2-13, 2-14, 2-16, 2-19, 2-21, 2-23, 2-24, 2-27) consists of two parts that are distinct throughout their length.

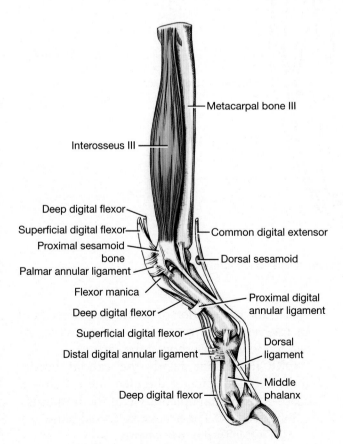

Metacarpal bone III

Interosseus III

Deep digital flexor

Superficial digital flexor

Proximal sesamoid bone

Palmar annular ligament

Flexor manica

Deep digital flexor

Superficial digital flexor

Distal digital annular ligament

Deep digital flexor

Common digital extensor

Dorsal sesamoid

Proximal digital annular ligament

Dorsal ligament

Middle phalanx

Fig. 2-26 Third digit, medial view.

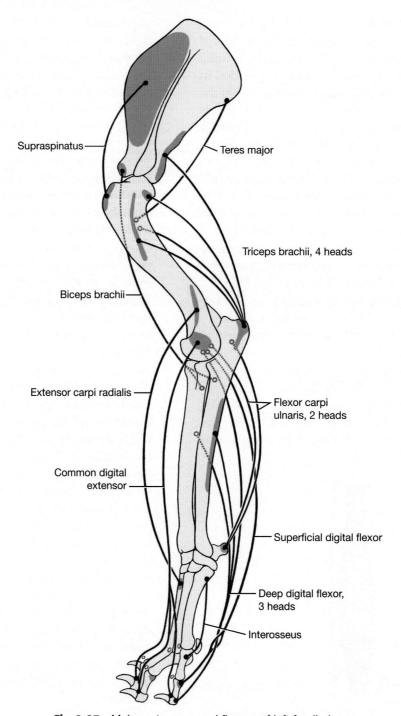

Supraspinatus

Teres major

Triceps brachii, 4 heads

Biceps brachii

Extensor carpi radialis

Flexor carpi
ulnaris, 2 heads

Common digital
extensor

Superficial digital flexor

Deep digital flexor,
3 heads

Interosseus

Fig. 2-27   Major extensors and flexors of left forelimb.

The **ulnar head** arises from the caudal border of the proximal end of the ulna. It is thin and wide proximally but narrow distally. It lies between the ulnaris lateralis and superficial digital flexor. The **humeral head** is large and fleshy and lies cranial to the ulnar head, except distally, where its tendon lies caudal to it. Dissect the insertion of this muscle on the accessory carpal bone and clean its origin. A subfascial bursa is present over

the tendon of insertion of the humeral head, and an intertendinous bursa is found between the two tendons of insertion at the carpus.

ORIGIN: Ulnar head—the caudal border and medial surface of the olecranon; humeral head—the medial epicondyle of the humerus.

INSERTION: The accessory carpal bone.

ACTION: To flex the carpus.

INNERVATION: Ulnar nerve.

5. The **deep digital flexor** (see Figs. 2-13, 2-14, 2-19, 2-21 through 2-24, 2-26, 2-27) has three heads of origin of dissimilar size, which arise from the humerus, radius, and ulna. Their bellies, along with the pronator quadratus, lie on the caudal surfaces of the radius and ulna. Transect both muscle bellies of the flexor carpi ulnaris in the middle of the antebrachium. Reflect the stumps to expose and identify the three heads of the deep digital flexor muscle. Notice that the **humeral head** of this muscle is much larger than the other two heads and has several bellies. The **ulnar head** is small and arises from the caudal border of the ulna. The **radial head** is the smallest and comes from the medial border of the radius. The tendons of all three heads fuse at the carpus to form a single tendon. This tendon is held in place in the carpal canal by the thick, deep part of the fibrous **flexor retinaculum**.

The **carpal canal** is formed by the accessory carpal bone laterally, the palmar carpal ligament and the carpal bones dorsally, and the flexor retinaculum on the palmar surface. Cut this retinaculum medially and reflect it laterally to the accessory carpal bone to expose the deep digital flexor tendon.

Distal to the carpus the deep digital flexor tendon divides into five branches. Each branch goes to the palmar surface of the base of the distal phalanx of its respective digit. There is a synovial bursa under the humeral head at the elbow and a carpal synovial sheath in the carpal canal. Dissect all of this digital flexor and the other digital muscles for digit III or IV. Observe all structures shown in Fig. 2-26. Digital synovial sheaths extend from proximal to the metacarpophalangeal joints to the insertion of the tendons on the distal phalanges of all the digits. The digital synovial sheaths, except that of the first digit, are common to both the superficial and the deep flexor tendons. Dissect the deep digital flexor tendon to its insertion on the distal phalanx of the third digit. It has already been exposed with the superficial digital flexor tendon at the metacarpophalangeal joint. Note the **annular digital ligaments** that support the deep digital flexor tendon proximal and distal to the palmar surface of the proximal interphalangeal joint.

ORIGIN: Humeral head—the medial epicondyle of the humerus; ulnar head—the proximal three fourths of the caudal border of the ulna; radial head—the middle third of the medial border of the radius.

INSERTION: The flexor tubercle on the palmar surface of the distal phalanx of each digit.

ACTION: To flex the carpal and metacarpophalangeal joints and the proximal and distal interphalangeal joints of the digits.

INNERVATION: Median and ulnar nerves.

6. The **pronator quadratus** (see Figs. 2-14, 2-21, 2-24, 2-25) fills in the space between the radius and ulna. Spread the flexor muscles and observe the pronator. The fibers of this muscle run transversely between the ulna and radius.

ATTACHMENTS: The apposed surfaces of the radius and ulna.

ACTION: To pronate the paw.

INNERVATION: Median nerve.

Muscles of the Forepaw (Manus)

There are several special muscles of the digits. Only the **interossei** will be dissected. The four interosseous muscles are fleshy and similar in size and shape (see Figs. 2-26, 2-27). They lie deep to the deep digital flexor tendons and cover the palmar surfaces of the four main metacarpal bones. Transect the deep digital flexor tendon at the proximal end of the carpus and reflect it distally. Dissect the interosseous muscle of the third digit. Each muscle arises from the base of its respective metacarpal bone and the carpal joint capsule. After a short course, each divides into two tendons, which attach to the base of the proximal phalanx. Imbedded in each tendon is a sesamoid bone that lies on the palmar surface of the metacarpophalangeal joint. There are thus two **proximal sesamoids** imbedded in the tendon of insertion at metacarpophalangeal joints II, III, IV, and V. In addition, each muscle at its termination at the metacarpophalangeal joint gives off a tendon on each side of the joint that extends dorsally on the first phalanx to join the common digital extensor tendon. This increases the ability of this muscle to support the metacarpophalangeal joint during weight bearing. The interosseous muscle is a flexor of the metacarpophalangeal (fetlock) joint and maintains the joint angle when the dog bears weight on the paw. Complete exposure of the tendon of insertion of an interosseous muscle can be accomplished by separating the third and fourth digits to the level of the carpometacarpal joint. Abduct the fourth and fifth digits to observe the full length of the interosseous muscle on the third digit. Transect the muscle at the middle of the metacarpal bone and reflect the distal portion to expose the sesamoid bones in the tendon at the metacarpophalangeal joint.

LIVE DOG

Palpate the lateral epicondyle of the humerus. Feel for the groove between the lateral supracondylar crest and the olecranon, where a needle can be inserted through the anconeus muscle into the elbow joint. Follow the extensor muscles distally in the forearm. Follow the tendons of the extensor carpi radialis and common digital extensor across the carpus. Flex the carpus and palpate the antebrachiocarpal joint on either side of these tendons where a needle puncture can be made.

Palpate the medial humeral epicondyle and the origins of the flexor muscles on it. At the carpus, palpate the terminations of the flexor carpi ulnaris and ulnaris lateralis on the accessory carpal. Palpate the tendon of the superficial digital flexor at the carpal canal. Flex the carpus and feel the tendon loosen. Extend it and feel the tendon become taut. Flex and extend the metacarpophalangeal and interphalangeal joints and appreciate the action of the digital extensors and flexors on these joints. Laceration of the digital flexors will cause overextension of the interphalangeal joints affected.

JOINTS OF THE THORACIC LIMB

The **humeral** or shoulder joint (Fig. 2-28) is a ball-and-socket joint between the glenoid cavity

of the scapula and the head of the humerus. It is capable of movements in any direction, but the chief movements it undergoes are flexion and extension. Transect the subscapularis medially and the teres minor laterally to gain access to the humeral joint capsule. The humeral joint capsule is a loose sleeve of synovial membrane and thin fibrous tissue that unites the scapula and humerus. Poorly developed thickenings of the fibrous part of the joint capsule on each side are called the **medial** and **lateral glenohumeral ligaments** (see Figs. 2-28, 2-29). There is a collagenous thickening across the tendon of origin of the biceps at the intertubercular groove; this is the **transverse humeral retinaculum** (see Fig. 2-28). The joint capsule surrounds the tendon of origin of the biceps brachii in the intertubercular groove, forming its tendon sheath.

The **cubiti** or elbow joint (Figs. 2-30, 2-31) is a hinge joint formed by the condyle of the humerus, the head of the radius, and the trochlear notch of the ulna. In addition, there is the proximal radioulnar articulation, although it is not weight bearing. The elbow joint capsule attaches to the articular margins; it extends distally a short distance between the radius and ulna. All compartments communicate with each other. The **lateral** and **medial collateral ligaments** are pronounced thickenings in the fibrous layer of the capsule. The biceps and brachialis tendons cover the distal portion of the medial collateral ligament. Transect and reflect these tendon insertions

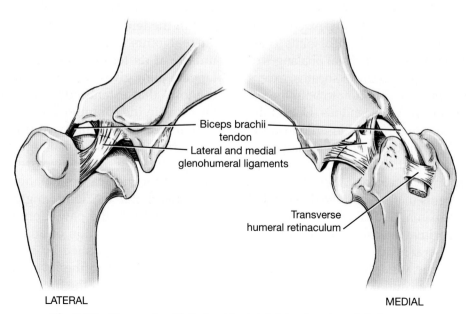

Biceps brachii tendon
Lateral and medial glenohumeral ligaments
Transverse humeral retinaculum

LATERAL   MEDIAL

Fig. 2-28 Ligaments of left shoulder joint, lateral and medial views.

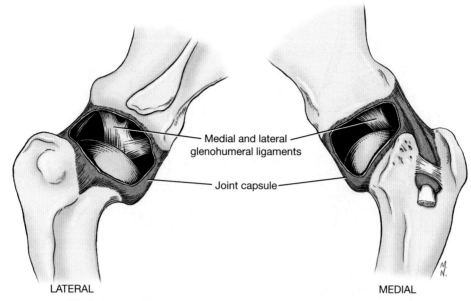

Fig. 2-29 Capsule of left shoulder joint, lateral and medial views.

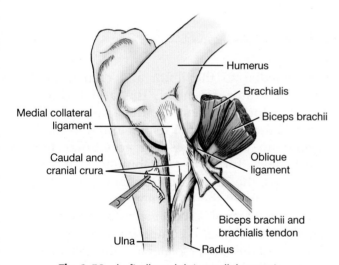

Fig. 2-30 Left elbow joint, medial aspect.

to expose the medial collateral ligament. Transect the medial collateral ligament to expose the medial coronoid process of the ulna that it covers. This is a site of osteochondrosis lesions. On the lateral side, transect and reflect the origin of the lateral digital extensor to expose the lateral collateral ligament (see Fig. 2-31). These taut ligaments prevent adduction or abduction of the elbow and restrict movement to the sagittal plane. Some rotational movement occurs at the radioulnar joint.

The **interosseous ligament** is a condensation of collagenous tissue that unites the radius and ulna proximally (see Fig. 2-31).

The carpal joint is a composite of three articular levels: (1) proximally an **antebrachiocarpal joint** between the radius and ulna articulating with the intermedioradial and ulnar carpal bones; (2) a **middle carpal joint** between the two rows of carpal bones; and (3) a **carpometacarpal joint** between the distal row of carpal bones and the metacarpals. The carpal joint capsule extends as a sleeve from the distal ends of the radius and ulna to the metacarpus. It attaches to the carpal bones in its course across the joint and forms separate compartments. The antebrachiocarpal joint compartment does not communicate with the middle carpal joint compartment. The middle carpal and carpometacarpal joint compartments communicate between the distal row of carpal bones.

The joint capsule of the carpus differs from that of typical hinge joints in that both the dorsal and palmar surfaces are heavily reinforced by the fibrous layer of the joint capsule. On the dorsal surface of the joint, the fibrous layer of the capsule contains grooves in which the extensor tendons lie. This layer is loose between the radius and ulna proximally and the proximal row of carpals distally because most of the movement of the carpus takes place there. Cut through the joint capsule of this antebrachiocarpal joint to observe its components and the degree of movement of the joint. On the palmar side the **palmar carpal ligament** is a thick fibrous layer that firmly attaches to the bones of the carpus.

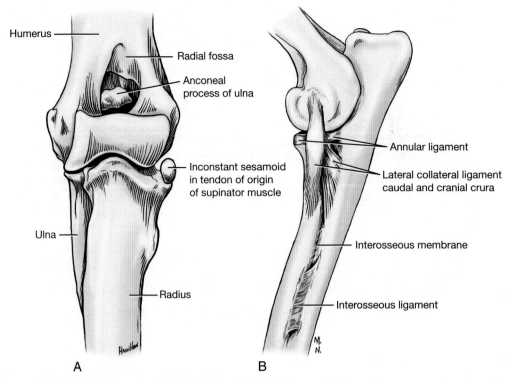

Fig. 2-31   Left elbow joint. **A**, Cranial aspect. **B**, Lateral aspect.

This is important in preventing collapse of the carpus when the limb bears weight. This layer of fibrocartilage forms the deep (dorsal) boundary of the carpal canal (Fig. 2-22). Numerous ligaments within the joint capsule connect the various bones of the carpus. These will not be dissected.

The **metacarpophalangeal, proximal interphalangeal**, and **distal interphalangeal** joints are the three articulations of each main digit. Medial and lateral collateral ligaments support these joints.

Each metacarpophalangeal joint includes two proximal sesamoids in the tendons of the interossei, which articulate with the flexor surface of the metacarpal head.

BONES OF THE PELVIC LIMB

The **pelvic girdle**, or pelvis, of the dog consists of two hip bones, which are united at the **symphysis pelvis** midventrally and join the sacrum dorsally. Each hip bone, or **os coxae**, is formed by the fusion of three primary bones and the addition of a fourth in early life (Fig. 2-32). The largest and most cranial of these is the **ilium**, which articulates with the sacrum. The **ischium** is the most caudal, whereas the **pubis** is located

ventromedial to the ilium and cranial to the large obturator foramen. The **acetabulum**, a socket, is formed where the three bones meet. It receives the head of the femur in the formation of the hip joint. The small **acetabular bone**, which helps form the acetabulum, is incorporated with the ilium, ischium, and pubis when they fuse (about the third month).

The **pelvic canal** is short ventrally but long dorsally. Its lateral wall is composed of the ilium, ischium, and pubis. Dorsolateral to the skeletal part of the wall, the pelvic canal is bounded by soft tissues. The **pelvic inlet** is limited laterally and ventrally by the arcuate line of the ilium. Its dorsal boundary is the promontory of the sacrum. The **pelvic outlet** is bounded ventrally by the **ischiatic arch** (the ischiatic arch is formed by the concave caudal border of the two ischii); mid-dorsally by the first caudal vertebra; and laterally by the superficial gluteal muscle, muscles of the pelvic diaphragm, and the sacrotuberous ligament.

Os Coxae

1. The **ilium** (Figs. 2-32, 2-33 through 2-35), a flat bone presenting two surfaces and three borders, forms the cranial one half to three fifths of the os coxae. It can be divided into a wide cranial part, which is concave laterally and known

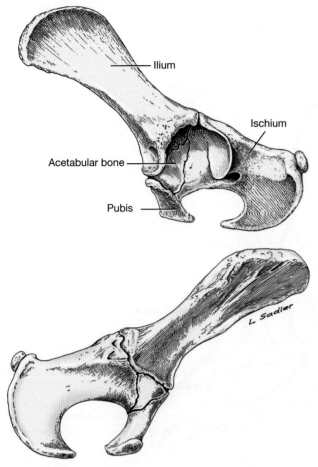

Fig. 2-32 Left hip bone, 15-week-old beagle.

as the **wing**, and a narrow, laterally compressed caudal part, the **body**.

The cranial border is arciform and usually roughened and is more commonly known as the **iliac crest**. It is thin but gradually increases in thickness dorsally. The angle of junction of the iliac crest with the ventral border is known as the cranial ventral iliac spine, which provides a place of origin for both bellies of the sartorius and a part of the tensor fasciae latae. The **tuber coxae** is composed of the cranial ventral iliac spine and the adjacent part of the ventral border of the wing of the ilium. The rest of the ventral border is concave. It ends in the **lateral area for the rectus** femoris (see Fig. 2-33) just cranial to the acetabulum.

The dorsal border of the ilium is broad and massive. The junction of the dorsal border with the iliac crest forms an obtuse angle that is a rounded prominence, the **cranial dorsal iliac spine**. Caudal to the cranial dorsal iliac spine is the wide but blunt **caudal dorsal iliac spine**. The two spines and intervening bone make up

the **tuber sacrale**, which occupies nearly half the length of the dorsal border of the ilium. The caudal half of the dorsal border is gently concave. It forms the **greater ischiatic notch** and also helps form the ischiatic spine, which is dorsal to the acetabulum.

The external or **gluteal surface** (see Fig. 2-33) of the wing of the ilium is nearly flat caudally and concave cranially, where it is limited by the iliac crest. The dorsal part of this concave area is bounded by a heavy ridge, the tuber sacrale. The gluteal surface is rough ventrocranially. The middle gluteal and a portion of the deep gluteal attach here.

The internal or **sacropelvic surface** (see Fig. 2-34) of the wing of the ilium presents a smooth, nearly flat area that provides attachment for the iliocostalis, longissimus, and the quadratus lumborum muscles. The **auricular surface** is rough and articulates with a similar surface of the sacrum, forming the sacroiliac joint. The **arcuate line** is located along the ventromedial edge of the sacropelvic surface of the body of the ilium and runs from the auricular surface to the iliopubic eminence of the pubis. The tendon of the psoas minor attaches along the medial aspect of this line.

2. The **ischium** (see Figs. 2-32 through 2-35) consists of tuberosity, body, table, and ramus. It forms the caudal part of the os coxae and enters into the formation of the acetabulum, obturator foramen, and symphysis pelvis. Its caudal border consists of the ischiatic tuberosity laterally and one half of the ischiatic arch medially. The **ischiatic tuberosity** is the thick caudolateral margin of the bone. The lateral angle of the tuber is enlarged and hooked; it furnishes attachment for the sacrotuberous ligament. The medial angle is rounded. The ventral surface is the place of origin for the biceps femoris, semitendinosus, and semimembranosus. The crus of the penis and the muscle that surrounds it also attach to the ischiatic tuberosity medially.

The **body of the ischium** is the part lateral to the obturator foramen. The **ischiatic spine** is a rounded crest dorsal to the acetabulum, where the body of the ischium meets the ilium. The coccygeus attaches here. Caudal to this spine the border of the ischium is depressed and marked by a series of low ridges produced by

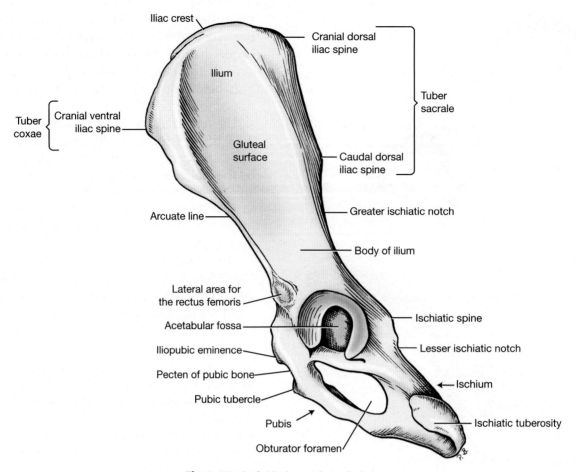

Fig. 2-33   Left hip bone, lateral view.

the tendon of the internal obturator. This area is known as the **lesser ischiatic notch** (see Figs. 2-33, 2-34). The gemelli arise from the lateral surface adjacent to the lesser ischiatic notch.

The **ramus** of the ischium is the thin and wide medial part of the ischium. It is bounded laterally by the obturator foramen and blends caudally with the body of the ischium. The ramus meets its fellow at the symphysis and is fused with the pubis cranially. The **ischiatic table** is the flat portion where the ramus meets the body (see Fig. 2-34). It faces dorsally and is the site of origin of the internal obturator muscle. The quadratus femoris and the external obturator arise from its ventral surface. The **ischiatic arch** is formed by the medial portion of the caudal border of each ischium.

3. The **pubis** (see Figs. 2-32 through 2-35) extends from the ilium and ischium laterally to the symphysis medially and consists of a body and two rami. The **body** is located cranial to the obturator foramen. The **cranial ramus** extends from the body to the ilium and enters into the formation of the acetabulum. The **caudal ramus** fuses with the ischial ramus at the middle of the pelvic symphysis. The ventral surface of the pubis and adjacent ischial ramus serve as origin for the gracilis, the adductor, and the external obturator. The dorsal surface gives rise to a small part of the internal obturator and the levator ani. The **obturator sulcus**, a groove for the obturator nerve, is located at the cranial end of the obturator foramen and passes dorsally over the pelvic surface of the body of the bone. The **iliopubic eminence** projects from the cranial border of the cranial ramus of the pubic bone. The pectineus attaches to it. The **pubic tubercle** projects cranially from the pubis on the midline. The roughened cranial border of the pubis between the iliopubic eminence and the pubic tubercle is the **pecten**, to which the abdominal muscles attach by means of a prepubic tendon to be dissected later. The prepubic tendon is composed primarily of the tendons of the paired rectus abdominis and pectineus muscles.

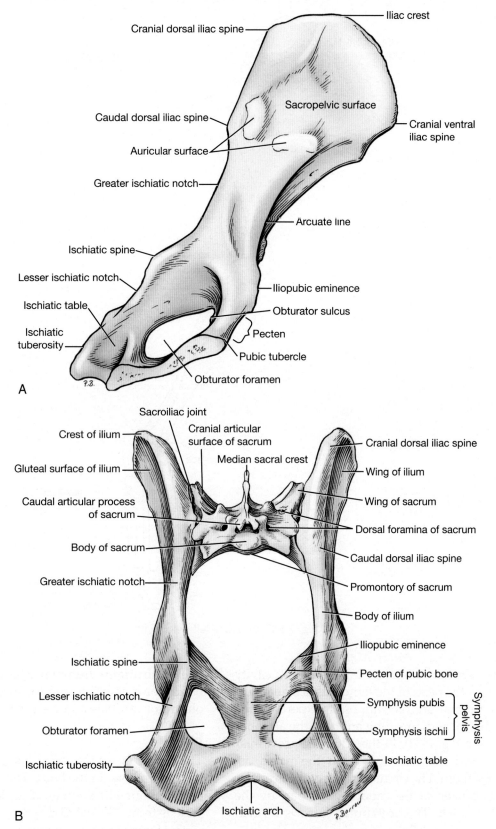

Fig. 2-34 **A,** Left hip bone, medial view. **B,** Pelvis and sacrum, caudodorsal view.

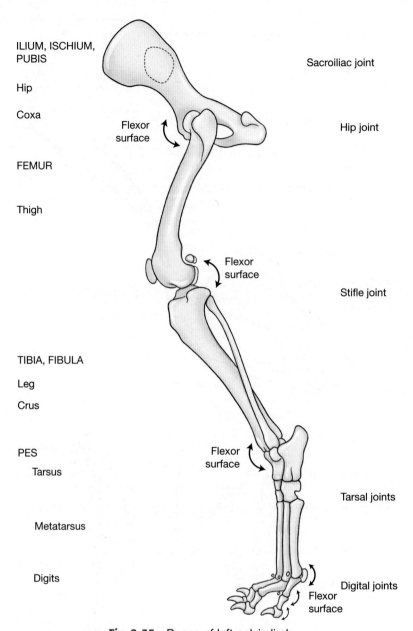

ILIUM, ISCHIUM,
PUBIS

Hip

Coxa

Flexor
surface

FEMUR

Thigh

TIBIA, FIBULA

Leg

Crus

PES

Tarsus

Metatarsus

Digits

Sacroiliac joint

Hip joint

Flexor
surface

Stifle joint

Flexor
surface

Tarsal joints

Digital joints
Flexor
surface

Fig. 2-35   Bones of left pelvic limb.

The **acetabulum** (see Figs. 2-32, 2-33) is a cavity that receives the head of the femur. Its articular surface is semilunar and is composed of parts of the ilium, ischium, and, in young animals, the acetabular bone (see Fig. 2-32). In the adult the acetabular bone is fused imperceptibly with the pubis, ischium, and ilium. The circumference of the articular surface is broken at the caudomedial part by the **acetabular notch**. The **acetabular fossa** is formed by the ischium and the acetabular bone. The ligament of the head of the femur attaches in this fossa. The fossa and the notch are the nonarticular parts of the acetabulum. The two sides of the notch are connected by the transverse acetabular ligament.

The **obturator foramen** is closed in life by the obturator membrane and the external and internal obturator muscles that the membrane separates.

Femur

The femur (see Figs. 2-35, 2-36), or thigh bone, is the largest bone in the body. The flexor angle of the hip is about 110 degrees. The flexor angle at the stifle is from 130 to 135 degrees.

The femur is a typical long bone with a cylindrical body and two expanded extremities. The proximal extremity presents on its medial side a smooth, nearly hemispherical **head**, most of which is articular except for a small shallow fossa beginning

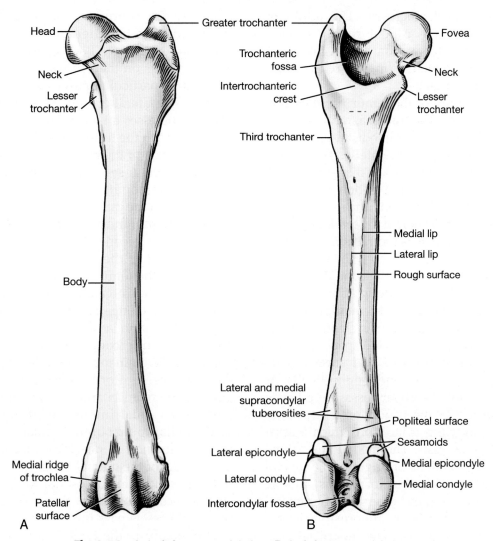

Fig. 2-36 A, Left femur, cranial view. **B,** Left femur, caudal view.

near the middle of the head and usually extending to its caudomedial margin. This fossa is the **fovea capitis femoris,** to which the ligament of the head of the femur attaches. The head is attached to the medial part of the proximal extremity by the **neck** of the femur. The neck is distinct but short and provides attachment for the joint capsule. The **greater trochanter,** the largest eminence of the proximal extremity, is located directly lateral to the head. To it attach the middle gluteal and deep gluteal. The **trochanteric fossa** is a deep cavity medial to the greater trochanter. The gemelli and the external and internal obturators insert in this fossa. The **lesser trochanter,** a pyramidal projection at the proximal end of the medial side of the body of the femur, serves for the insertion of the iliopsoas. A ridge of bone extends from the summit of the greater trochanter to the lesser trochanter. This, the **intertrochanteric crest,** represents the caudolateral

boundary of the trochanteric fossa. The quadratus femoris inserts on the crest at the level of the lesser trochanter. The **third trochanter** is poorly developed. It appears at the base of the greater trochanter as a small, rough area on which the superficial gluteal inserts. The third and lesser trochanters are located in about the same transverse plane. The vastus parts of the quadriceps femoris attach to the smooth proximal cranial part of the femur.

The **body** of the femur is slightly convex cranially. Viewed cranially, the body presents a smooth, rounded surface. The caudal surface is rough and is limited by **medial** and **lateral lips**. The lips, closest together in the middle of the body, diverge as they approach each extremity. The proximal part of the medial lip ends in the lesser trochanter, the distal part at the medial supracondylar tuberosity. The proximal part of the lateral lip ends in the third trochanter, the distal part at the lateral supracondylar tuberosity. The adductor inserts on most of the caudal rough surface, whereas a tendon extends from the pectineus to the distal part of the medial lip, where the semimembranosus also attaches.

The distal extremity of the femur presents several articular surfaces. The **trochlea,** with ridges, is the smooth groove on the craniodistal part of the bone for articulation with the **patella**. The medial trochlear ridge is usually thicker than the lateral. The patella is a sesamoid in the tendon of insertion of the large quadriceps femoris that extends the stifle. It aids in the protection of the tendon and the joint, but its chief purpose is redirection of the tendon of insertion of the quadriceps. The trochlea of the femur is continuous with the condyles, which articulate, both directly and through fibrocartilaginous menisci, with the tibia. The **medial and lateral condyles** are separated from each other by the **intercondylar fossa**, a deep, wide space. The two condyles are similar in shape and surface area. Each is convex transversely and longitudinally. At the depth of the intercondylar fossa the cruciate ligaments attach. On the caudodorsal aspect of each femoral condyle is a facet on which a sesamoid bone (fabella) rests. The medial and lateral fabellae are in the tendons of origin of the medial and lateral heads of the gastrocnemius muscle. Proximal to these sesamoid facets are the **medial** and **lateral supracondylar tuberosities** from which the gastrocnemii arise. The superficial digital flexor also arises from the lateral tuberosity. The **popliteal surface** is a large, flat, triangular area on the caudal surface of the distal extremity proximal to the condyles and intercondylar fossa. The **medial and lateral epicondyles** are rough areas on each side, proximal to the condyles. They serve for the attachment of the collateral ligaments of the stifle. The lateral epicondyle also gives rise to the popliteus. The small **extensor fossa** is located on the lateral epicondyle at the junction of the lateral condyle and the lateral lip of the trochlea; from it arises the long digital extensor. The semimembranosus is inserted just proximal to the medial epicondyle.

Tibia

The tibia (Fig. 2-37), the shin or leg bone, has a proximal articular surface that flares out transversely and is also broad craniocaudally. It is wider than the distal end of the femur, with which it articulates, and is formed largely by two relatively flat condyles. The **medial condyle** is separated from the **lateral condyle** by the **intercondylar eminence**. Both condyles include the articular areas on their proximal surfaces and the adjacent nonarticular parts of the proximal extremity. The lateral condyle is particularly prominent. It possesses a facet on its lateral side for articulation with the head of the fibula and provides origin for part of the peroneus longus and cranial tibial muscles. A sesamoid bone in the tendon of origin of the popliteus (seen in radiographs) articulates with the caudolateral condyle of the tibia. The semimembranosus is inserted on the medial condyle. Two biconcave fibrocartilages, the **menisci**, fill part of the space between the apposed condyles of the femur and tibia, making the joint congruent. The **intercondylar eminence** consists of two small, elongated tubercles, which form its highest part, and a shallow intercondylar area. The **cranial intercondylar area** is a depression cranial to the eminence and in large part between the condyles. It affords attachment to the cranial parts of the menisci and the cranial cruciate ligament. The **caudal intercondylar area** occupies a place similar to that of the cranial area but caudal to the eminence. It provides attachment for the caudal part of the medial meniscus. The **popliteal notch** is caudal to the caudal intercondylar area and is located between the two condyles. The popliteal vessels pass through the notch. The **tibial tuberosity** is the large quadrangular process on the proximal cranial surface of the tibia. The quadriceps femoris, the biceps femoris, and the sartorius attach to this tuberosity by means of the patella and patellar ligament. The tibial tuberosity is continued distally by the **cranial border of the tibia**. It inclines laterally on the body. The following muscles attach wholly or in part to the cranial border of the tibia: biceps femoris, semitendinosus, gracilis, and sartorius. The **extensor groove** is a small, smooth groove located at the junction of the lateral condyle and the tibial tuberosity. The long digital extensor passes through it.

The **body** is triangular proximally, nearly cylindrical in the middle, and four-sided distally. The semitendinosus and gracilis are inserted on the proximal medial surface. The proximal third of the caudal surface serves for the insertion of the popliteus medially and for the origins of the deep digital flexor laterally.

The distal extremity of the tibia is quadrilateral in transverse section. The **tibial cochlea,** the

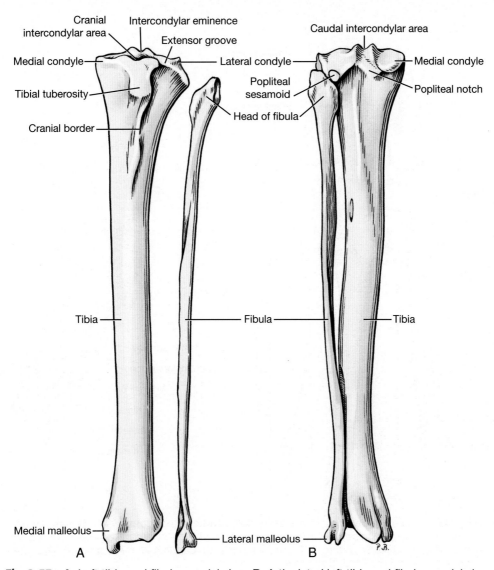

Fig. 2-37 **A,** Left tibia and fibula, cranial view. **B,** Articulated left tibia and fibula, caudal view.

articular surface, consists of two grooves that receive the ridges of the proximal trochlea of the
talus. The medial part of the distal extremity of the
tibia is the **medial malleolus**. The lateral surface
of the distal extremity articulates with the fibula
by a small facet. No muscles arise from the distal
half of the tibia.

Fibula

The fibula (see Figs. 2-35, 2-37) has proximal and
distal extremities and an intermediate **body**. The
proximal extremity, or **head**, articulates with the
lateral condyle of the tibia. The distal extremity,
the **lateral malleolus**, has two grooves that contain the tendons of the fibularis longus, fibularis
brevis, and the lateral digital extensor. These
grooves redirect the force of contraction. On the
medial surface of the tibia is a distinct facet for

articulation with the distolateral surface of the
tibia and with the talus.

Tarsal Bones

The **tarsus** (see Figs. 2-35, 2-38), between the metatarsals and the leg, is composed of seven tarsal
bones and the related soft tissues. It is also called the
hock. The bones are arranged in three irregular rows.
The proximal row is composed of a long, laterally
located **calcaneus** and a shorter, medially located
talus. The talus has a **trochlea** on its proximal end
with two ridges separated by a groove for articulation with the tibial cochlea. This is the tarsocrural
joint where flexion and extension occur between the
leg and hindpaw. The talus articulates with the calcaneus laterally and the central tarsal bone distally.
The calcaneus articulates with the adjacent talus
and distally with the fourth tarsal bone.

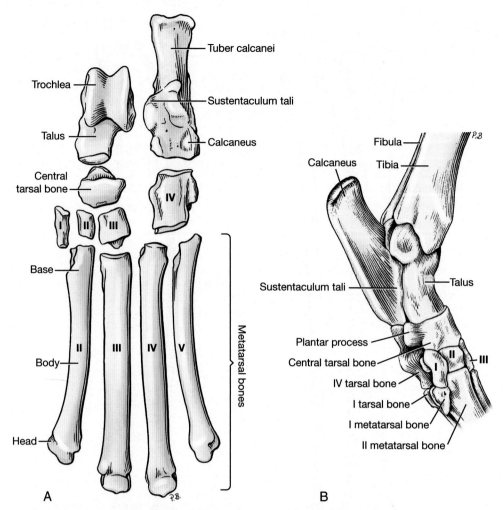

Fig. 2-38 **A,** Left tarsal and metatarsal bones disarticulated, dorsal view. **B,** Left tarsus, articulated, medial aspect. (**A** From Evans HE: *Miller's anatomy of the dog*, ed 3, Philadelphia, 1993, Saunders. **B** From Evans HE, de Lahunta A: *Miller's anatomy of the dog*, ed 4, St Louis, 2013, Saunders.)

The **tuber calcanei** is a traction process of the calcaneus that projects proximally and caudally. The extensor muscles of the tarsus insert on this process via the common calcanean tendon. On the medial side of the calcaneus is a bony process, the **sustentaculum tali.** The tendon of the lateral digital flexor glides over the plantar surface of this process.

The distal row consists of four bones. Three small bones, the **first, second,** and **third tarsal** bones, are located side by side and are separated from the proximal row by the **central tarsal bone.** The large **fourth tarsal bone,** which completes the distal row laterally, articulates with the calcaneus proximally. The fourth tarsal is as long as the combined lengths of the third and central tarsal bones against which it lies. The fourth tarsal bone is grooved on the distal half of its lateral surface for the passage of the tendon of the fibularis longus.

Metatarsal Bones

The metatarsal bones (see Fig. 2-38) resemble the metacarpal bones except for the first, which may be divided, rudimentary, or absent.

Phalanges

The phalanges (Fig. 2-39) and sesamoids form the skeleton of the digit. Those of the hindpaw, or **pes**, are similar to those of the forepaw, or **manus**.

The first digit, or **hallux**, is frequently absent. When present, it is called a *dewclaw* and may vary from a fully developed digit, articulating with a normal first metatarsal bone, to a vestigial structure composed only of a terminal phalanx.

LIVE DOG

Palpate the iliac crests beside the sacrum at the cranial aspect of the pelvis, the entire length of

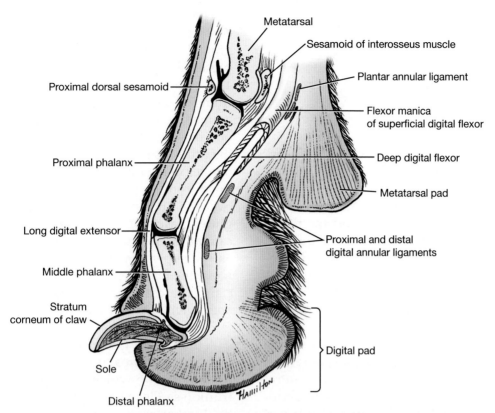

Metatarsal

Sesamoid of interosseus muscle

Plantar annular ligament

Flexor manica
of superficial digital flexor

Deep digital flexor

Metatarsal pad

Proximal dorsal sesamoid

Proximal phalanx

Long digital extensor

Middle phalanx

Proximal and distal
digital annular ligaments

Stratum
corneum of claw

Digital pad

Sole

Distal phalanx

Fig. 2-39 Median section of the third digit of the hindpaw.

the tuber ischii caudolaterally, and the ischiatic arch between these tuberosities. Note their symmetry. Pelvic fractures and sacroiliac luxation are common and result in palpable asymmetry.

Palpate the greater trochanter of the femur lateral to the hip. Place your thumb in the groove between the greater trochanter and the ischial tuberosity. Rotate the thigh laterally and note the displacement of your thumb by the greater trochanter. This will not occur when there is a hip luxation.

At the distal end of the femur, palpate the trochlea and the edges of the patella that articulate with it. Palpate the condyles of the femur and tibia. Flex, extend, and rotate the stifle to appreciate the level of this articulation. The tibial tuberosity and cranial border are palpable on the proximal tibia. Feel the body of the tibia where it is subcutaneous on the medial side. Palpate the narrow distal tibia and fibula. Flex and extend the tarsocrural joint, and on the dorsal aspect feel the ridges of the trochlea of the talus and the intermediate ridge of the cochlea of the tibia that participate in this joint. Palpate the tuber calcanei and note how a proximal pull on this lever will extend the joint. A

fracture of this will cause the joint to overflex, and the dog will walk partly plantigrade.

MUSCLES OF THE PELVIC LIMB

Caudal thigh
 Biceps femoris
 Semitendinosus
 Semimembranosus
Medial thigh
 Sartorius
 Gracilis
 Pectineus
 Adductor
Lateral pelvis (rump)
 Tensor fasciae latae
 Superficial gluteal
 Middle gluteal
 Deep gluteal
Caudal hip
 Internal obturator
 Gemelli
 Quadratus femoris
 External obturator
Cranial thigh
 Quadriceps femoris

Iliopsoas
Sartorius
Craniolateral leg
  Cranial tibial
  Long digital extensor
  Fibularis longus
Caudal leg
  Gastrocnemius
  Superficial digital flexor
  Deep digital flexors
  Popliteus

Remove the skin from the caudal part of the left half of the trunk, the pelvis, and the thigh. Continue the midventral incision from the umbilicus to the root of the tail. In making this incision, closely circle the external genital parts and the anus. Extend an incision distally on the medial surface of the left thigh to the tarsus. Encircle the tarsus with a skin incision. First, reflect the skin from the medial surface of the thigh and crus and then, starting at the tarsus, reflect the whole flap of skin from the lateral surface of the leg, stifle, thigh, pelvis, and abdomen to the mid-dorsal line. The cutaneous trunci may be removed with the skin because it is more intimately attached to the skin than to the underlying structures.

There are superficial and deep fasciae of the pelvic limb. They cannot always be separated, and, in general, the deep fascia is more dense than the superficial fascia.

The **superficial fascia of the trunk** (Fig. 2-40) continues dorsally on the pelvis as the **superficial gluteal fascia**. In obese specimens much fat is present between this fascia and the deep fascia. The cutaneous trunci arises as an aponeurosis from the superficial gluteal fascia. It may be examined in the skin just reflected and in the previous dissection. Its fibers run cranioventrally to the caudal part of the axilla. Its most ventral border lies in the fold of the flank; dorsally, it is separated from its fellow by a narrow band of fascia over the lumbar area and pelvis. The **superficial gluteal fascia** passes to the tail as the **superficial caudal fascia** and continues distally on the limb as the superficial lamina of the fascia lata. Remove the fat-laden areolar tissue and the superficial fascia covering the caudal part of the trunk and pelvis. Do not cut into the glistening deep fascia underneath.

A thick deep fascia covers the dorsal muscles of the lumbar area, pelvis, and tail. The **thoracolumbar fascia**, which is the **deep fascia of the trunk** (see Figs. 2-40, 2-41), is well developed in the lumbar region and is continued caudally at the iliac crest by the **deep gluteal fascia**. This distinct glistening fascia covers the muscles of the pelvis and serves in part as origin for the middle and superficial gluteals. The deep gluteal fascia is continued caudally on the tail by the **deep caudal fascia**. The latter follows the irregularities of the caudal muscles and closely

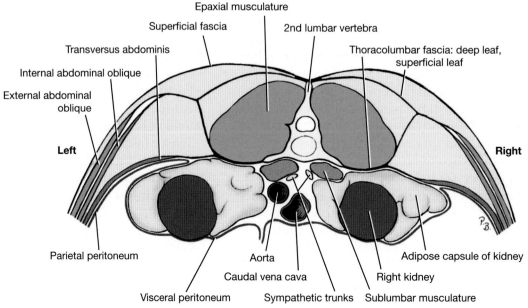

Fig. 2-40   Schematic transection in the lumbar region showing fascial layers.

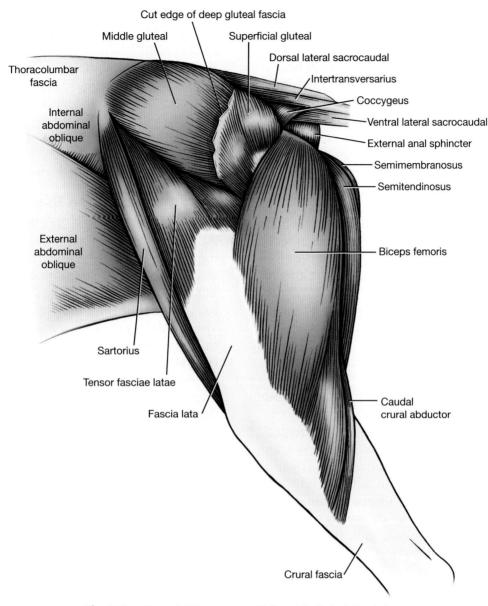

Middle gluteal

Cut edge of deep gluteal fascia

Superficial gluteal

Dorsal lateral sacrocaudal

Thoracolumbar fascia

Intertransversarius

Coccygeus

Internal abdominal oblique

Ventral lateral sacrocaudal

External anal sphincter

Semimembranosus

Semitendinosus

External abdominal oblique

Biceps femoris

Sartorius

Tensor fasciae latae

Caudal crural abductor

Fascia lata

Crural fascia

Fig. 2-41 Superficial muscles of left pelvic limb, lateral view.

binds these to the vertebrae of the tail. Distally, the deep gluteal fascia blends with the fascia of the thigh, where it becomes the **medial** and **lateral femoral fasciae**. The medial fascia is thin, whereas the lateral femoral fascia, the **fascia lata**, is thick and serves as an aponeurotic insertion for thigh muscles. The femoral fascia is continued on the leg as the **crural fascia**. Clean but do not cut any of the deep fascia until instructed to do so.

Caudal Muscles of the Thigh

This group consists of three primary muscles: biceps femoris, laterally; semitendinosus, caudally; and semimembranosus, medially. (A slender

caudal crural abductor muscle is closely associated with the mediocaudal surface of the biceps femoris [see Figs. 2-41, 2-43].)

1. The **biceps femoris** (see Figs. 2-41, 2-44, 2-45, 2-47, 2-52, 2-54 through 2-57) is the longest and widest of the muscles of the thigh. The bulk of its fibers run craniodistally, although caudally there are fibers that run directly distally. Identify the lateral aspect of the tuber ischii and the sacrotuberous ligament that extends from it to the sacrum. The biceps femoris arises from these structures. Cranially, it inserts by means of the fascia lata and crural fascia. Carefully clean the caudal border and the adjacent surface of the muscle. The lymph node lying in the

fat at its caudal border directly caudal to the stifle is the **popliteal lymph node**. Do not cut the cranially lying fascia lata, which serves as part of its insertion. Caudally, a strand of heavy fascia runs to the tuber calcanei and helps to form the **common calcanean tendon**. Transect the biceps femoris. The sciatic nerve is interposed between the biceps femoris and the adductor. Observe the insertions of the biceps femoris.

ORIGIN: The sacrotuberous ligament and the ischiatic tuberosity.

INSERTION: By means of the fascia lata and crural fascia to the patella, patellar ligament, and cranial border of the tibia; by means of the crural fascia to the subcutaneous part of the tibial body; the tuber calcanei.

ACTION: To extend the hip, stifle, and tarsal joints. The caudal part of the muscle flexes the stifle joint.

INNERVATION: Sciatic nerve.

2. The **semitendinosus** (see Figs. 2-41 through 2-47, 2-52, 2-54, 2-55, 2-57), near its origin, lies between the biceps femoris and semimembranosus. Near its insertion it lies on the medial head of the gastrocnemius and is covered by the gracilis. It is nearly as wide as it is thick and extends principally from the ischiatic tuberosity to the tibial body. By means of the crural fascia, it also attaches to the tuber calcanei. Completely free this muscle from surrounding structures but do not transect it.

ORIGIN: The ischiatic tuberosity.

INSERTION: The distocranial border of the tibia. The medial surface of the body of the tibia and the tuber calcanei by means of the crural fascia.

ACTION: To extend the hip joint, flex the stifle joint, and extend the tarsal joints.

INNERVATION: Sciatic nerve.

3. The **semimembranosus** (see Figs. 2-41 through 2-47, 2-50, 2-52, 2-57) is greater in transverse sectional area than the semitendinosus but is not as long. It is wedged between the semitendinosus and biceps femoris laterally and the gracilis and adductor medially. It has two bellies of nearly equal size. This short but thick muscle extends from the ischiatic tuberosity to the medial side of the distal end of the femur and the proximal end of the tibia. The insertions may be seen more adequately after the sartorius and gracilis muscles have been dissected.

ORIGIN: The ischiatic tuberosity.

INSERTION: The distal medial lip of the caudal rough surface of the femur and the medial condyle of the tibia.

ACTION: To extend the hip joint. The part that attaches to the femur extends the stifle joint; the part that attaches to the tibia flexes or extends the stifle joint, depending on the position of the limb.

INNERVATION: Sciatic nerve.

Medial Muscles of the Thigh

1. The **sartorius** (see Figs. 2-41 through 2-45, 2-47, 2-52) consists of two straplike parts that lie on the cranial and craniomedial surfaces of the thigh. These parts extend from the ilium to the tibia. The **cranial part** forms the cranial contour of the thigh and may be nearly 1 cm thick. The **caudal part** is on the medial side of the thigh and is thinner, wider, and longer than the cranial part. Both muscle parts lie predominantly on the medial side of the large quadriceps femoris. Transect both parts and reflect the distal parts to their insertions on the patella and cranial border of the tibia.

ORIGIN: Cranial part—the crest of the ilium and the thoracolumbar fascia; caudal part—the cranial ventral iliac spine and the adjacent ventral border of the ilium.

INSERTION: Cranial part—the patella, in common with the rectus femoris of the quadriceps; caudal part—the cranial border of the tibia, in common with the gracilis.

ACTION: To flex the hip joint. The cranial part extends the stifle joint; the caudal part flexes the stifle joint.

INNERVATION: Femoral nerve.

2. The **gracilis** (see Figs. 2-42, 2-44, 2-45, 2-47, 2-52, 2-54, 2-55) arises from the **symphysial tendon**, a thick, flat tendon attached ventrally to the symphysis pelvis. The aponeurosis of the gracilis covers the adductor. Transect the gracilis through its aponeurotic origin. Reflect it distally and observe its insertion as well as that of the semitendinosus on the cranial border of the tibia.

ORIGIN: The pelvic symphysis by means of the symphysial tendon.

INSERTION: The cranial border of the tibia and, with the biceps femoris and semitendinosus, the tuber calcanei.

ACTION: To adduct the limb, flex the stifle joint, and extend the hip and tarsal joints.

INNERVATION: Obturator nerve.

The **femoral triangle** (see Fig. 2-79) is the shallow triangular space through which the femoral vessels run to and from the pelvic limb. It is located on the proximal medial surface of the thigh with its base at the abdominal wall. The triangle lies between the caudal belly of the sartorius cranially and the pectineus and adductor caudally. The iliopsoas and rectus femoris form the proximal lateral part of the triangle (see Fig. 2-49). The vastus medialis forms the distal lateral part. This triangle contains, among other structures, the femoral artery and vein. Remove the medial femoral fascia and adipose tissue that covers and fills in around the femoral artery and vein. Notice that the vein lies caudal to the artery. The pulse is usually taken from the femoral artery here.

3. The **pectineus** (see Figs. 2-42, 2-44 through 2-47, 2-49, 2-50) is a small, spindle-shaped muscle that belongs to the deep medial muscles of the thigh.

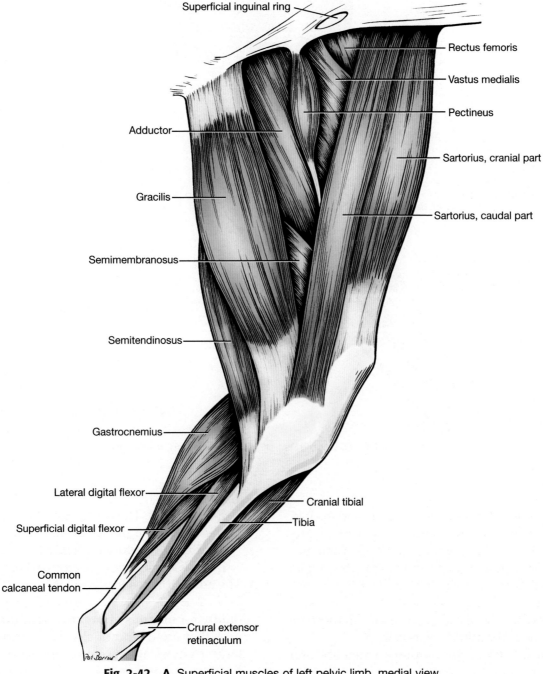

Fig. 2-42   A, Superficial muscles of left pelvic limb, medial view.

Continued

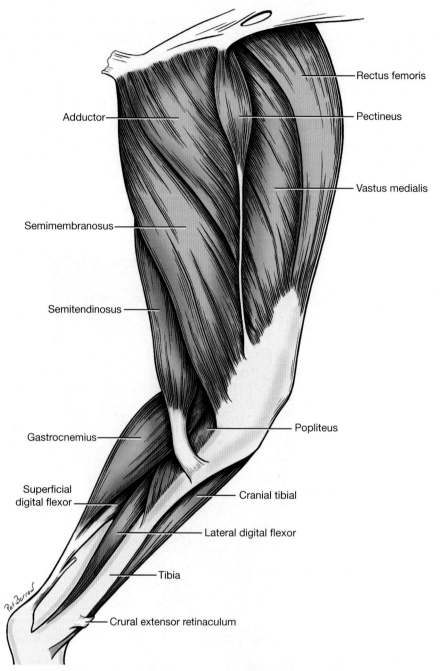

Adductor

Semimembranosus

Semitendinosus

Gastrocnemius

Superficial
digital flexor

Rectus femoris

Pectineus

Vastus medialis

Popliteus

Cranial tibial

Lateral digital flexor

Tibia

Crural extensor retinaculum

Pat Barrow

Fig. 2-42, cont'd   B, Deep muscles of left pelvic limb, medial view.

It lies between the adductor caudally and the vastus medialis cranially. It has an origin on the prepubic tendon and iliopubic eminence. There is a small cartilage imbedded in the iliopubic origin. By blunt dissection with the handle of the scalpel, isolate the tendon of insertion on the caudomedial surface of the distal end of the femur. Transect the pectineus in the middle of its belly.

ORIGIN: From the iliopubic eminence and the pubic tubercle via the prepubic tendon.

INSERTION: The distal end of the medial lip of the caudal rough face of the femur.

ACTION: To adduct the limb.

INNERVATION: Obturator nerve.

4. The **adductor** (see Figs. 2-42 through 2-44, 2-46, 2-47, 2-49, 2-50, *A*) consists of two muscles (**adductor magnus et brevis** and **adductor longus**) that are often not clearly divisible. It is a large pyramidal muscle compressed between the semimembranosus and pectineus, and it

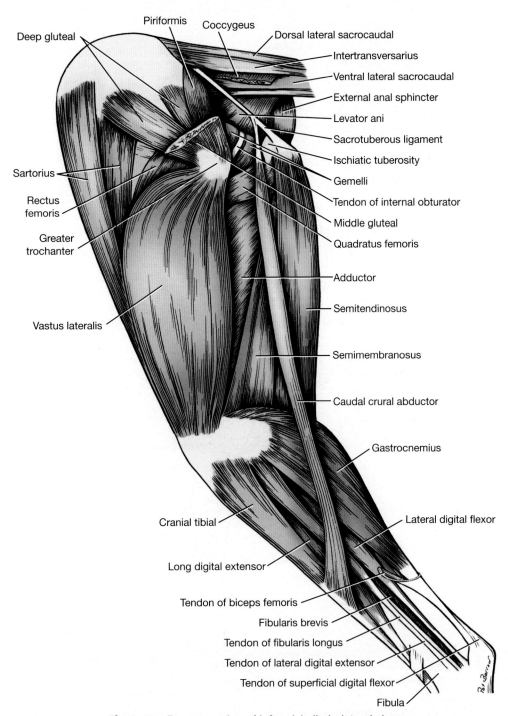

Piriformis
Coccygeus
Deep gluteal
Dorsal lateral sacrocaudal
Intertransversarius
Ventral lateral sacrocaudal
External anal sphincter
Levator ani
Sacrotuberous ligament
Ischiatic tuberosity
Gemelli
Tendon of internal obturator
Middle gluteal
Quadratus femoris
Adductor
Semitendinosus
Semimembranosus
Caudal crural abductor
Gastrocnemius
Lateral digital flexor
Sartorius
Rectus femoris
Greater trochanter
Vastus lateralis
Cranial tibial
Long digital extensor
Tendon of biceps femoris
Fibularis brevis
Tendon of fibularis longus
Tendon of lateral digital extensor
Tendon of superficial digital flexor
Fibula

Fig. 2-43 Deep muscles of left pelvic limb, lateral view.

extends from the pelvic symphysis to the caudal aspect of the femur. It is partly covered by the biceps femoris laterally and gracilis medially. Transect the adductor at its origin along the symphysis. Do not transect the external obturator, which lies even deeper.

ORIGIN: The entire pelvic symphysis by means of the symphysial tendon, the adjacent part of the ischiatic arch, and the ventral surface of the pubis and ischium.

INSERTION: The entire lateral lip of the caudal rough face of the femur.

ACTION: To adduct the limb and extend the hip joint.

INNERVATION: Obturator nerve.

Lateral Muscles of the Pelvis

1. The **tensor fasciae latae** (see Figs. 2-41, 2-44) is a triangular muscle that attaches proximally to the tuber coxae. It lies between the sartorius

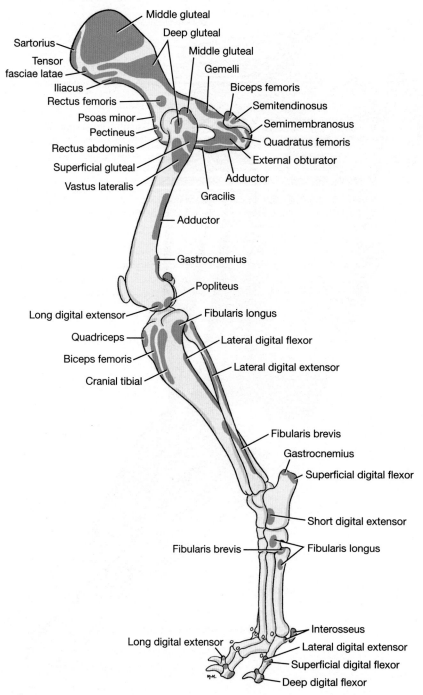

Fig. 2-44   Muscle attachments on pelvis and left pelvic limb, lateral view.

cranially, the middle gluteal caudodorsally, and the quadriceps distomedially. Part of its caudodorsal surface is attached to the middle gluteal near its origin. The muscle can be divided into two portions. The cranial, more superficial portion is inserted on the lateral femoral fascia, which radiates over the quadriceps and blends with the fascial insertion of the biceps femoris. The deeper caudal portion is inserted on a layer of lateral femoral fascia that runs deep to the biceps toward the stifle

on the lateral surface of the vastus lateralis. Transect the tensor fasciae latae across its middle and reflect the two halves toward their attachments.

ORIGIN: The tuber coxae and adjacent part of the ilium; the aponeurosis of the middle gluteal muscle.

INSERTION: The lateral femoral fascia.

ACTION: To tense the lateral femoral fascia, flex the hip joint, and extend the stifle joint.

INNERVATION: Cranial gluteal nerve.

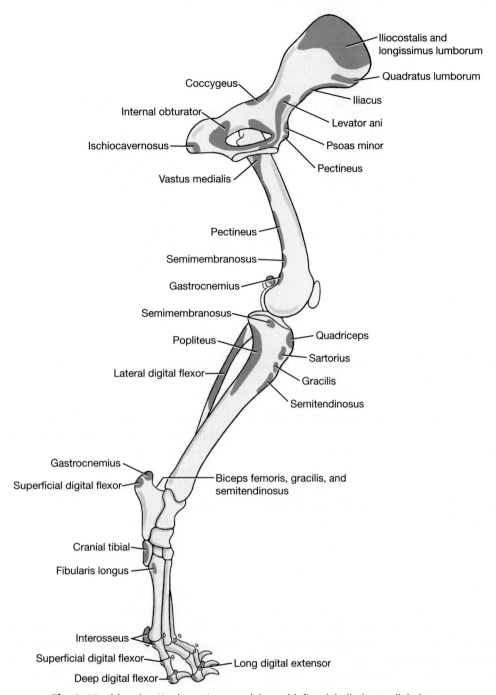

Iliocostalis and
longissimus lumborum

Quadratus lumborum

Coccygeus

Iliacus

Internal obturator

Levator ani

Ischiocavernosus

Psoas minor

Pectineus

Vastus medialis

Pectineus

Semimembranosus

Gastrocnemius

Semimembranosus

Popliteus

Quadriceps

Sartorius

Lateral digital flexor

Gracilis

Semitendinosus

Gastrocnemius

Superficial digital flexor

Biceps femoris, gracilis, and
semitendinosus

Cranial tibial

Fibularis longus

Interosseus

Superficial digital flexor

Long digital extensor

Deep digital flexor

Fig. 2-45 Muscle attachments on pelvis and left pelvic limb, medial view.

2. The **superficial gluteal** (see Figs. 2-41, 2-44, 2-50) is small and lies caudal to the middle gluteal. Its fibers run distally, from the deep gluteal fascia that covers the middle gluteal and from the sacrum and the first caudal vertebra to the level of the greater trochanter of the femur, where they converge before forming an aponeurosis that runs under the biceps to the third trochanter. Clean the superficial gluteal and transect it 1 cm from the beginning of its aponeurosis of insertion. Do not transect the caudally lying **sacrotuberous ligament**

(Figs. 2-43, 2-58). This is a collagenous band that runs from the sacrum to the lateral angle of the ischiatic tuberosity. Notice that the superficial gluteal arises from the proximal half of this ligament. Sever the deep gluteal fascia 1 cm cranial to its junction with the muscle fibers of the superficial gluteal.

ORIGIN: The lateral border of the sacrum and the first caudal vertebra, partly by means of the sacrotuberous ligament; the cranial dorsal iliac spine by means of the deep gluteal fascia.

INSERTION: The third trochanter.

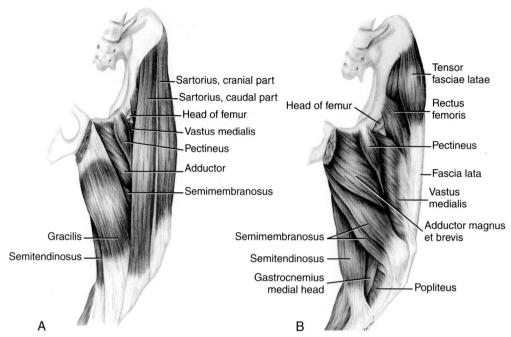

Fig. 2-46 Muscles of thigh. **A,** Superficial muscles, medial aspect. **B,** Deep muscles, medial aspect. (From Evans HE, de Lahunta A: *Miller's anatomy of the dog,* ed 4, St Louis, 2013, Saunders.)

ACTION: To extend the hip joint and abduct the limb.

INNERVATION: Caudal gluteal nerve.

3. The **middle gluteal** (see Figs. 2-41, 2-43, 2-44, 2-50, 2-57) is a large, ovoid muscle that lies between the tensor fasciae latae and the superficial gluteal. Clean the surface of the muscle by reflecting the deep gluteal fascia and its attached transected superficial gluteal muscle dorsocranial to the iliac crest. This reveals that the fibers of the middle gluteal for the most part parallel its long axis. Carefully separate the cranioventral part of the middle gluteal from the underlying deep gluteal. The entire caudodorsal border of the middle gluteal is covered by the superficial gluteal. The deep caudal portion of the middle gluteal is readily separated from the main muscle mass and is called the **piriformis muscle** (see Fig. 2-43). Starting at the middle of the cranioventral border of the middle gluteal, transect the entire muscle and reflect the distal half toward its insertion on the apex of the greater trochanter of the femur.

ORIGIN: The crest and gluteal surface of the ilium.

INSERTION: The greater trochanter.

ACTION: To extend and abduct the hip joint and to rotate the pelvic limb medially.

INNERVATION: Cranial gluteal nerve.

4. The **deep gluteal** (see Figs. 2-43, 2-44, 2-48, 2-50) is fan-shaped and completely covered by the middle gluteal. Its fibers converge to insert on the cranial face of the greater trochanter.

ORIGIN: The body of the ilium; the ischiatic spine.

INSERTION: The cranial aspect of the greater trochanter.

ACTION: To extend and abduct the hip joint and to rotate the pelvic limb medially.

INNERVATION: Cranial gluteal nerve.

The **articularis coxae** (Fig. 2-50, *B*) is a small, spindle-shaped muscle lying on the craniolateral aspect of the hip joint capsule. It is covered by the deep gluteal muscle. It arises from the lateral surface of the ilium along with the rectus femoris and inserts on the neck of the femur. (No dissection is necessary.)

Caudal Hip Muscles

The four muscles of this group are important because of their proximity to the hip. They lie caudal to the hip and extend from the inner and outer surfaces of the ischium to the femur. All rotate the limb laterally. This action opposes the medial rotation by the gluteals so that the thigh moves in a sagittal plane at the hip.

1. The **internal obturator** (see Figs. 2-43, 2-45, 2-48, 2-50) is fan-shaped on the dorsal surface

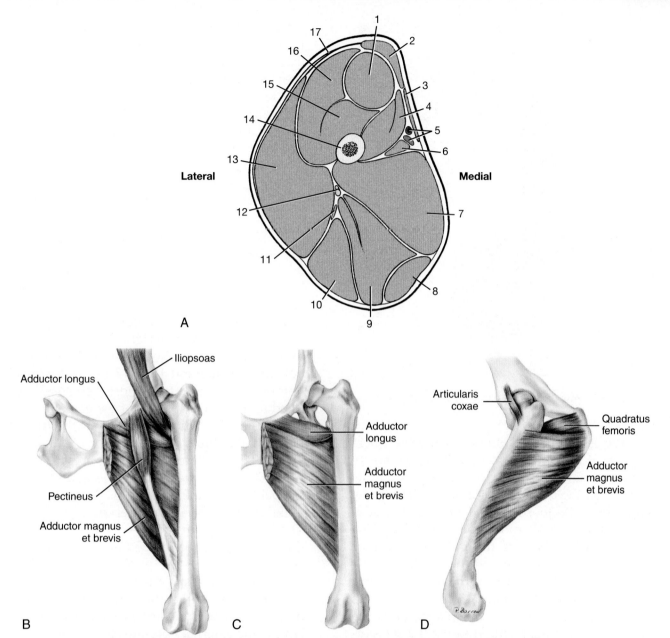

Fig. 2-47 A, Transverse section of left thigh. **B,** Adductor magnus et brevis, adductor longus, pectineus, and iliopsoas, cranial aspect. **C,** Adductor magnus et brevis and adductor longus, cranial aspect. **D,** Adductor magnus et brevis, quadratus femoris, and articularis coxae, lateral aspect. (Parts B-D from Evans HE, de Lahunta A: *Miller's anatomy of the dog,* ed 4, St Louis, 2013, Saunders.)

1. Rectus femoris
2. Sartorius, cranial part
3. Sartorius, caudal part
4. Vastus medialis
5. Femoral a. and v.
6. Pectineus
7. Adductor
8. Gracilis
9. Semimembranosus
10. Semitendinosus
11. Caudal crural abductor
12. Sciatic n.
13. Biceps femoris
14. Femur
15. Vastus intermedius
16. Vastus lateralis
17. Fascia lata

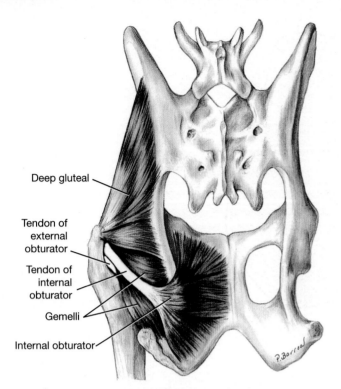

Deep gluteal

Tendon of external obturator

Tendon of internal obturator

Gemelli

Internal obturator

Fig. 2-48   Muscles of left hip joint, dorsal aspect.

of the ischium and pubis. Its muscle fibers converge toward the lesser ischiatic notch. The body of the muscle may be exposed at its origin on the dorsal surface of the ischium by removing the loose fat and the fascia caudomedial to the sacrotuberous ligament. The most caudal fibers of the internal obturator run craniolaterally toward the lesser ischiatic notch, where the tendon of the muscle begins. The tendon of the internal obturator passes over the lesser ischiatic notch ventral to the sacrotuberous ligament. Transect the sacrotuberous ligament and reflect the adjacent soft tissues to expose the tendon of insertion of the internal obturator muscle running to the trochanteric fossa. Transect the tendon of the internal obturator as it crosses the gemelli and reflect it to observe the bursa that lies between the tendon and the lesser ischiatic notch.

ORIGIN: The symphysis pelvis and the dorsal surface of the ischium and pubis.

INSERTION: The trochanteric fossa of the femur.

ACTION: To rotate the pelvic limb laterally at the hip joint.

INNERVATION: Sciatic nerve.

2. The **gemelli** (see Figs. 2-43, 2-44, 2-48, 2-50), two muscles fused together, lie under the

tendon of the internal obturator. They are interposed between the quadratus femoris and external obturator distally and the deep gluteal proximally. The gemelli are deeply grooved by the tendon of the internal obturator so that their edges overlap this tendon.

ORIGIN: The lateral surface of the ischium, caudal to the acetabulum and ventral to the lesser ischiatic notch.

INSERTION: The trochanteric fossa.

ACTION: To rotate the pelvic limb laterally at the hip joint.

INNERVATION: Sciatic nerve.

3. The **quadratus femoris** (see Figs. 2-43, 2-44, 2-49, 2-50) is short and thick. It lies deep to the biceps femoris, where it is interposed between the adductor medially, the biceps femoris laterally, and the external obturator and gemelli dorsally. Its fibers are at right angles to the long axis of the thigh. It should be examined from both the medial and lateral sides. The dorsal border of the quadratus femoris lies closely applied to the ventral border of the gemelli.

ORIGIN: The ventral surface of the caudal part of the ischium.

INSERTION: Intertrochanteric crest.

ACTION: To extend the hip joint and rotate the pelvic limb laterally.

INNERVATION: Sciatic nerve.

4. The **external obturator** (see Figs. 2-44, 2-48 through 2-50) is fan-shaped and arises on the ventral surface of the pubis and ischium. It covers the obturator foramen. Its caudal border is covered by the quadratus femoris, whereas its cranial border is hidden by the adductor. Follow the external obturator to its insertion.

ORIGIN: The ventral surface of the pubis and ischium.

INSERTION: The trochanteric fossa.

ACTION: To rotate the pelvic limb laterally at the hip joint.

INNERVATION: Obturator nerve.

Cranial Muscles of the Thigh

1. The **quadriceps femoris** (see Figs. 2-42 through 2-47, 2-49, 2-50, 2-52, 2-57) is divided into four heads of origin, which are fused distally. It arises from the femur and the ilium and is inserted on the tibial tuberosity. The patella lies in the tendon of insertion. This muscle is the most powerful extensor of the stifle joint and is necessary for the animal to support its weight.

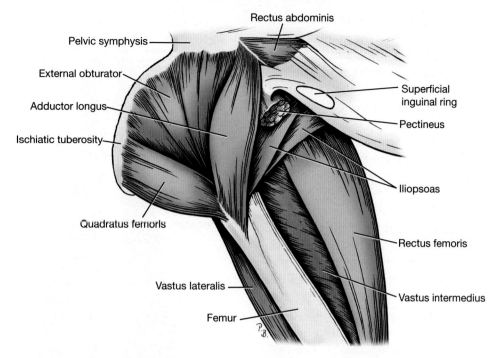

Fig. 2-49 Deep muscles medial to left hip joint.

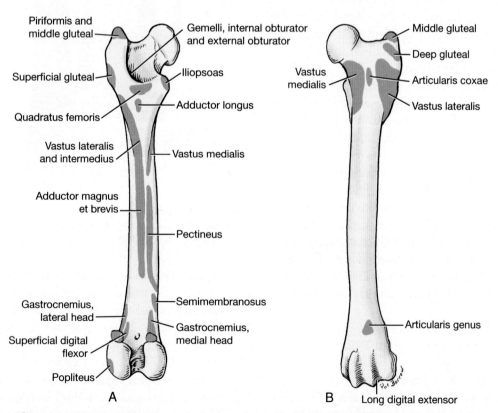

Fig. 2-50 **A,** Left femur with muscle attachments, caudal view. **B,** Left femur with muscle attachments, cranial view.

The **patella**, a sesamoid bone, is intercalated in the large tendon of insertion of the quadriceps. It articulates with the trochlea of the femur.

The **patellar ligament** extends from the patella to the tibial tuberosity. It is the tendon of insertion of the quadriceps femoris.

The **rectus femoris** (see Figs. 2-42 through 2-44, 2-46, 2-47, 2-49) is the most cranial component of the quadriceps femoris and the only one to arise from the ilium. Proximally, it is circular in transverse section and passes between the vastus medialis and the vastus lateralis. Uncover the rectus femoris near its origin. Transect and reflect the proximal part. The rectus arises from the ilium cranial to the acetabulum and inserts on the tibial tuberosity. It is a flexor of the hip joint as well as an extensor of the stifle joint.

The **vastus lateralis** (see Figs. 2-43, 2-44, 2-47, 2-49, 2-50) lies lateral and caudal to the rectus femoris, to which it is fused distally. The vastus lateralis is partly separated from the vastus intermedius by a scantily developed intermuscular septum. Notice that the vastus lateralis arises from the proximal part of the lateral lip of the caudal rough surface of the femur. It is inserted with the rectus femoris on the tibial tuberosity.

The **vastus intermedius** (see Figs. 2-47, 2-49, 2-50) lies directly on the smooth cranial surface of the femur and is quite intimately fused with the other two vasti. It arises with the vastus lateralis, which covers it, from the lateral side of the proximal end of the femur. It inserts on the tibial tuberosity with the other members of the group.

The **vastus medialis** (see Figs. 2-42, 2-45 through 2-47, 2-50) arises from the medial side of the proximal end of the cranial surface of the femur and the proximal end of the medial lip of the caudal rough surface. It is inserted with the other heads of the quadriceps on the tibial tuberosity.

ORIGIN: Rectus femoris—ilium; vasti muscles—proximal femur.

INSERTION: Tibial tuberosity.

ACTION: To extend the stifle joint and flex the hip joint (rectus).

INNERVATION: Femoral nerve.

2. The **iliopsoas** (see Figs. 2-49 through 2-51, 2-57), a sublumbar muscle, is now visible at its insertion on the lesser trochanter of the femur. This end of the muscle lies between the pectineus medially and the rectus femoris laterally. The iliopsoas represents a fusion of the psoas major and iliacus muscles. The **psoas major** (see

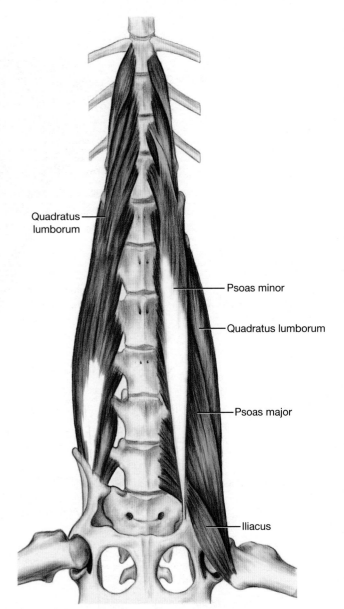

Fig. 2-51 Sublumbar muscles, deep dissection, ventral aspect. The psoas major and psoas minor have been removed on the right side.

Fig. 2-51) is long and arises from the ventral aspect of the transverse processes and bodies of lumbar vertebrae. It passes caudally and ventrally under the cranioventral aspect of the ilium, where it joins the iliacus. The **iliacus** (see Figs. 2-44, 2-45, 2-51) is short and arises from the smooth ventral surface of the ilium between the arcuate line and the lateral border of the ilium. The two muscle masses continue caudoventrally as the iliopsoas to their conjoined insertion on the lesser trochanter. The action of the iliopsoas is to flex the hip joint and the lumbar vertebral column. It is the major flexor of the hip joint. Do not dissect it at this time but study the illustration of the deep dissection of sublumbar muscles.

ORIGIN: Psoas major—lumbar vertebrae; iliacus—cranioventral ilium.

INSERTION: Lesser trochanter.

ACTION: To flex the hip joint.

INNERVATION: Ventral branches of lumbar spinal nerves; femoral nerve.

The **quadratus lumborum** is partially hidden from ventral view by the psoas major and psoas minor (see Fig. 2-51).

Muscles of the Leg (Crus)

The muscles of the leg, or crus, the region between the stifle and hock, are divided into craniolateral and caudal groups. Note that the leg is not the pelvic limb. Remove the skin that remains on the distal part of the pelvic limb to the level of the proximal interphalangeal joints.

The **superficial crural, tarsal, metatarsal**, and **digital fasciae** are similar to the superficial fasciae of the corresponding regions of the forelimb. Cutaneous vessels and nerves course in the superficial fascia. One such vessel is the cranial branch of the lateral saphenous vein, which is used for venipuncture.

The medial and lateral femoral fasciae blend over the stifle and are continued distally in the leg as the **deep crural fascia**. The deep crural fascia covers the muscles of the leg and the free-lying surfaces of the crural skeleton. Septa from this fascia extend between the muscles to attach to the bone. Laterally, the fibers of the caudal branch of the biceps femoris radiate into it. Medially, the semitendinosus and gracilis are continuous with this fascia. These connections are located caudally where the crural fascia contributes to the common calcanean tendon.

Just proximal to the flexor surface of the tarsus, the deep crural fascia is thickened to form an oblique band of about 0.5 cm, the **crural extensor retinaculum**. As it stretches obliquely from the distal third of the fibula to the medial malleolus of the tibia, it binds down the tendons of the long digital extensor and the cranial tibial muscles.

The deep crural fascia decreases in thickness as it passes over the tarsus, where it becomes the deep tarsal fascia. A fibrous loop that attaches to the calcaneus wraps around the tendon of the long digital extensor. This is the **tarsal extensor retinaculum** (see Fig. 2-53). The deep fascia extends into the metatarsal and digital pads and closely joins these pads with the overlying skeletal and ligamentous parts. Make an incision through the cranial crural fascia and reflect it to the common calcanean tendon and the tibia.

Craniolateral Muscles of the Leg

1. The **cranial tibial** (see Figs. 2-42 through 2-45, 2-52 through 2-57) is the most cranial muscle of this group. Its medial margin is in contact with the tibia. It arises from the cranial border and the adjacent proximal articular margin of the tibia. Its tendon inserts on the plantar surface of the base of the first and second metatarsals. The tendon of the cranial tibial runs under the **crural extensor retinaculum** (see Fig. 2-53) and is provided with a synovial sheath over most of the flexor surface of the tarsus.

   ORIGIN: The extensor groove and the adjacent articular margin of the tibia; the lateral edge of the cranial tibial border.

   INSERTION: The plantar surface of the base of metatarsals I and II.

   ACTION: To flex the tarsocrural joint and to rotate the paw laterally so that the plantar surface faces medially.

   INNERVATION: Fibular nerve.

2. The **long digital extensor** (see Figs. 2-43 through 2-45, 2-53, 2-54, 2-56, 2-57) is a spindle-shaped muscle that is partly covered by the cranial tibial medially and the fibularis longus laterally. Expose the muscle and its tendon of origin from the extensor fossa of the femur. The tendon runs over the articular margin of the tibia in the extensor groove and is lubricated by an extension of the stifle joint capsule. In the distal crus it runs under the **crural extensor retinaculum** along with the cranial tibial tendon. Observe the four tendons of insertion of the long digital extensor. As the tendons pass over the tarsus, they are surrounded by a synovial sheath and are held in place by the **tarsal extensor retinaculum** (see Fig. 2-53). In the metatarsus the four tendons diverge toward their respective digits, where they insert on the extensor process of the distal phalanx.

   ORIGIN: The extensor fossa of the femur.

   INSERTION: The extensor processes of the distal phalanges of digits II, III, IV, and V.

   ACTION: To extend the digital joints and flex the tarsal joints.

   INNERVATION: Fibular nerve.

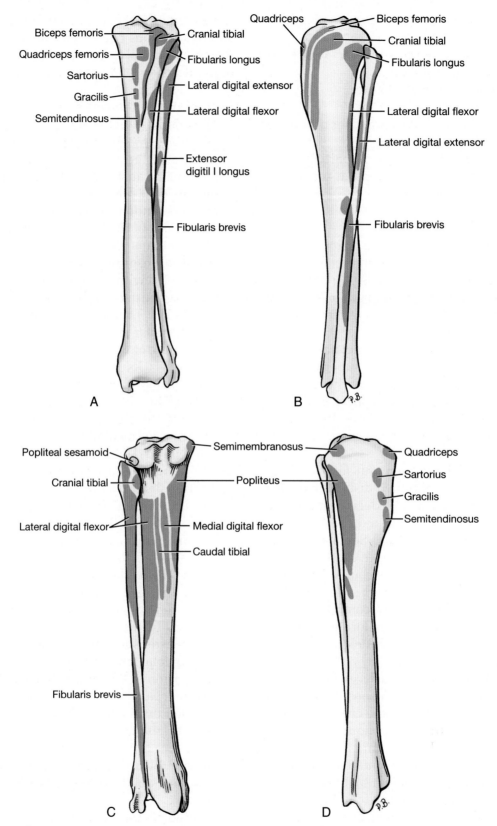

Fig. 2-52   **A,** Left tibia and fibula with muscle attachments, cranial view. **B,** Left tibia and fibula with muscle attachments, lateral view. **C,** Left tibia and fibula with muscle attachments, caudal view. **D,** Left tibia and fibula with muscle attachments, medial view.

plane through the crural extensor retinaculum and extends to its insertion on the fourth tarsal and the plantar surfaces of the base of all metatarsals. Open the synovial sheath at its proximal end. Preserving all ligaments and tendons that lie superficial to the tendon, trace it to its insertion on the fourth tarsal. Do not dissect the tendon beyond this attachment. Notice that it lies in a sulcus of the lateral malleolus of the fibula and that at the distal end of the tarsus it makes nearly a right angle as it turns medially around a groove in the fourth tarsal bone and courses to the plantar side.

ORIGIN: The lateral condyle of the tibia, the proximal end of the fibula, and the lateral epicondyle of the femur by means of the lateral collateral ligament of the stifle.

INSERTION: The fourth tarsal bone; the plantar aspect of the base of the metatarsals.

ACTION: To flex the tarsal joints and rotate the paw medially so that the plantar surface faces laterally.

INNERVATION: Fibular nerve.

The lateral digital extensor and the fibularis brevis (see Figs. 2-43, 2-44, 2-52, 2-54, 2-55) are located beneath the peroneus longus on the lateral aspect of the leg and need not be dissected.

Caudal Muscles of the Leg

1. The **gastrocnemius muscle** (see Figs. 2-42 through 2-46, 2-50, 2-53 through 2-57) consists of two heads that enclose the superficial digital flexor between them. These muscles form the caudal bulge of the leg (calf) and contribute the major component of the **common calcanean tendon**.

The two heads of the gastrocnemius arise from the medial and lateral supracondylar tuberosities of the femur. In each tendon of origin there is a sesamoid bone (fabella) that articulates with the caudodorsal aspect of the femoral condyle.

Identify the lateral and medial heads of the gastrocnemius and follow them to their union as a common tendon that inserts on the proximal dorsal surface of the tuber calcanei. The superficial digital flexor muscle, which is hidden proximally between the two heads of the gastrocnemius, emerges distally as a superficial tendon that passes over the medial surface of the gastrocnemial tendon, caps the tuber calcanei, and continues over the plantar surface of the calcaneus. With a probe, separate the

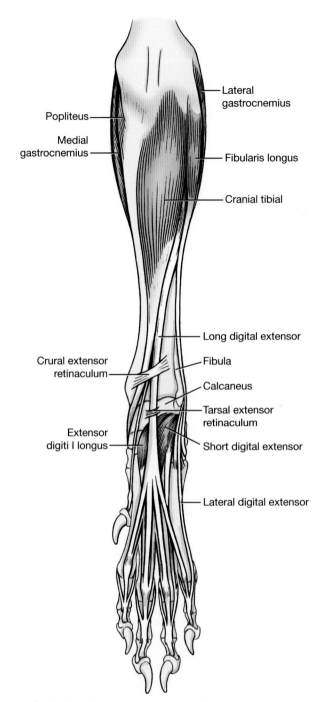

Fig. 2-53   Muscles of left pelvic limb, cranial view.

Labels in figure:
- Popliteus
- Medial gastrocnemius
- Lateral gastrocnemius
- Fibularis longus
- Cranial tibial
- Long digital extensor
- Crural extensor retinaculum
- Fibula
- Calcaneus
- Tarsal extensor retinaculum
- Extensor digiti I longus
- Short digital extensor
- Lateral digital extensor

3. The **fibularis longus** (see Figs. 2-43 through 2-45, 2-52, 2-53, 2-56) lies just caudal to the long digital extensor, where a triangular portion of its short belly lies directly under the crural fascia. It is a short, thick, wedge-shaped muscle that lies in large part cranial to the fibula. It arises from the lateral collateral ligament of the stifle and the adjacent parts of the tibia and fibula. Its stout tendon courses distally on the lateral side of the fibula caudal to the crural extensor retinaculum. It has a long synovial sheath that begins at a

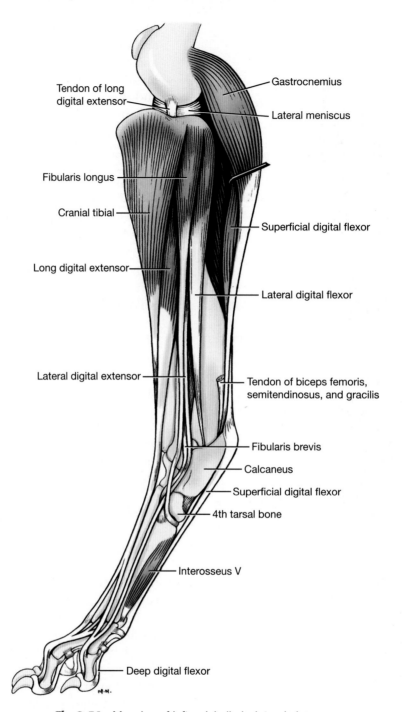

Fig. 2-54   Muscles of left pelvic limb, lateral view.

gastrocnemius from the superficial digital flexor by entering between their tendons. Proximally, bluntly separate the superficial digital flexor from the heads of the gastrocnemius.

The superficial digital flexor has a common origin with the lateral head of the gastrocnemius—the lateral supracondylar tuberosity of the femur—and is closely adherent to that head. Transect each head of the gastrocnemius and reflect them proximally to see their origin and the associated sesamoid bones.

ORIGIN: The medial and lateral supracondylar tuberosities of the femur.

INSERTION: The proximal dorsal surface of the tuber calcanei.

ACTION: To extend the tarsal joints and flex the stifle joint.

INNERVATION: Tibial nerve.

2. The **superficial digital flexor** (see Figs. 2-42 through 2-45, 2-50, 2-54 through 2-57) is a spindle-shaped

muscle that arises from the lateral supracondylar tuberosity of the femur with the lateral head of the gastrocnemius. Its deep surface is in apposition to the deep digital flexor and the popliteus, whereas its other surfaces are largely covered by the gastrocnemius. Proximal to the calcaneal process, its tendon passes from deep to superficial by crossing the medial surface of the gastrocnemius tendon. Farther distally the tendon widens, caps the tuber calcanei, attaches on each side, and continues distally. Make a median plane incision through the superficial digital flexor tendon from the place where it gains the caudal side of the gastrocnemius to the tuber calcanei. Continue the incision distal to the tuber calcanei for an equal distance. Observe the large **calcaneal bursa** of the superficial digital flexor that lies under its tendon as it crosses the tuber calcanei. Notice the distinct medial and lateral attachments of

the tendon on the tuber calcanei. Opposite the distal plantar surface of the tarsus, the tendon bifurcates; each of these branches in turn bifurcates, thus forming four tendons of nearly equal size. Each tendon is disposed in its digit as the corresponding tendon in the forepaw. They need not be dissected.

ORIGIN: The lateral supracondylar tuberosity of the femur.

INSERTION: The tuber calcanei and the bases of the middle phalanges of digits II, III, IV, and V.

ACTION: To flex the first two digital joints of the four principal digits; flex the stifle joint; extend the tarsal joints.

INNERVATION: Tibial nerve.

3. The **deep digital flexor** (see Figs. 2-42 through 2-45, 2-52, 2-54 through 2-57) and the popliteus are the principal muscles yet to be dissected on the caudal surface of the leg. The separation between

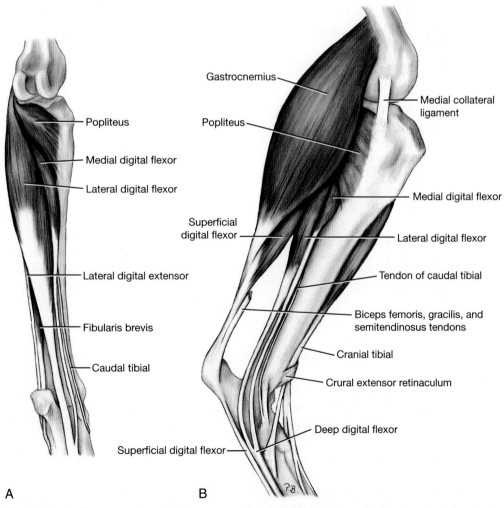

Fig. 2-55 **A,** Deep muscles of left crus, caudal view. **B,** Muscles of left crus, medial aspect.

Continued

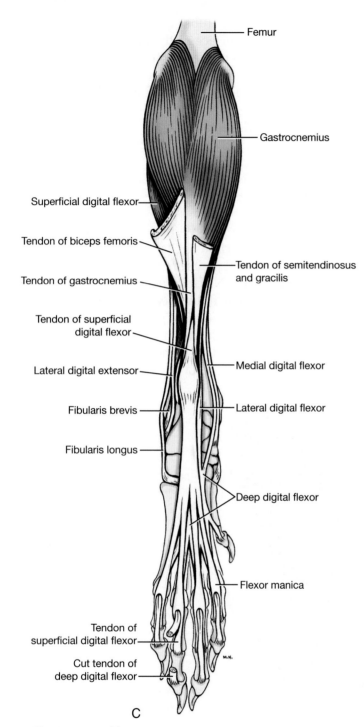

C

Fig. 2-55, cont'd   C, Muscles of left pelvic limb, caudal view.

Labels on figure C:
- Femur
- Gastrocnemius
- Superficial digital flexor
- Tendon of biceps femoris
- Tendon of semitendinosus and gracilis
- Tendon of gastrocnemius
- Tendon of superficial digital flexor
- Lateral digital extensor
- Medial digital flexor
- Fibularis brevis
- Lateral digital flexor
- Fibularis longus
- Deep digital flexor
- Flexor manica
- Tendon of superficial digital flexor
- Cut tendon of deep digital flexor

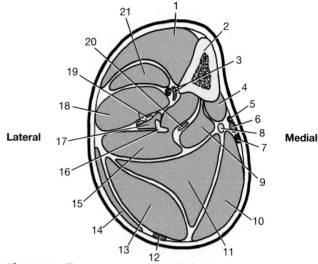

Fig. 2-56   Transverse section of left crus.
1. Cranial tibial
2. Tibia
3. Cranial tibial a. and v.
4. Popliteus
5. Saphenous a., cranial branch
6. Medial saphenous v.
7. Saphenous a., caudal branch
8. Tibial n.
9. Medial digital flexor
10. Gastrocnemius, medial head
11. Superficial digital flexor
12. Lateral saphenous v.
13. Gastrocnemius, lateral head
14. Biceps femoris
15. Lateral digital flexor
16. Fibula
17. Lateral digital extensor
18. Fibularis longus
19. Fibular nerves
20. Caudal tibial
21. Long digital extensor

Figure labels: Lateral, Medial

them runs distomedially. Transect the superficial digital flexor proximal to its tendon to expose these muscles. The two muscles that compose the deep digital flexor are now exposed.

The **lateral digital flexor** (formerly the flexor hallucis longus) (see Figs. 2-43, 2-45, 2-52, 2-54 through 2-56) arises from the caudolateral border of the proximal two thirds of the tibia, most of the proximal half of the fibula, and the

adjacent interosseous membrane. Its tendon begins as a wide expanse on the caudal side of the muscle but condenses distally. Medial to the tuber calcanei, it is surrounded by the tarsal synovial sheath and bound in the groove over the sustentaculum tali of the calcaneus by the **flexor retinaculum**. At the level of the distal row of tarsal bones, observe the tendon of the lateral digital flexor joining that of the medial digital flexor to form a common tendon. The courses, relations, and attachments of the tendons distal to the tarsus are similar to those of the deep flexor tendon of the forelimb. Their dissection is not necessary.

The **medial digital flexor** (see Figs. 2-52, 2-55, 2-56) is smaller and lies between the lateral digital flexor and the popliteus. From the proximal end of the tibia, it runs distomedially. Its tendon lies on the caudomedial side of the

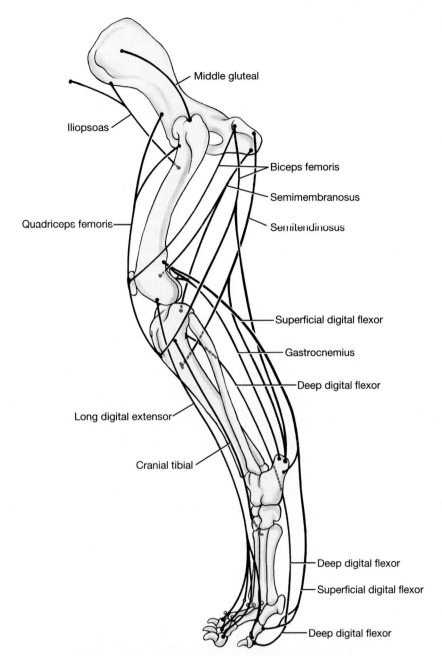

Fig. 2-57 Major flexors and extensors of pelvic limb.

Labels on figure: Middle gluteal; Iliopsoas; Quadriceps femoris; Biceps femoris; Semimembranosus; Semitendinosus; Superficial digital flexor; Gastrocnemius; Deep digital flexor; Long digital extensor; Cranial tibial; Deep digital flexor; Superficial digital flexor; Deep digital flexor

tibia. At the distal row of tarsal bones, it unites with the tendon of the lateral digital flexor.

ORIGIN: The caudal aspect of the proximal two thirds of the tibia, the proximal half of the fibula, and the adjacent interosseous membrane.

INSERTION: The flexor tubercle on the plantar surface of the base of each of the distal phalanges.

ACTION: To flex the digits and extend the tarsal joints.

INNERVATION: Tibial nerve.

4. The **popliteus** (see Figs. 2-44 through 2-46, 2-50, 2-52, 2-53, 2-55, 2-56) is covered by the

gastrocnemius and the superficial digital flexor and lies on the stifle joint capsule and caudal surface of the proximal tibia. It arises from the lateral epicondyle of the femur by a long tendon that should be isolated just cranial to the lateral collateral ligament of the stifle. It courses caudally, medial to the lateral collateral ligament. At the junction of the tendon with the muscle, there is a **sesamoid** that articulates with the caudal aspect of the lateral condyle of the tibia. The muscle portion starts at the lateral tibial condyle and extends to the proximal third of the tibia on the medial side of the leg. Transect the popliteus at the tendomuscular junction and reflect it proximally to observe the sesamoid. The popliteus inserts on the proximal third of the tibia.

ORIGIN: The lateral epicondyle of the femur.

INSERTION: The proximal third of the caudal surface of the tibia.

ACTION: To rotate the leg medially.

INNERVATION: Tibial nerve.

LIVE DOG

Palpate the middle gluteal on the lateral side of the wing of the ilium. Follow it to its termination on the greater trochanter. Palpate the quadriceps femoris cranially in the thigh and feel the straplike sartorius along its cranial edge. Follow the quadriceps distally to its patella and the patellar ligament with its termination on the tibial tuberosity. Proximally, in the thigh feel the tensor fasciae latae between the sartorius and the quadriceps. Palpate the muscle mass in the caudal thigh. This includes, from lateral to medial, the biceps femoris, semitendinosus, semimembranosus, and gracilis. Feel the spindle-shaped pectineus proximally in the medial thigh on the caudal border of the femoral triangle. Abduct the limb and feel this muscle tighten. Palpate the pulse in the femoral artery just cranial to this muscle. The pulse rate and quality are usually determined here.

Grasp the tail and press down on the floor of the pelvis just cranial to the ischial arch. The muscle here is the internal obturator. The depression here between the tail and anus medially, superficial gluteal laterally, and internal obturator ventrally is the ischiorectal fossa, where perineal hernias occur.

Caudal to the stifle, feel for the popliteal lymph node between the distal ends of the biceps femoris and semitendinosus. In the leg, feel the craniolateral muscles that are the flexors of the tarsus and extensors of the digits. Proximally, their muscle bellies fill the concave surface of the body of the tibia. Caudally, feel the two gastrocnemius muscles proximally. Trace them from their origin on the distal femur to where their tendons join and form part of the common calcanean tendon. Follow this common tendon to the tuber calcanei. Feel the division between the gastrocnemius tendon and the tendon of the superficial digital flexor. Follow the latter on the plantar side of the tuber calcanei. Palpate the digital flexors distally in the caudal leg area and plantar aspect of the tarsus.

JOINTS OF THE PELVIC LIMB

The ischium and pubis of the right and left sides are joined on the median plane at the **symphysis pelvis**.

The **sacroiliac joint** (Figs. 2-58, 2-59) is an articulation of stability rather than mobility. The right and left wings of the ilia articulate with the broad right and left wings of the sacrum. In the adult most of the apposed articular surfaces are united by fibrocartilage that surrounds a small area of articulating hyaline cartilage with synovial fluid. Around the periphery of the articular areas, bands of strong collagenous tissue, the **dorsal** and **ventral sacroiliac ligaments**, reinforce the fibrocartilage. Do not dissect this joint.

The **sacrotuberous ligament** (see Figs. 2-58, 2-59) runs from the transverse processes of the last sacral and first caudal vertebrae to the lateral angle of the ischiatic tuberosity. It serves as an origin for several muscles that have been dissected.

The **hip joint** (see Figs. 2-58, 2-59) is a ball-and-socket joint whose main movements are flexion and extension. This joint can move in any direction, but the opposed action of the medial and lateral rotator muscles limits the movement to primarily flexion and extension. The joint capsule passes from the neck of the femur to a line peripheral to the acetabular lip. Transect the deep gluteal and iliopsoas muscles at their insertions. Cut the hip joint capsule to expose the joint and associated ligaments. Consider the various muscles that may be encountered by surgical approaches to the hip from different directions.

The **ligament of the femoral head** (see Fig. 2-59) is a thick band of collagenous tissue that extends from the acetabular fossa to the fovea capitis. At its acetabular attachment it may blend slightly with the transverse acetabular ligament. A synovial membrane covers it. Transect this ligament.

The **transverse acetabular ligament** (see Fig. 2-59) is a small band that extends from one side of the acetabular notch to the opposite side. It is located at the ventrocaudal aspect of the acetabulum and continues as the **acetabular lip**, which deepens the acetabulum by forming a fibrocartilaginous border around it.

The joint capsule of the **stifle** (Figs. 2-60 through 2-64) forms three sacs. Two of these are between the femoral and tibial condyles (femorotibial joint sacs), and the third is beneath the patella (femoropatellar joint sac). All three sacs communicate with one another. The femorotibial joint sacs

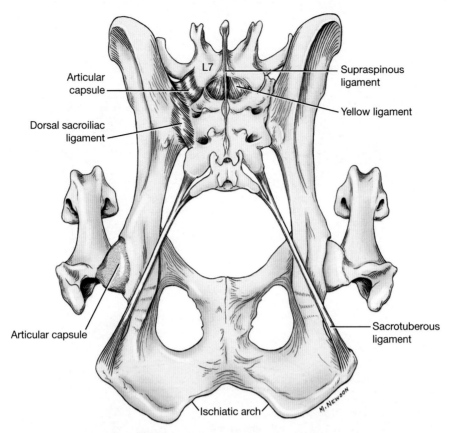

Fig. 2-58   Ligaments of pelvis, dorsal view.

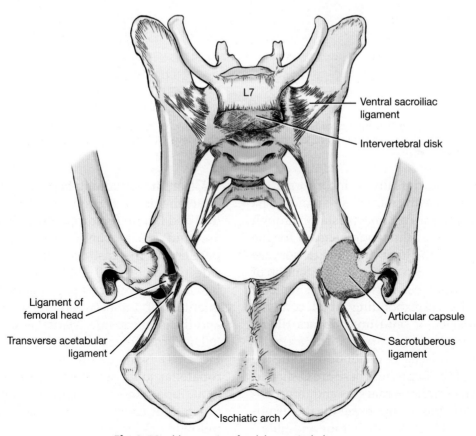

Fig. 2-59   Ligaments of pelvis, ventral view.

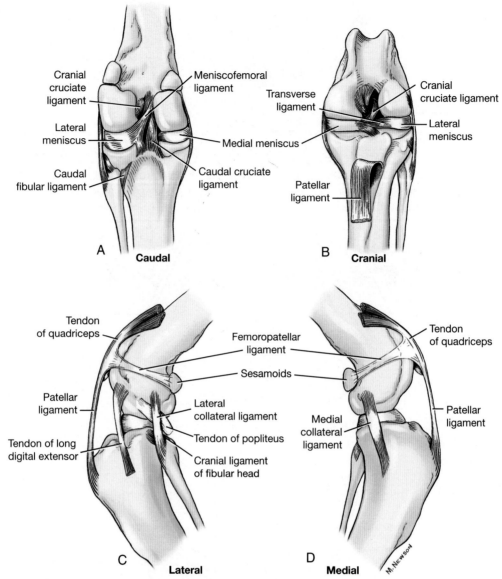

Fig. 2-60 **A,** Ligaments of left stifle joint, caudal view. **B,** Ligaments of left stifle joint, cranial view. **C,** Ligaments of left stifle joint, lateral view. **D,** Ligaments of left stifle joint, medial view.

extend caudally and dorsally to incorporate the articulation of the gastrocnemial sesamoids. The lateral femorotibial sac continues distally through the extensor groove as the tendon sheath for the tendon of origin of the long digital extensor (see Figs. 2-60, *C*, 2-61). It also surrounds the tendon of origin of the popliteus. Between each femoral condyle and the corresponding tibial condyle, there is a **meniscus**, or **semilunar fibrocartilage**, that develops in the joint capsule. The articular surface of the meniscus is continuous with the synovial layer of the joint sac. These are C-shaped discs with thick peripheral margins and thin, concave central areas that compensate for the incongruence that exists between the femur and tibia.

Clean the remaining fascia and related muscle attachments away from the stifle. Note the **medial** and **lateral femoropatellar ligaments**, which are thin fascial bands extending between the patella and the gastrocnemial sesamoid on each side (see Figs. 2-60, 2-61). Transect the patellar ligament and reflect it proximally. Note the large quantity of fat between the patellar ligament and the joint capsule. Medial and lateral parapatellar fibrocartilages extend from the patella (see Fig. 2-64). Note the proximal extent of the femoropatellar joint sac. Remove the fat around the joint, open the joint capsule, and remove as much joint capsule as necessary to observe the following ligaments.

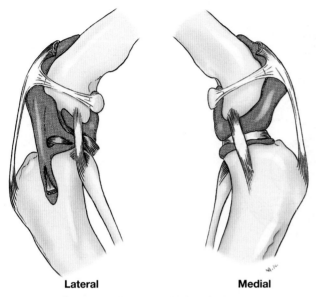

Lateral **Medial**

Fig. 2-61 Capsule of left stifle joint.

Each meniscus attaches to the cranial and caudal intercondylar areas of the tibia (see Fig. 2-63) via the **cranial and caudal meniscotibial ligaments**. A **transverse ligament** connects the cranial ends of the menisci. The caudal part of the lateral meniscus is attached to the intercondylar fossa of the femur by a **meniscofemoral ligament** (see Figs. 2-60, 2-62, 2-63). The medial meniscus is attached to the medial collateral ligament and moves only slightly when the stifle is flexed. The lateral meniscus is separated from the lateral collateral ligament by the tendon of origin of the popliteus. When the stifle joint is flexed, the tibia rotates medially and the lateral meniscus moves caudally on the tibial condyle.

The **femorotibial ligaments** are the collateral and cruciate ligaments. The **medial collateral ligament** extends from the medial epicondyle of the femur to the medial side of the tibia distal to the medial condyle. It fuses with the lateral aspect of the medial meniscus.

The **lateral collateral ligament** extends from the lateral epicondyle of the femur over the tendon of origin of the popliteus to the head of the fibula and adjacent lateral condyle of the tibia. Clean these ligaments to observe their attachments. With the stifle extended, these ligaments prevent abduction, adduction, and rotation of the stifle. When the stifle joint is flexed, the lateral ligament is loosened.

The **cruciate ligaments** pass between the intercondylar areas of the tibia and femur and limit craniocaudal motion of these bones. The ligaments cross each other near their attachments in the intercondylar fossa of the femur.

The **cranial cruciate ligament** attaches within the intercondylar fossa of the femur to the caudomedial part of the lateral condyle. It extends distocranially to attach to the cranial intercondylar area of the tibia. This attachment is just caudal to the cranial attachment of the medial meniscus.

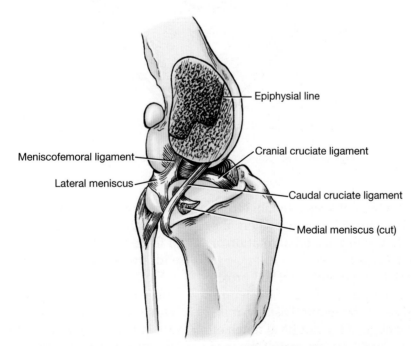

Epiphysial line

Meniscofemoral ligament

Cranial cruciate ligament

Lateral meniscus

Caudal cruciate ligament

Medial meniscus (cut)

Fig. 2-62 Cruciate and meniscal ligaments of left stifle joint, medial aspect.

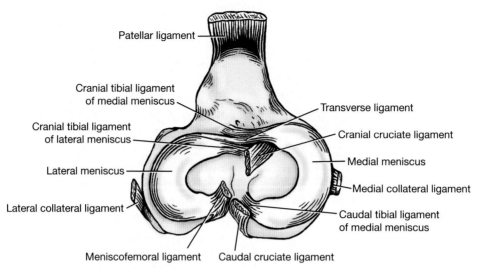

Fig. 2-63 Menisci and ligaments, proximal end of left tibia.

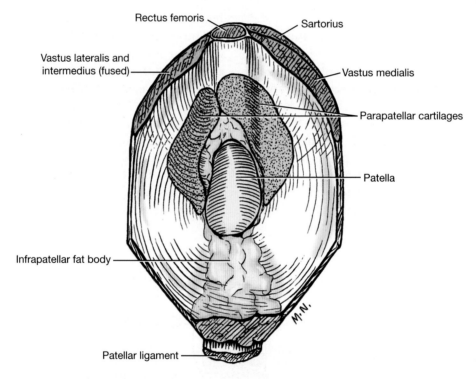

Fig. 2-64 Left patella and fibrocartilages, articular surface.

The cranial cruciate ligament keeps the tibia from sliding cranially beneath the femur when the limb bears weight. It also limits medial rotation of the tibia when the stifle is flexed.

The **caudal cruciate ligament** attaches proximally within the intercondylar fossa of the femur to the medial condyle of the femur. Distally, it attaches to the medial edge of the popliteal notch of the tibia behind the caudal attachment of the medial meniscus. This ligament prevents caudal

movement of the tibia beneath the femur when the limb bears weight. Observe the attachments of these ligaments. They are named in accordance with the position of their tibial attachments.

Flex the stifle and, while holding the femur firmly in one hand, try to move the tibia cranially with the other. In the normal dog there is no movement. Transect the tibial attachment of the cranial cruciate ligament and repeat the procedure. The excessive cranial excursion of the tibia that results is diagnostic for a ruptured cranial cruciate ligament.

Transect the collateral ligaments to observe the effect on the joint. Note the menisci and their attachments.

The two **tibiofibular joints** are a proximal joint between the head of the fibula and the lateral condyle of the tibia and a distal joint between the lateral malleolus of the fibula and the lateral surface of the distal end of the tibia. Throughout the length of the interosseous space between the tibia and fibula is a sheet of fibrous tissue uniting the two bones, the **interosseous membrane** of the crus.

The **tarsal joint** is a composite of several articulations and joint sacs. The tarsocrural joint sac is the largest and incorporates the articulations of the distal tibia and fibula with that of the talus and calcaneus. Greatest movement in the tarsus occurs between the cochlea of the tibia and the trochlea of the talus. Puncture to obtain synovia is made into this joint sac. Other joint sacs include the proximal and distal intertarsal sacs and the tarsometatarsal sac. Medial and lateral collateral ligaments cross the tarsus from the tibia and fibula to the metatarsal bones. Numerous ligaments join the individual tarsal bones to each other. These will not be dissected.

LIVE DOG

Place the thumb of one hand behind the greater trochanter. With the other hand, grasp the femur and flex and extend and rotate the hip. Try to lift the femoral head out of the acetabulum. This will be prevented by the ligament of the femoral head and joint capsule. To enter the hip joint with a needle, first palpate the cranial surface of the greater trochanter. Insert the needle here and pass it through the gluteal muscles in a medial and slightly ventral direction.

Stand behind the dog and palpate each stifle. Feel the patellar ligament and notice the normal slight depression caudal to it on the medial side. When the joint is swollen, this is less evident. Remember that there is fat between the patellar ligament and the stifle joint capsule.

With the dog recumbent, extend the stifle and palpate the patella. Move it laterally and medially. You should not be able to luxate the normal patella. Palpate the ridges of the trochlea. Follow them distally to the femoral condyles. Palpate the tibial condyles and the collateral ligaments of the stifle. With the stifle extended, rotate the tibia medially and laterally to test the integrity of the collateral ligaments. Flex the stifle, repeat this rotation, and note the normal increase in rotation, especially medially. This medial rotation is limited by the cranial cruciate ligament. Keep the stifle flexed and hold the femur with one hand while attempting to move the tibia cranially and caudally with the other hand to determine the integrity of the cruciate ligaments. To enter the stifle joint with a needle, pass the needle caudally on either side of the patellar ligament through the fat pad.

Palpate the tarsus. Flex and extend the tarsocrural joint and feel the ridges of the trochlea of the talus on the dorsal aspect. Inflammation of this joint will cause this joint sac to enlarge. To enter the tarsocrural joint with a needle, extend the joint and palpate the lateral ridge of the trochlea of the talus. Pass the needle through the fascia into the joint on either side of this ridge.

BONES OF THE VERTEBRAL COLUMN AND THORAX

The **vertebral column** (see Fig. 2-1) consists of approximately 50 irregular bones. The vertebrae are arranged in five groups: **cervical, thoracic, lumbar, sacral**, and **caudal**. The first letter or abbreviation of the word designating each group followed by the number of vertebrae in each group expresses a vertebral formula. That of the dog is $C_7T_{13}L_7S_3Cd_{20}$. The number of caudal vertebrae may vary. The three sacral vertebrae fuse to form what is considered a single bone, the **sacrum**.

A typical vertebra consists of a body; a vertebral arch consisting of right and left pedicles and laminae; and transverse, spinous, and articular processes (see Figs. 2-68, 2-69).

The **body** of a vertebra is constricted centrally. The cranial extremity is convex, and the caudal extremity is concave. Adjacent vertebral bodies are connected by intervertebral discs, each of which is a fibrocartilaginous structure composed of a soft center, the **nucleus pulposus** (see Fig. 2-71), surrounded by concentric layers of dense fibrous tissue, the **anulus fibrosus**. These intervertebral discs will be dissected when the spinal cord is studied.

The **vertebral arch** is subdivided into basal parts, the **pedicles**, and the dorsal portion, formed by two **laminae**. Together with the body the vertebral arch forms a short tube, the **vertebral foramen**. All the vertebral foramina join to form the **vertebral canal**. The pedicles of each vertebra extend from the dorsolateral surface of the body. They present smooth-surfaced notches. The **cranial vertebral notches** are shallow; the **caudal vertebral notches** are deep. When the vertebral column is articulated, the notches of adjacent vertebrae and the intervening fibrocartilage form the right and left **intervertebral foramina.** Through these pass the spinal nerves and blood vessels. The dorsal part of the vertebral arch is composed of right and left laminae, which unite to form a **spinous process** or spine. Each typical vertebra has, in addition to the dorsally located **spinous process**, or spine, paired **transverse processes** that project laterally from the region where the arch joins the vertebral body. Farther dorsally on the arch, at the junction of pedicle and lamina, are located the **articular processes**. There are two of these on each side of the vertebra: a cranial pair whose articulating surfaces point dorsally or medially and a caudal pair whose surfaces are directed ventrally or laterally.

Cervical Vertebrae

There are seven cervical vertebrae in most mammals. The **atlas** (Figs. 2-65, 2-67), or first cervical vertebra, is atypical in both structure and function. It articulates with the skull cranially. Its chief peculiarities are modified articular processes, a lack of a spinous process, and a reduction of its body. The lateral shelflike transverse processes are thick, forming the **wings of the atlas**. These are united by the **body** (ventral arch) ventrally and **arch** dorsally. The two **cranial articular foveae** articulate with the occipital condyles of the skull to form the **atlanto-occipital joint**, of which the main movement is flexion and extension. The **caudal articular foveae** consist of two shallow glenoid cavities that form a freely movable articulation with the second cervical vertebra. Rotatory movement occurs at this atlantoaxial joint. Examine the caudal part of the dorsal surface of the body for the **fovea dentis**. This is concave from side to side and articulates

with the dens of the second cervical vertebra. This articular area blends laterally with the caudal articular fovea. Besides the large vertebral foramen through which the spinal cord passes, there are two pairs of foramina in the atlas. The **transverse foramina** are actually short canals that pass obliquely through the transverse processes of the atlas and contain the vertebral artery and vein. The **lateral vertebral foramina** perforate the cranial part of the vertebral arch. The first cervical spinal nerves pass through these foramina.

The **axis**, or second cervical vertebra (Figs. 2-66, 2-67), presents an elongated, ridgelike spinous process as its most prominent characteristic. It is also unlike other vertebrae in that cranially the body projects forward in a peglike eminence, the **dens**. The ventral surface of the dens is articular, whereas the tip and dorsal surface may be rough because of ligamentous attachment. The **cranial articular surface** is located on the body and is continuous with the articular area of the dens. The caudal part of the vertebral arch has two articular processes that face ventrolaterally. At the root of the transverse process is the small transverse foramen. The cranial vertebral notch concurs with that of the atlas to form the first

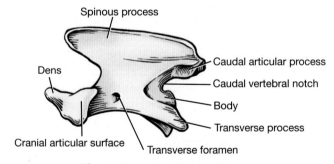

Fig. 2-66   Axis, left lateral view.

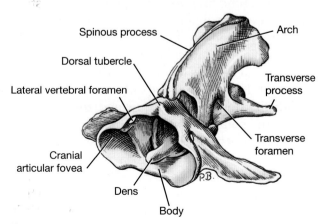

Fig. 2-67   Atlas and axis articulated, craniolateral aspect.

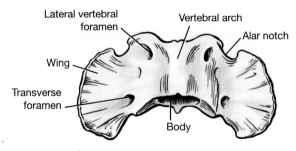

Fig. 2-65   Atlas, dorsal view.

intervertebral foramen for the transmission of the second cervical nerve (Fig. 2-67). The caudal notch concurs with that of the third cervical vertebra to form the second intervertebral foramen, through which the third cervical nerve passes. Other features of this bone are similar to those of a typical vertebra.

The middle three cervical vertebrae (Fig. 2-68) differ little from a typical vertebra. The spinous processes are low but gradually increase in height from third to fifth. The transverse processes are two pronged and are perforated at the base by a transverse foramen.

The sixth cervical vertebra has a high spine and an expanded **ventral lamina** of the transverse process. The seventh cervical vertebra (Fig. 2-69) lacks transverse foramina and has the highest cervical spine.

The **cranial articular processes** of cervical vertebrae 3 to 7 face dorsally and cranially in apposition to the **caudal articular processes** of adjacent vertebrae. There is a prominent **ventral crest** on the caudal midventral aspect of the vertebral body.

Thoracic Vertebrae

There are 13 thoracic vertebrae (Fig. 2-70); the first 9 are similar. The bodies of the thoracic vertebrae

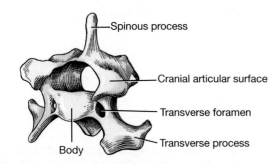

Fig. 2-68 Fifth cervical vertebra, craniolateral aspect.

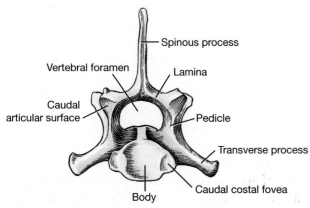

Fig. 2-69 Seventh cervical vertebra, caudal aspect.

are short. The first through the tenth have a **cranial** and a **caudal costal fovea** on each side for rib articulation. Because the foveae of two adjacent vertebrae form the articular surface for the head of one rib, they are sometimes called *demifacets.* The body of the tenth vertebra frequently lacks caudal foveae, whereas the eleventh through the thirteenth have only one complete cranial costal fovea on each side. The head of the first rib articulates between the last cervical and first thoracic vertebrae. The tubercles of the ribs articulate with the transverse processes of the thoracic vertebrae of the same number in all instances.

The **spine** is the most conspicuous feature of each of the first nine thoracic vertebrae. The massiveness of the spines gradually decreases with successive vertebrae, but there is little change in length and direction until the seventh or eighth vertebra is reached. The spines then become progressively shorter and incline caudally through the ninth and tenth. The spine of the eleventh thoracic vertebra is nearly perpendicular to the long axis of that bone. This vertebra is designated the **anticlinal vertebra**. All spines caudal to the eleventh vertebra point cranially; all spines cranial to the eleventh vertebra point caudally (see Fig. 2-75).

The transverse processes are short, blunt, and irregular. All contain costal foveae for articulation with the tubercles of the ribs.

The **articular processes** are located at the junctions of the pedicles and the laminae. The cranial pair are nearly confluent at the median plane on thoracic vertebrae 3 through 10. Similar to cervical vertebrae 3 through 7, the cranial articular surfaces of thoracic vertebrae 1 through 10 face dorsally and slightly craniomedially. Because the caudal articular processes articulate with the cranial ones of the vertebra behind, they are similar in shape but face in the opposite direction. The joints between thoracic vertebrae 10 and 13 are conspicuously modified because the articular surfaces of the caudal articular processes are located on the lateral side and the articular surfaces of the cranial articular processes of thoracic vertebrae 11 through 13 face medially. A similar arrangement is seen in all lumbar vertebrae. This type of interlocking articulation allows flexion and extension of the caudal-thoracic and lumbar region while limiting lateral movement.

The **accessory process** (see Fig. 2-70, *B*) projects caudally from the pedicle ventral to the caudal articular process and over the dorsal aspect of the

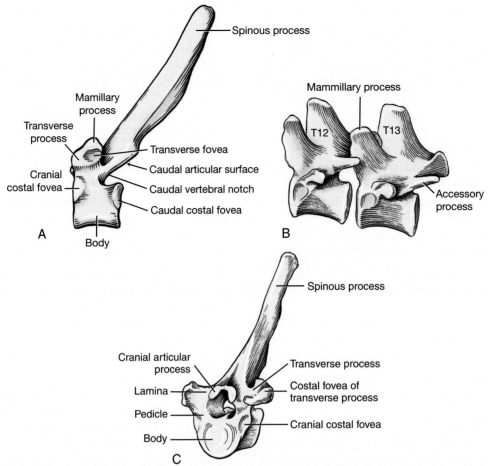

Fig. 2-70 A, Sixth thoracic vertebra, left lateral view. **B,** Twelfth and thirteenth thoracic vertebrae, left lateral view. **C,** Sixth thoracic vertebra, cranial lateral aspect. (Part **C** from Evans HE, de Lahunta A: *Miller's anatomy of the dog,* ed 4, St Louis, 2013, Saunders.)

intervertebral foramen. It is present from the midthoracic region to the fifth or sixth lumbar vertebra. The **mamillary process** is a knoblike dorsal projection of the transverse processes of the second through tenth thoracic vertebrae and cranial articular processes of the eleventh thoracic through the caudal vertebrae. Epaxial muscles of the transversospinalis system attach to these processes.

Lumbar Vertebrae

The **lumbar vertebrae** (Fig. 2-71) have longer bodies than the thoracic vertebrae. The **transverse processes** are directed cranially as well as ventrolaterally. The **articular processes** lie mainly in sagittal planes. The **caudal processes** protrude between the cranial ones of succeeding vertebrae. The prominent blunt **spinous processes** are largest in the midlumbar region and have a slight cranial direction. The seventh lumbar vertebra is slightly shorter than the other lumbar vertebrae.

Sacrum

The **sacrum** (Fig. 2-72) results from the fusion of the bodies and processes of three vertebrae. This bone lies between the ilia and firmly articulates with them.

The **body** of the first segment is larger than the combined bodies of the other two segments. The three are united to form a concave ventral surface.

The dorsal surface presents several markings that result from the fusion of the three sacral vertebrae. The **median sacral crest** represents the fusion of the three spinous processes. The dorsal surface also bears two pairs of **dorsal sacral foramina**, which transmit the dorsal branches of the first two sacral spinal nerves.

The pelvic (ventral) surface has two pairs of **pelvic sacral foramina**. They transmit the ventral branches of the first two sacral spinal nerves. The wing of the sacrum is the enlarged lateral part that bears a large, rough surface, the **auricular face**, which articulates with the ilium.

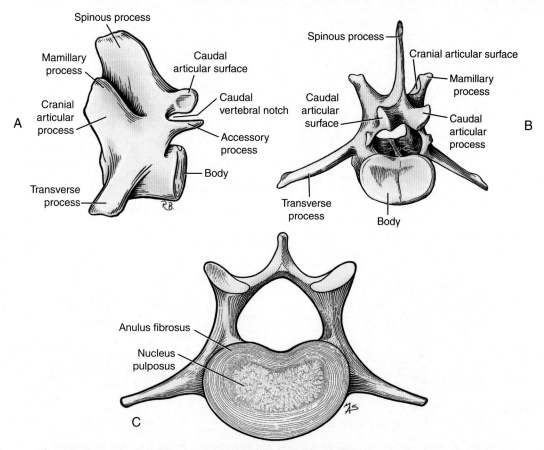

Fig. 2-71 A, Fourth lumbar vertebra, left lateral view. **B,** Fifth lumbar vertebra, caudola-teral view. **C,** Intervertebral disc in lumbar region of 10-week-old pup, cranial view. (From Evans HE, de Lahunta A: *Miller's anatomy of the dog,* ed 4, St Louis, 2013, Saunders.)

The **base** of the sacrum faces cranially. The ventral part of the base has a transverse ridge, the **promontory**. This, with the ilia, forms the dorsal boundary of the pelvic inlet.

Caudal Vertebrae

The average number of caudal vertebrae (Fig. 2-73) in the dog is 20. These lose their distinctive features as one proceeds caudally.

Ribs

All 13 pairs of ribs (Figs. 2-74, 2-75) have dorsal bony and ventral cartilaginous parts that meet at a costochondral junction. This junction may be expanded in rapidly growing animals. The cartilaginous parts are called **costal cartilages**. The first nine pairs of ribs articulate directly with the sternum. The costal cartilages of the tenth, eleventh, and twelfth unite with one another to form the **costal arch**. The thirteenth rib often ends freely in the flank. The bony part of a typical rib presents a head, neck, tuberculum, and body.

The **head** of ribs 1 through 10 articulates with the costal foveae of 2 contiguous vertebrae and the intervening fibrocartilage. For ribs 11 through 13, the head articulates only with the cranial costal fovea on the body of the vertebra of the same number. The **tubercle** of the rib articulates with the costal fovea of the transverse process of the vertebra of the same number. Between the head and tuberculum of the rib is the **neck**.

Sternum

The sternum is composed of eight unpaired segments, the **sternebrae** (see Figs. 2-74, 2-75). Consecutive sternebrae are joined by the **intersternebral cartilages**. The first sternebra, also known as the **manubrium**, ends cranially in a clublike enlargement. The last sternebra is flattened dorsoventrally and is called the **xiphoid process**. The caudal end of this process is continued by a thin plate, the xiphoid cartilage.

LIVE DOG

Palpate the wings of the atlas. While holding these firmly, move the head up and down to extend and flex the atlanto-occipital joint. The point at which a transverse line drawn across the

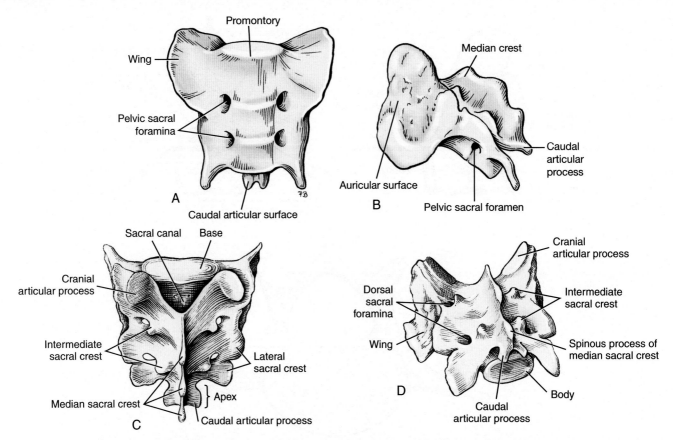

Fig. 2-72   **A,** Sacrum, ventral view. **B,** Sacrum, left lateral view. **C,** Sacrum, dorsal aspect. **D,** Sacrum, caudal lateral aspect. (Parts **C** and **D** from Evans HE, de Lahunta A: *Miller's anatomy of the dog,* ed 4, St Louis, 2013, Saunders.)

cranial edge of the wings of the atlas intersects the median plane is the site for puncture to obtain cerebrospinal fluid.

Palpate the spine of the axis. Move each wing of the atlas up and down to rotate the atlantoaxial joint. Palpate the transverse processes of cervical vertebrae 3 through 6. Note their relative positions in the neck and the large volume of epaxial muscles dorsal to them. Feel the ventral edge of the broad transverse processes of the sixth cervical vertebra.

Palpate the prominent spines of thoracic and lumbar vertebrae. Palpate the transverse processes

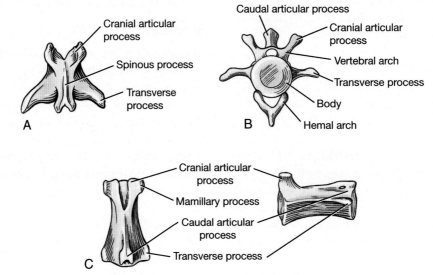

Fig. 2-73   **A,** Third caudal vertebra, dorsal view. **B,** Fourth caudal vertebra, cranial view. **C,** Sixth caudal vertebra, dorsal and lateral views.

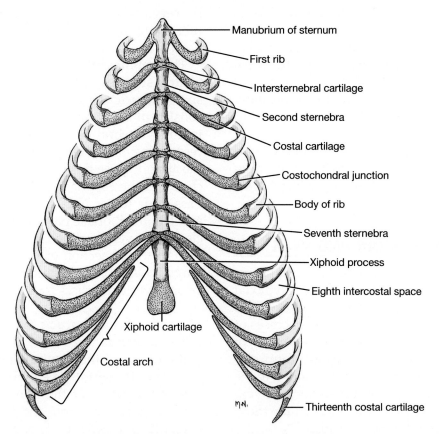

Manubrium of sternum

First rib

Intersternebral cartilage

Second sternebra

Costal cartilage

Costochondral junction

Body of rib

Seventh sternebra

Xiphoid process

Eighth intercostal space

Xiphoid cartilage

Costal arch

Thirteenth costal cartilage

Fig. 2-74 Rib cage and sternum, ventral view.

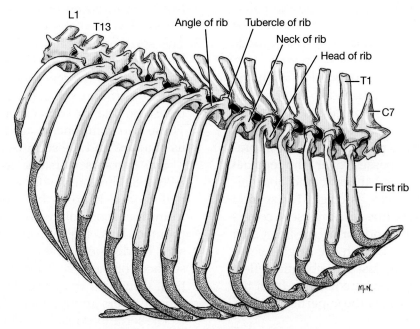

L1

T13

Angle of rib

Tubercle of rib

Neck of rib

Head of rib

T1

C7

First rib

Fig. 2-75 Rib cage and sternum, right lateral view.

of the lumbar vertebrae. Locate the iliac crests and feel the spine of the seventh lumbar vertebra between them. This spine is shorter than that of the sixth vertebra and is used to locate the site for lumbosacral puncture for epidural anesthesia. Lumbar myelography is usually done between the spines of the sixth and fifth lumbar vertebrae.

Palpate the ribs and compress the thorax, noting the flexibility of the ribs. Palpate the sternum from manubrium to the xiphoid cartilage. Note the costal arch.

MUSCLES OF THE TRUNK AND NECK

The muscles of the trunk and neck, or **axial muscles**, are classified morphologically into **hypaxial** and **epaxial** groups. The epaxial muscles (see Fig. 2-81) lie dorsal to the transverse processes of the vertebrae and function mainly as extensors of the vertebral column. The hypaxial group embraces all other trunk muscles not included in the epaxial division. These muscles are located ventral to the transverse processes and include those of the abdominal and thoracic walls.

The **superficial fascia of the trunk** covers the thorax and abdomen subcutaneously. It is continuous cranially and caudally with the superficial fasciae of the thoracic limb, the neck, and the pelvic limb. Clean this fascia and fat from the thorax and abdomen. It contains the cutaneous trunci muscle and numerous cutaneous vessels and nerves.

The **deep fascia of the trunk** (see Fig. 2-40), the thoracolumbar fascia, is attached to the ends of the spinous and transverse processes of the thoracic and lumbar vertebrae. From its dorsal attachment to the spinous processes and the supraspinous ligament, it passes over the epaxial musculature to the lateral thoracic and abdominal walls, where it serves as origin for several muscles. On each side this fascia closely covers the abdominal muscles and forms the linea alba on the ventral midline. Detach the origin of the latissimus dorsi from the last few ribs and reflect it to the mid-dorsal line, where it arises from the lumbar vertebral spines via the superficial leaf of the thoracolumbar fascia.

Hypaxial Muscles

Muscles of the Neck

The **longus capitis** (see Fig. 2-82) lies on the lateral surface of the cervical vertebrae, lateral to the longus colli. It arises from the transverse processes of the cervical vertebrae and inserts on the muscular tubercle on the ventral surface of the basioccipital bone of the skull.

The **longus colli** (see Figs. 3-8, 3-20) covers the ventral surfaces of the vertebral bodies from the sixth thoracic vertebra cranially to the atlas. It consists of many overlapping fascicles that attach to the vertebral bodies or the transverse processes. The most cranial cervical bundles attach to the atlas. Expose this muscle by reflecting the trachea and the esophagus and related soft tissues. Pass your finger into the thoracic inlet dorsally and feel the thoracic part of the longus colli muscle on the vertebral bodies. This portion will be seen in the dissection of the thoracic cavity. The longus colli must be reflected to expose the cervical intervertebral discs for surgical purposes.

Muscles of the Thoracic Wall

1. The **scalenus** (Figs. 2-76, 2-82) lies ventral to the origin of the cervical and cranial thoracic parts of the serratus ventralis. It attaches to the first few ribs and the transverse processes of the cervical vertebrae and is divided into several slips. It is a muscle of inspiration.
2. The **serratus ventralis cervicis** and **thoracis** (see Figs. 2-16, 2-76, 2-82) form a large, fan-shaped muscle with an extensive origin on the neck and trunk. Its insertion on the serrated face of the scapula has been observed (see Fig. 2-14).
3. The **serratus dorsalis** consists of cranial and caudal components that arise by a broad aponeurosis from the tendinous raphe of the neck and from the thoracic and lumbar spines and insert on the proximal portions of the ribs. These two components are the serratus dorsalis cranialis and the serratus dorsalis caudalis.

The **serratus dorsalis cranialis** (see Figs. 2-76, 2-82) lies on the dorsal surface of the cranial thorax. It arises by a broad aponeurosis from the thoracolumbar fascia deep to the rhomboideus. It runs caudoventrally and inserts by distinct serrations on the craniolateral surfaces of the ribs. It lifts the ribs for inspiration. Transect this muscle at the beginning of its muscle fibers and reflect both portions.

The **serratus dorsalis caudalis** is smaller and is found on the dorsal surface of the caudal thorax. It consists of distinct muscle leaves that arise by an aponeurosis from the thoracolumbar fascia, course cranioventrally, and insert on the caudal borders of the last three ribs. It functions in drawing the last three ribs caudally in expiration.

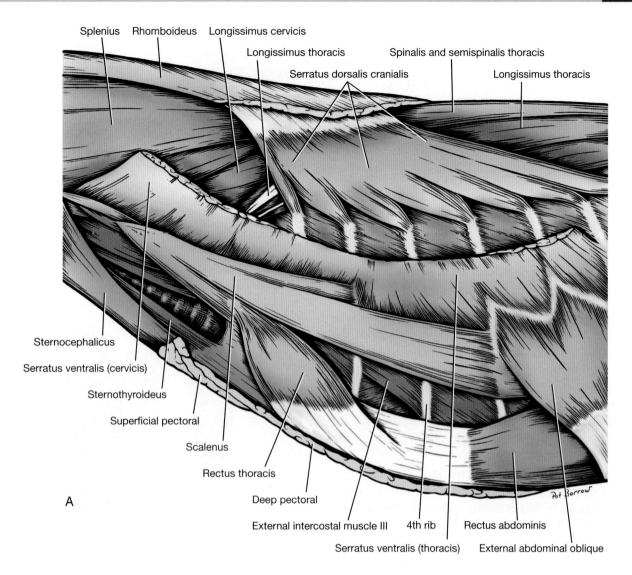

A

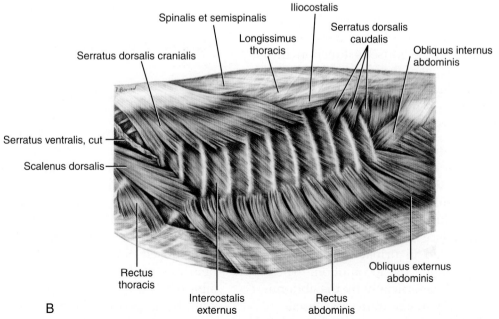

B

Fig. 2-76 **A,** Muscles of neck and thorax, lateral view. **B,** Superficial muscles of thoracic cage, lateral aspect. (M. serratus ventralis [thoracis] has been removed.)

Continued

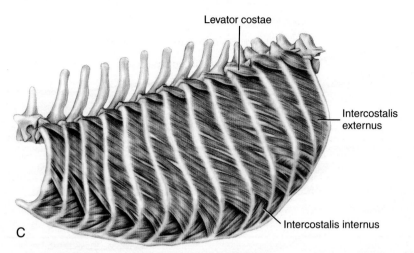

Fig. 2-76, cont'd   **C,** Deep muscles of thorax, lateral aspect. (Parts **B** and **C** from Evans HE, de Lahunta A: *Miller's anatomy of the dog,* ed 4, St Louis, 2013, Saunders.)

4. There are 12 **external intercostal muscles** (see Figs. 2-76, 3-4 through 3-6) on each side of the thoracic wall. Their fibers run caudoventrally from the caudal border of one rib to the cranial border of the rib caudal to it. Their ventral border is near the costochondral junction. They function in respiration by drawing the ribs together, and their overall effect depends on the fixation of the rib cage.

5. The **internal intercostal muscles** (see Figs. 3-4 to 3-6) are easily differentiated from the external intercostal muscles because their fibers run cranioventrally from the cranial border of one rib to the caudal border of the rib cranial to it. Medial to most of the internal intercostal muscles is the pleura, which attaches to the muscles and ribs by the endothoracic fascia. The internal intercostal muscles extend the whole distance of the intercostal spaces. These muscles function in a manner similar to that of the external intercostal muscles by drawing the ribs together.

Expose the fifth external intercostal muscle and reflect it to observe the internal intercostal.

Muscles of the Abdominal Wall

The four abdominal muscles (Figs. 2-76 through 2-80), named from external to internal, are the **external abdominal oblique**, the **internal abdominal oblique,** the **rectus abdominis**, and the **transversus abdominis** (see Figs. 2-77, 2-78). When they contract, they aid in urination, defecation, parturition, respiration, or locomotion. These muscles are covered superficially by the abdominal fasciae and deeply by the transverse fascia.

1. The **external abdominal oblique** (see Fig. 2-76 through 2-80) covers the ventral half of the

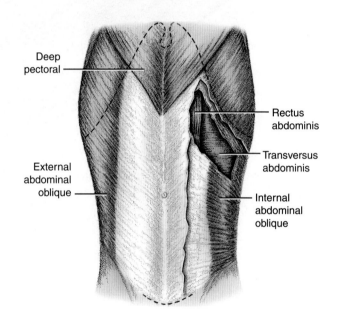

Fig. 2-77   Muscles of abdominal wall, ventral view.

lateral thoracic wall and the lateral part of the abdominal wall. The costal part arises from the last ribs. The lumbar part arises from the last rib and from the thoracolumbar fascia. The fibers of this muscle run caudoventrally. In the ventral abdominal wall, this muscle forms a wide aponeurosis that inserts on the **linea alba** and the prepubic tendon. The linea alba (see Fig. 2-78) is the midventral raphe that consists of the fused thoracolumbar fascia and the aponeuroses of the abdominal muscles. The linea alba extends from the xiphoid process to the symphysis pelvis. The aponeurosis of the external abdominal oblique, combined with that of the internal abdominal oblique, forms most

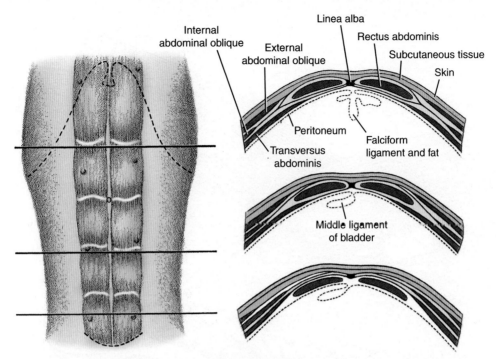

Fig. 2-78 Abdominal wall in ventral view with transections at three levels.

of the external lamina of the sheath of the rectus abdominis.

Caudoventrally, just cranial to the iliopubic eminence and lateral to the midline, the aponeurosis of the external abdominal oblique separates into two parts, which then come together to form the **superficial inguinal ring** (see Figs. 2-79, 2-80). This is the external opening of a very short natural passageway through the abdominal wall, the **inguinal canal**. The superficial inguinal ring is a slit in this aponeurosis with a cranial and caudal angle. The caudal angle is attached to the small palpable iliopubic cartilage that is located in the tendon of origin of the pectineus. Abduct the pelvic limb and follow the pectineus to its origin, where this cartilage can be palpated. The superficial inguinal ring is indistinct because it is covered by thoracolumbar fascia. The internal opening and the boundaries of the canal will be seen when the abdominal cavity is opened. A blind extension of peritoneum protrudes through the inguinal canal to a subcutaneous position outside the body wall. This is the **vaginal tunic** (see Figs. 2-79, 2-80, 4-4, 4-5) in the male and the **vaginal process** in the female (see Figs. 4-2, 4-4). In the male it is accompanied by the testis and spermatic cord, which it envelops. In the female the vaginal process envelops the round ligament of the uterus

and a varying amount of fat and ends blindly a short distance from the vulva. In both sexes the external pudendal artery and vein and the genitofemoral nerve also pass through the inguinal canal (see Figs. 2-79, 4-2).

Clean the surface of the aponeurosis of the external abdominal oblique and identify the superficial inguinal ring and vaginal tunic or process. Be careful not to destroy the ring and tunic or process in cleaning this muscle. The vaginal tunic or process is covered by the spermatic fascia, which is continuous with the abdominal fascia at this ring.

Transect the external abdominal oblique close to its costal and lumbar origin. Reflect this muscle ventrally from the internal abdominal oblique to the line of fusion between their aponeuroses. The fused aponeuroses cover the external surface of the rectus abdominis.

The **inguinal ligament** (see Fig. 2-80) is the caudal border of the aponeurosis of the external abdominal oblique. It terminates on the iliopubic eminence and prepubic tendon. The ventral portion of the ligament is interposed between the **superficial inguinal ring** and the **vascular lacuna** (see Figs. 2-79, 4-82). The vascular lacuna is the base of the femoral triangle, the space that contains the femoral vessels that run to and from the hindlimb. The inguinal ligament thus forms

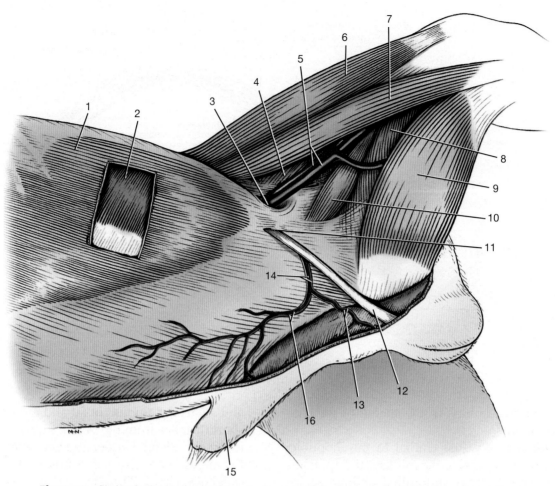

Fig. 2-79 Abdominal muscles and inguinal region of the male, superficial dissection, left side.
1. External abdominal oblique
2. Internal abdominal oblique
3. Vascular lacuna
4. Vastus medialis
5. Femoral artery and vein in femoral triangle
6. Cranial part of sartorius
7. Caudal part of sartorius
8. Adductor
9. Gracilis
10. Pectineus
11. Superficial inguinal ring
12. Parietal vaginal tunic
13. Cranial scrotal artery and vein
14. External pudendal artery and vein
15. Prepuce
16. Caudal superficial epigastric artery and vein

part of the cranial border of the vascular lacuna and the caudal border of the inguinal canal. Transect the aponeurosis of insertion of the external abdominal oblique 2 cm cranial to its caudal border and the superficial inguinal ring and reflect the muscle ventrally. Identify these structures.

2. The **internal abdominal oblique** (see Figs. 2-79, 2-80) arises from the superficial leaf of the thoracolumbar fascia caudal to the last rib, in common with the lumbar part of the external abdominal oblique, and from the tuber coxae and adjacent portion of the inguinal ligament. Its fibers run cranioventrally. It inserts by a wide aponeurosis on the costal arch, on the rectus abdominis, and on the linea alba and prepubic tendon. At the rectus abdominis it is fused with the aponeurosis of the external abdominal oblique to form the external sheath of

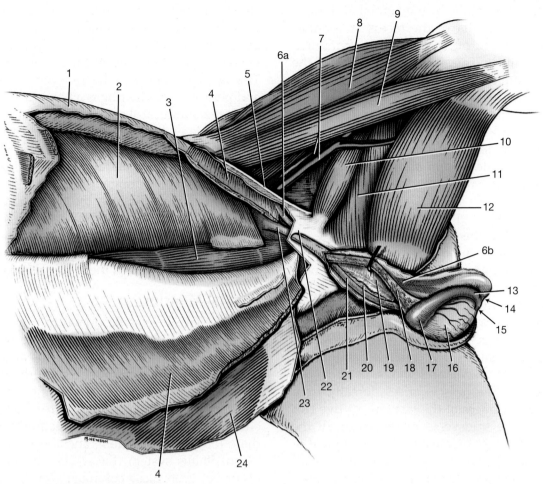

Fig. 2-80 Abdominal muscles and inguinal region of the male, deep dissection, left side.
1. Thoracolumbar fascia
2. Transversus abdominis
3. Rectus abdominis
4. Internal abdominal oblique (transected and reflected)
5. Inguinal ligament (caudal border of aponeurosis of external abdominal oblique muscle)
6a. Cremaster muscle at its origin
6b. Cremaster muscle on external surface of parietal layer of vaginal tunic
7. Femoral artery and vein
8. Cranial part of sartorius
9. Caudal part of sartorius
10. Pectineus
11. Adductor
12. Gracilis
13. Tail of epididymis
14. Ligament of tail of epididymis
15. Proper ligament of testis
16. Testis in visceral vaginal tunic
17. Head of epididymis
18. Testicular artery and vein in visceral vaginal tunic (mesorchium)
19. Mesorchium
20. Mesoductus deferens
21. Ductus deferens in visceral vaginal tunic
22. Superficial inguinal ring, lateral crus
23. Parietal vaginal tunic in the inguinal canal
24. External abdominal oblique (reflected)

the rectus abdominis. In the cranial abdomen, at the lateral border of the rectus abdominis, the aponeurosis of the internal abdominal oblique splits and passes on both sides of the rectus abdominis to insert on the linea alba (see Figs. 2-78 and 2-80).

Transect the muscle 2 cm from its origin (Fig. 2-80) and reflect it ventrally to the rectus abdominis. In doing so, detach its insertions on the ribs. Separate it from all underlying structures except the rectus abdominis. Study the aponeurosis of the internal abdominal oblique, which contributes to the external lamina of the sheath of the rectus abdominis. Note how the caudal border of the muscle forms the cranial border of the inguinal canal. In the male, note that fibers from the caudal border of the internal oblique form the **cremaster muscle,** which accompanies the vaginal tunic (see Fig. 2-80).

3. The **transversus abdominis** (see Figs. 2-40, 2-80) is medial to the internal abdominal oblique and the rectus abdominis. Its fibers run transversely. The muscle arises dorsally from the medial surfaces of the last four or five ribs and from the transverse processes of all the lumbar vertebrae by means of the deep leaf of the thoracolumbar fascia. Its aponeurosis attaches to the linea alba after crossing the internal surface of the rectus abdominis. Except for its most caudal part, the aponeurosis of the transversus abdominis forms the internal sheath of the rectus abdominis. The most caudal portion joins the external sheath and fuses with the linea alba and prepubic tendon.

4. The **rectus abdominis** (see Figs. 2-76 through 2-78, 2-80) extends from the pecten of the pubis, as the prepubic tendon, to the sternum. It flexes the thoracolumbar part of the vertebral column. Observe its cranial aponeurosis from the first few ribs and sternum. The rectus abdominis has distinct transverse tendinous intersections. In the umbilical region the external lamina of the sheath of the rectus abdominis is formed by the fused aponeuroses of the oblique muscles. The internal lamina is formed by the aponeurosis of the transversus abdominis.

Inguinal Canal

The **inguinal canal** is a slit between the abdominal muscles. It extends from the deep to the superficial inguinal ring (see Figs. 2-80, 4-5). The **superficial inguinal ring** in the aponeurosis of the external abdominal oblique has already been dissected. The **deep inguinal ring** is formed on the inside of the abdominal wall by the annular reflection of transversalis fascia onto the vaginal tunic or process. This fascia lies between the transversus abdominis and peritoneum. The ring is a boundary and not a distinct anatomical structure. The inguinal canal is bounded laterally by the aponeurosis of the external abdominal oblique, cranially by the internal abdominal oblique, caudally by the caudal border of the external abdominal oblique (the inguinal ligament), and medially by the lateral border of the rectus abdominis and by the transversalis fascia and peritoneum. The vaginal tunic and the **spermatic cord** or the vaginal process pass obliquely caudoventrally through the inguinal canal.

Epaxial Muscles

The epaxial muscles lie dorsal to the transverse processes of the vertebrae. They are associated with the vertebral column and ribs and may be divided into three parallel longitudinal muscle masses on each side. Each is composed of many overlapping fascicles. These three columns include the lateral iliocostalis system, the intermediate longissimus system, and the medial transversospinalis system (Fig. 2-81). Various fusions occur between these columns, giving rise to different muscle patterns that are difficult to separate. These muscles act as extensors of the vertebral column and also produce lateral movements of the trunk when contracting on only one side.

Iliocostalis System

1. The **iliocostalis lumborum** (Fig. 2-81) arises from the wing of the ilium in common with the longissimus lumborum and inserts on the transverse processes of the lumbar vertebrae and the last four or five ribs. In the lumbar region this muscle is fused medially with the longissimus lumborum. The thoracolumbar fascia covers these muscles. Remove this fascia and any underlying fat to expose the glistening aponeurosis of these fused muscles, which attaches to the crest of the ilium and the spines of the lumbar and last four or five thoracic vertebrae. The cranial end of this iliocostalis muscle is distinctly separated from the longissimus lumborum as it inserts on the ribs. Expose this insertion.

2. The **iliocostalis thoracis** (see Figs. 2-81, 2-82) is a long, narrow muscle mass extending from the twelfth rib to the transverse process of the

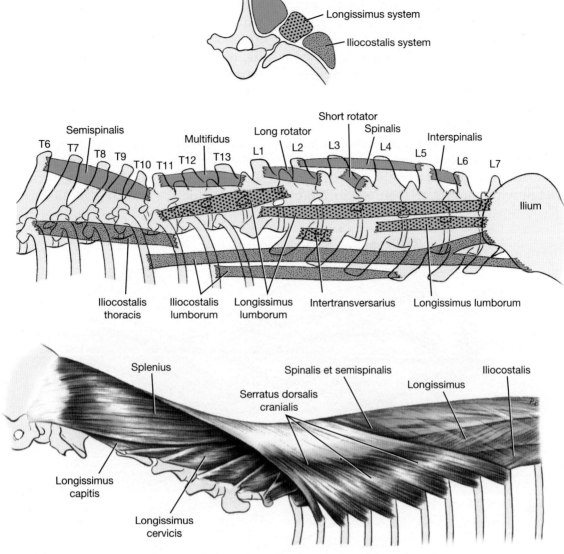

Fig. 2-81 Schema of epaxial muscles. Each of the named muscles shown can be present, spanning other vertebrae, thus overlapping and obscuring their individual nature.

seventh cervical vertebra. Individual components of the muscle extend between and overlap the ribs. Identify the boundaries of this muscle mass.

Longissimus System

The longissimus is the intermediate portion of the epaxial musculature. Lying medial to the iliocostalis, its overlapping fascicles extend from the ilium to the head. It consists of three major regional divisions: **thoracolumbar, cervical,** and **capital.**

1. The **longissimus thoracis et lumborum** (see Figs. 2-76, 2-81, 2-82) arises from the crest and medial surface of the wing of the ilium and, by means of an aponeurosis, from the supraspinous ligament and the spines of the lumbar and thoracic vertebrae. Its

fibers course craniolaterally. Superficially, only a shallow furrow is seen to separate the longissimus and iliocostalis muscles in the lumbar region. This division of the longissimus inserts on various processes of the lumbar and thoracic vertebrae. The thoracic portion may be seen inserting on the ribs and the seventh cervical vertebra, just medial to the iliocostalis thoracis.

2. The **longissimus cervicis** (see Figs. 2-76, 2-81, 2-82), the cranial continuation of the longissimus muscle into the neck, consists of four fascicles arranged so that the caudal fascicles partially cover those that lie directly cranioventral to them. They lie in the angle between the cervical and thoracic vertebrae and insert on the transverse processes of the last few cervical vertebrae.

3. The **longissimus capitis** (see Figs. 2-81, 2-82) is a distinct muscle medial to the longissimus cervicis and splenius muscles. It extends from the first three thoracic vertebrae to the mastoid part of the temporal bone. It is firmly united with the splenius as it passes over the wing of the atlas to its insertion.

Transversospinalis System

The transversospinalis system, the most medial and deep epaxial muscle mass, consists of a number of different groups of muscles that join one vertebra with another or span one or more vertebrae. This complex system extends from the sacrum to the head. Included are muscles whose names depict their attachments or the functions of their fascicles: **spinalis, semispinalis, multifidus, rotatores, interspinalis,** and **intertransversarius**. These muscles must be reflected to perform a surgical laminectomy. Only a few of these muscles will be dissected in the neck.

The **splenius** (see Figs. 2-76, 2-81, 2-82) is a rather large muscle on the dorsolateral surface of the neck, deep to the rhomboideus capitis and the serratus dorsalis cranialis. Its fibers extend in a

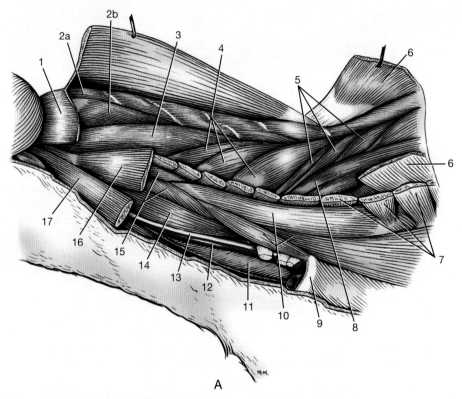

A

Fig. 2-82   A, Deep muscles of neck, left side.
1. Splenius
2. Semispinalis capitis:
   a. Biventer cervicis
   b. Complexus
3. Longissimus capitis
4. Longissimus cervicis
5. Longissimus thoracis
6. Serratus dorsalis cranialis
7. Serratus ventralis
8. Iliocostalis thoracis
9. First rib
10. Scalenus
11. Esophagus
12. Common carotid a.
13. Vagosympathetic trunk
14. Longus capitis
15. Intertransversarius
16. Omotransversarius
17. Mastoid part of cleidocephalicus

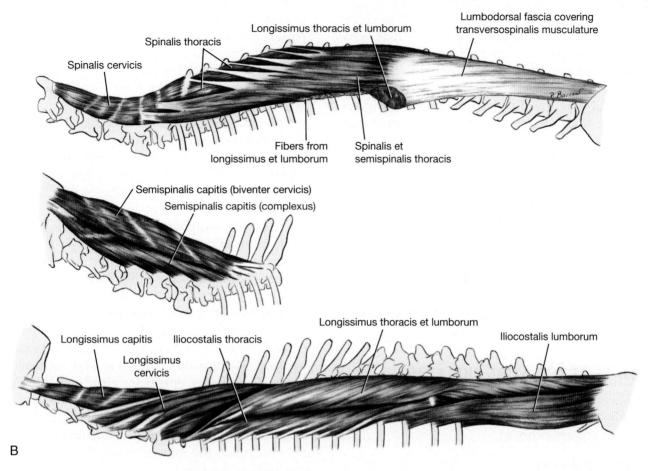

Spinalis cervicis

Spinalis thoracis

Longissimus thoracis et lumborum

Lumbodorsal fascia covering transversospinalis musculature

Fibers from longissimus et lumborum

Spinalis et semispinalis thoracis

Semispinalis capitis (biventer cervicis)
Semispinalis capitis (complexus)

Longissimus capitis   Iliocostalis thoracis

Longissimus cervicis

Longissimus thoracis et lumborum

Iliocostalis lumborum

B

Fig. 2-82, cont'd   B, Topography of the epaxial muscles.

slightly cranioventral direction from the third thoracic vertebra to the skull. The muscle arises from the cranial border of the thoracolumbar fascia, the spines of the first three thoracic vertebrae, and the entire median raphe of the neck. It inserts on the nuchal crest and mastoid part of the temporal bone. Transect the splenius 2 cm caudal to its insertion and reflect the muscle mass to the median plane.

The **semispinalis capitis** (see Fig. 2-82) is a member of the cervical portion of the transversospinalis group. It lies deep to the splenius and extends from the thoracic vertebrae to the head. It consists of two muscles, the dorsal **biventer cervicis** and the ventral **complexus**.

The **biventer cervicis** is dorsal to the complexus and has tendinous intersections. It arises from thoracic vertebrae and inserts on the caudal surface of the skull. Transect the muscle and reflect it.

The **complexus** is ventral to the biventer and arises from cervical vertebrae. It inserts on the nuchal crest. Transect this muscle and reflect it.

The **nuchal ligament** (see Fig. 2-84) may now be seen extending from the tip of the spinous process of the first thoracic vertebra to the broad caudal end of the spine of the axis. It is a laterally compressed, paired, yellow elastic band lying between the medial surfaces of the two semispinalis capitis muscles.

The **supraspinous ligament** continues the nuchal ligament caudally and extends from the spinous process of the first thoracic vertebra to the caudal vertebrae. It passes from one spinous process to another.

LIVE DOG

Palpate the cervical epaxial muscles and note the volume of these muscles dorsal to the cervical vertebrae. Continue caudally and feel the symmetry of the epaxial muscles on either side of the vertebral spines. In racing greyhounds these thoracolumbar epaxial muscles are extremely well developed. Palpate the abdominal wall and visualize the individual layers, the direction of their muscle fibers, and the extent of the aponeuroses of these muscles. Occasionally, the peritoneal cavity is opened by a surgical approach that separates the abdominal muscles in the plane of their fibers—the grid technique. Palpate the rectus abdominis and visualize the aponeuroses that sheath it and the direction of the rectus fibers. Feel the linea alba, where most abdominal incisions are made.

With the dog in lateral recumbency, abduct one pelvic limb. Follow the pectineus muscle proximally toward its origin from the prominent iliopubic eminence. Palpate the iliopubic cartilage just cranial to this eminence. The medial crus of the superficial inguinal ring extends cranially from this cartilage. This crus has a slightly firm feeling, and the spermatic cord in the male and external pudendal vessels in both sexes may be felt passing over this medial crus as the structures emerge from the inguinal canal.

JOINTS OF THE AXIAL SKELETON

Some of these joints will be seen now and others will be observed when the vertebral column and spinal cord are exposed.

Vertebral Joints

The **atlanto-occipital joint** (Fig. 2-83) is continuous with the **atlantoaxial joint** through the articulation of the dens with the body of the atlas. The dens is held against the fovea dentis by the **transverse ligament of the atlas**, which passes dorsal

to it and is attached to the body on both sides. **Apical** and **alar ligaments** pass from the cranial end of the dens to the basioccipital bone between the occipital condyles. The spine of the axis is joined to the arch of the atlas by a thick **dorsal atlantoaxial ligament** (Fig. 2-84).

The remaining vertebrae articulate by synovial joints between articular processes and by fibrous joints between the bodies. The latter are **intervertebral discs** (Figs. 2-85 through 2-86), which consist of outer circumferential collagenous fibers, the **anulus fibrosus**, and an inner gelatinous core, the **nucleus pulposus**. The anulus is usually thicker ventrally.

Narrow longitudinal ligaments, one within the vertebral canal and the other beneath the vertebrae, extend across all of the vertebral bodies. The **ventral longitudinal ligament** (see Fig. 2-85) is on the ventral surface of the vertebral bodies and extends from the sacrum to the axis. It is best developed in the caudal thoracic and lumbar regions. The thicker **dorsal longitudinal ligament** (see Fig. 2-86) is on the midline of the floor of the vertebral canal ventral to the spinal cord. It widens where it passes over and attaches to the anulus fibrosus of the intervertebral discs. It extends cranially to the axis.

Yellow ligaments extend between vertebral arches to cover the epidural interarcuate space between the articular processes. **Interspinous ligaments** (see Fig. 2-84) connect adjacent spines above the arches. The **supraspinous ligament** is a longitudinal band of fibrous connective tissue that connects the apices of all spinous processes from the level of the third caudal vertebra to the first thoracic vertebra. The cranial continuation of this ligament into the cervical region is called the **nuchal ligament** (see Fig. 2-84). The nuchal ligament is elastic and paired. In the dog it extends from the apex of the first thoracic spine to the spine of the axis.

Ribs

The head of each rib articulates in a synovial joint with the craniodorsal aspect of the vertebral body of the same number. For the first 10 ribs this articulation includes the caudodorsal portion of the next cranial vertebral body. These adjacent vertebral articular surfaces are **cranial** and **caudal costal foveae**. The tuberculum of each rib except the last few has a fibrous articulation with the transverse process.

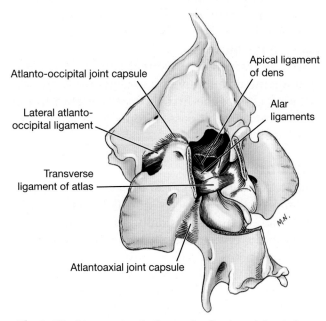

Atlanto-occipital joint capsule

Apical ligament of dens

Lateral atlanto-occipital ligament

Alar ligaments

Transverse ligament of atlas

Atlantoaxial joint capsule

Fig. 2-83   Ligaments of atlas and axis, dorsolateral view.

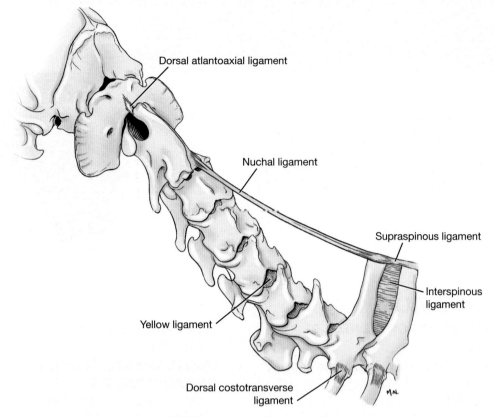

Fig. 2-84 Nuchal ligament.

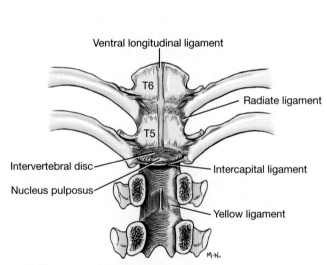

Fig. 2-85 Ligaments of vertebral column and ribs, ventral view.

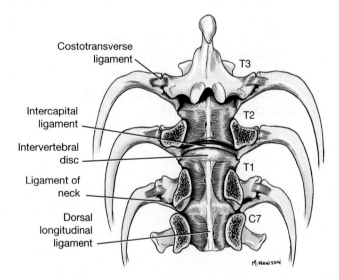

Fig. 2-86 Ligaments of vertebral column and ribs, dorsal view.

From the second through the tenth ribs, where the rib heads articulate between vertebral bodies, an **intercapital ligament** (see Figs. 2-85, 2-86) connecting right and left rib heads extends across the dorsal aspect of the anulus fibrosus ventral to the dorsal longitudinal ligament. This intercapital ligament holds the head of the rib in its joint and may provide additional containment for the intervertebral disc, which has a lower incidence of extrusion in this region.

The sternal part of each rib is cartilaginous. The second to seventh ribs join the sternum at modified synovial joints. Other ribs join the sternum as continuous fibrocartilages.

The Neck, Thorax, and Thoracic Limb

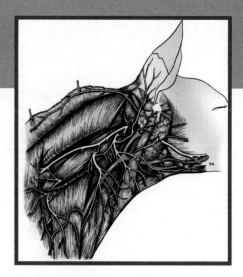

CHAPTER OUTLINE

Make a skin incision from the midventral line at the level of the right thoracic limb to the medial side of the right elbow joint. Make a circular skin incision at the elbow joint. Make transverse skin incisions from midventral to mid-dorsal lines at the level of the umbilicus and at the cranial part of the neck. Reflect the skin flap to the dorsal median plane, leaving the cutaneous muscles, superficial fascia, and veins on the dog (see Fig. 3-2). Leave the skin attached to the dorsal midline.

In the following dissection of vessels and nerves, the arteries can be recognized by the red latex that was injected into the arterial system. The veins sometimes contain dark clotted blood. Nerves are white and will stretch when bluntly dissected rather than tear as does fascia.

VESSELS AND NERVES OF THE NECK

There are eight pairs of cervical spinal nerves in the dog. The first cervical spinal nerve passes through the lateral vertebral foramen of the atlas. The remaining nerves pass through succeeding intervertebral foramina. The eighth cervical spinal nerve emerges from the intervertebral foramen between the seventh cervical and first thoracic vertebrae. Immediately on leaving the foramina, the nerves divide into large ventral and small dorsal branches. The dorsal branches supply structures dorsal to the vertebrae (see Fig. 3-6) and will not be dissected. When nerves are being dissected, it is helpful to separate the tissue bluntly by inserting a scissors and opening it to spread the tissue. Fascial strands of connective tissue will break, but nerves usually stretch.

Palpate the wing of the atlas and dissect the fascia near its caudoventral border to uncover the ventral branch of the **second cervical spinal nerve** (Figs. 3-1 and 3-2). This lies along or deep to the middle of the caudoventral border of the platysma, which is dorsal to the external jugular vein. Separate the overlying fascia until the nerve is found. It emerges between the mastoid part of the cleidocephalicus (cleidomastoideus) and the omotransversarius. The ventral branch of the second cervical spinal nerve divides into two cutaneous branches: (1) The **great auricular nerve** (see Figs. 3-2, 3-3, 5-41) extends toward the ear. It branches and supplies the skin of the neck, the ear, and the back of the head with sensory branches. Trace the nerve as far as present muscle and skin reflections will allow. (2) The **transverse cervical nerve** (see Figs. 3-2, 3-3) branches to the skin of the cranioventral part of the neck and need not be dissected.

The **external jugular vein** (see Figs. 3-2, 3-3), on the side of the neck, is formed by the **linguofacial** and **maxillary** veins (see Figs. 3-15, 5-41, 5-42). The ovoid body that lies in the fork formed by these veins is the **mandibular salivary gland** (see Fig. 3-2). The **mandibular lymph nodes** (see Figs. 2-12, 3-2) lie on both sides of the linguofacial vein, ventral to the mandibular salivary gland.

Ligate and transect the external jugular vein at its approximate middle and reflect each end. In some specimens the omobrachial and cephalic veins (see Figs. 3-3, 3-35) may be observed entering the external jugular vein after crossing the shoulder. These may be transected and reflected. Free the sternocephalicus and transect it 3 cm from its origin. Reflect it craniodorsally to a point cranial to the place where the second cervical nerve crosses the muscle. Transect the cleidocephalicus 1 cm cranial to the clavicular intersection. Reflect it toward its cervical and mastoid attachments.

The **superficial cervical lymph nodes** (see Fig. 3-26) lie in the areolar tissue cranial to the shoulder. They lie deep to the cervical part of the cleidocephalicus and the omotransversarius and receive lymph drainage from the cutaneous area of the head, neck, and thoracic limb.

The **accessory** or **eleventh cranial nerve** (see Figs. 3-1, 3-3, 5-54) is a large nerve found deep to the occipital part of the sternocephalicus and the cervical part of cleidocephalicus. As it emerges from the neck, it crosses the second cervical spinal nerve, runs along the dorsal border of the omotransversarius, and terminates in the thoracic part of the trapezius. Dissect between the trapezius and cleidocephalicus and identify this nerve coursing caudally to the trapezius. The accessory nerve is the only motor nerve to the trapezius. In addition, it supplies in part the omotransversarius, the mastoid and cervical portions of the cleidocephalicus, and the sternocephalicus.

Free the ventral border of the omotransversarius and lift it. Look for the ventral branches of the **third, fourth, and fifth cervical spinal nerves** (see Fig. 3-1), which are distributed in a segmental manner to the muscles and skin of the neck. The third and fourth nerves, after emerging from the intervertebral foramina, pass through the deep fascia and the omotransversarius. It may be difficult to identify each cervical nerve, and it is not necessary to do so.

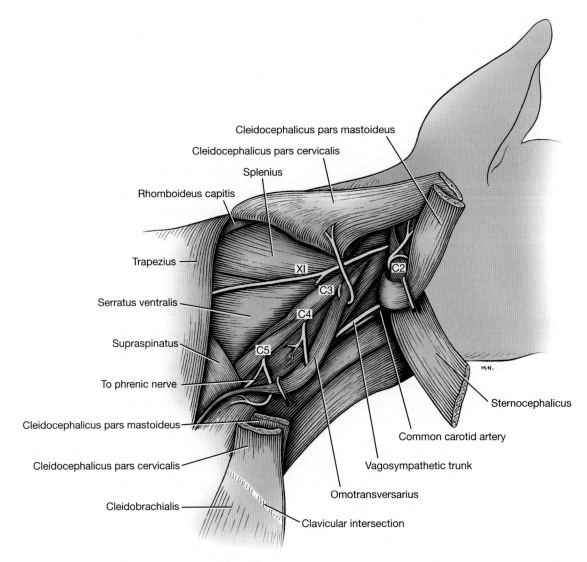

Fig. 3-1   Ventral branches of cervical spinal nerves emerging through the lateral musculature.

Transect the fused sternohyoideus and sterno-thyroideus 2 cm from their origin and reflect them to their insertions. Parts of the trachea, larynx, thyroid gland, esophagus, and carotid sheath are exposed. Identify these structures on your specimen. Note the common carotid artery dorsal to the sternothyroideus. Bound to its medial side is the **vagosympathetic nerve trunk**. The **medial retropharyngeal lymph node** (see Figs. 2-12, 5-44) lies opposite the larynx, ventrolateral to the carotid sheath.

THORAX
Superficial Vessels and Nerves of the Thoracic Wall

Before dissecting the thoracic nerves and vessels, study Figs. 3-4 through 3-7, which show the pattern of distribution of these structures. Notice that the artery and nerve of each intercostal space divide into dorsal and ventral branches. The dorsal branches enter the epaxial muscles. The ventral branches descend in the intercostal spaces along the caudal border of each rib. The dorsal and ventral arterial branches are derived from the **dorsal intercostal arteries** (see Figs. 3-4, *A*, 3-5). The first three dorsal intercostal arteries come from a branch of the costocervical trunk; the remaining nine come from the aorta. The dorsal intercostal arteries and veins have lateral cutaneous branches that perforate the intercostal and adjacent muscles to supply cutaneous structures, including the thoracic mammary glands. The dorsal intercostal artery and vein pass ventrally, where they anastomose with **ventral intercostal branches from the internal thoracic artery and vein**. At the ventral

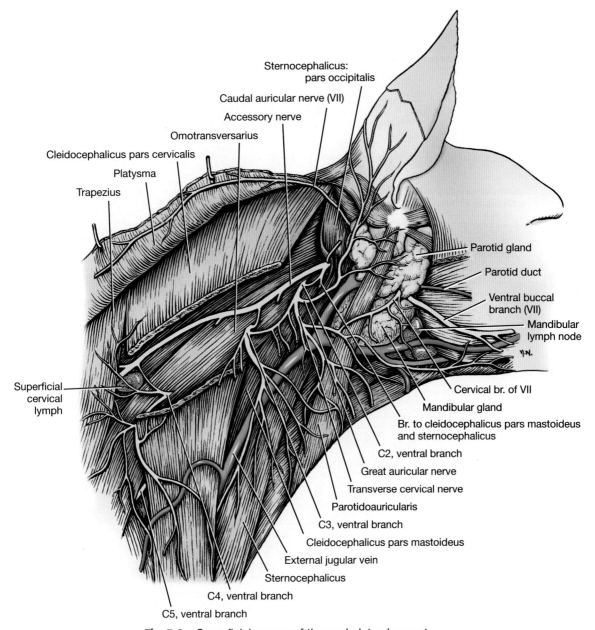

Sternocephalicus:
pars occipitalis

Caudal auricular nerve (VII)

Accessory nerve

Omotransversarius

Cleidocephalicus pars cervicalis

Platysma

Trapezius

Parotid gland

Parotid duct

Ventral buccal
branch (VII)

Mandibular
lymph node

Superficial
cervical
lymph

Cervical br. of VII

Mandibular gland

Br. to cleidocephalicus pars mastoideus
and sternocephalicus

C2, ventral branch

Great auricular nerve

Transverse cervical nerve

Parotidoauricularis

C3, ventral branch

Cleidocephalicus pars mastoideus

External jugular vein

Sternocephalicus

C4, ventral branch

C5, ventral branch

Fig. 3-2 Superficial nerves of the neck, lateral aspect.

aspect of each intercostal space, perforating branches of the internal thoracic vessels emerge and supply cutaneous structures and the thoracic mammary glands. The dorsal and ventral nerve branches are derived from the spinal nerve as it emerges from the intervertebral foramen (see Fig. 3-6). The ventral branches of the first 12 thoracic spinal nerves are **intercostal nerves** and have lateral and ventral cutaneous branches and branches medial to these that mostly innervate muscles.

Dorsal and lateral rows of lateral cutaneous branches of intercostal nerves, arteries, and veins

emerge at regular intervals between the ribs and supply the cutaneous muscle, subcutaneous tissue, and skin (see Fig. 3-6). The nerves of the dorsal row arise from the dorsal branches of the thoracic spinal nerves. A row of ventral cutaneous branches emerges through the origin of the deep pectoral muscle after having penetrated the ventral ends of the intercostal spaces. These vessels are perforating branches of the internal thoracic artery and vein. The nerves are terminal branches of the intercostal nerves. Although these emerge at regular intervals, not all will be seen in the dissection.

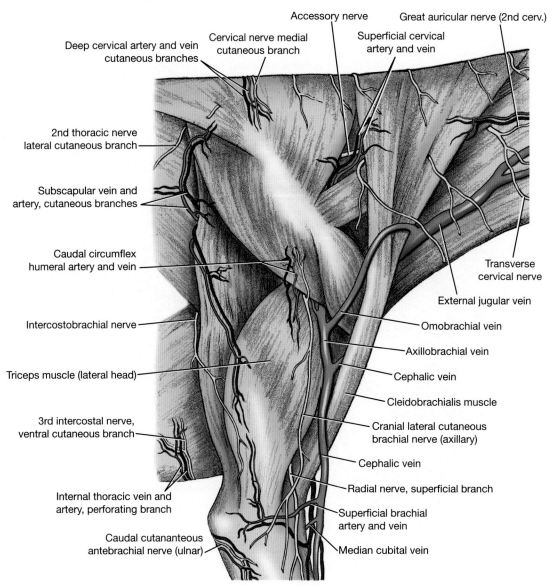

Accessory nerve   Great auricular nerve (2nd cerv.)

Deep cervical artery and vein
cutaneous branches

Cervical nerve medial
cutaneous branch

Superficial cervical
artery and vein

2nd thoracic nerve
lateral cutaneous branch

Subscapular vein and
artery, cutaneous branches

Caudal circumflex
humeral artery and vein

Transverse
cervical nerve

External jugular vein

Omobrachial vein

Intercostobrachial nerve

Axillobrachial vein

Cephalic vein

Triceps muscle (lateral head)

Cleidobrachialis muscle

Cranial lateral cutaneous
brachial nerve (axillary)

3rd intercostal nerve,
ventral cutaneous branch

Cephalic vein

Radial nerve, superficial branch

Internal thoracic vein and
artery, perforating branch

Superficial brachial
artery and vein

Caudal cutananteous
antebrachial nerve (ulnar)

Median cubital vein

Fig. 3-3   Superficial structures of scapula and brachium, lateral view.

The **cranial thoracic mamma** is supplied by the fourth, fifth, and sixth ventral and lateral cutaneous vessels and nerves and by branches of the lateral thoracic vessels. The latter are from the axillary vessels, which will be dissected later.

The **caudal thoracic mamma** is supplied in a similar manner from the sixth and seventh cutaneous nerves and vessels. In addition, mammary branches of the cranial superficial epigastric vessels supply this mamma.

The **axilla** is the space between the thoracic limb and the thoracic wall. It is bounded ventrally by the pectoral muscles and dorsally by the attachment of the serratus ventralis to the scapula. Cranially, it extends under the muscles that course from the arm to the neck. Caudally, a similar extension is found under the latissimus dorsi and cutaneous trunci.

The **lateral thoracic artery, vein,** and **nerve** emerge from the axilla between the latissimus dorsi and deep pectoral muscles. The nerve is motor to the cutaneous trunci and may be found on its ventral border. It consists of axons from the ventral branches of the eighth cervical and first thoracic spinal nerves. The vessels are branches of the axillary artery and vein that supply the muscle, skin, and subcutaneous tissues, including the cranial thoracic mamma. If these vessels and this nerve are not readily identified in your dissection, you may find them later when the axillary vessels and the brachial plexus are dissected.

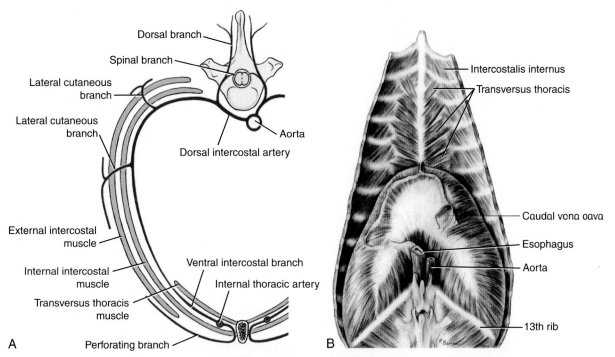

Fig. 3-4 A, Schematic transection of thoracic wall to show distribution of an intercostal artery. **B,** Diaphragm, thoracic surface. (Part **B** from Evans HE, de Lahunta A: *Miller's anatomy of the dog,* ed 4, St Louis, 2013, Saunders.)

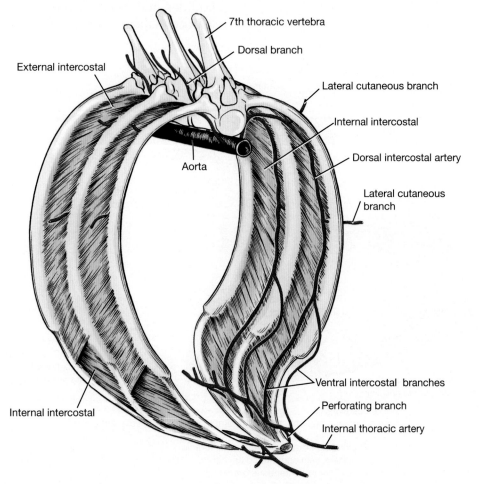

Fig. 3-5 Intercostal arteries as seen within rib cage.

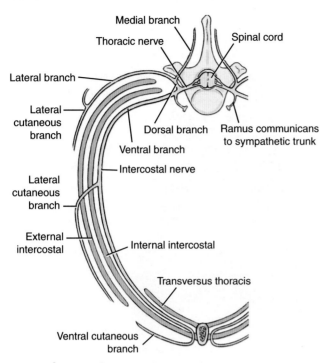

Fig. 3-6   Schema of a thoracic spinal nerve.

Transect the pectoral muscles close to the sternum. Reflect them toward the forelimb to expose the axilla.

The **axillary lymph node** lies dorsal to the deep pectoral muscle and caudal to the large axillary vein coming from the arm. Most of the afferent lymph vessels of the thoracic wall and deep structures of the limb drain into this node.

LIVE DOG

Palpate the structures in the neck ventral to the cervical vertebrae. The larynx and trachea are readily palpable. The esophagus is usually too soft to feel but should be on the left of the trachea in the middle and caudal cervical region. Try to palpate a pulse in the common carotid artery. It usually courses along the dorsolateral side of the trachea but is too deep to allow a pulse to be felt regularly. Cranially, feel the firm oval mandibular salivary gland and the smaller, looser mandibular lymph nodes. The latter can be felt subcutaneously at the angle of the mandible. Caudally in the neck, feel the superficial cervical lymph nodes cranial to the shoulder and deep to the omotransversarius or cleidocephalicus muscle. Extend the neck and

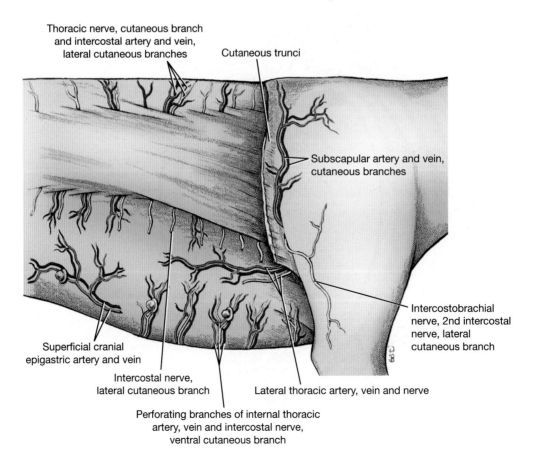

Fig. 3-7   Superficial vessels and nerves of thorax, right lateral view.

compress the vessels that enter the thorax at the thoracic inlet to try to distend the external jugular vein so that it is visible. This is more difficult to observe in long-haired breeds without removing the hair.

Deep Vessels and Nerves of the Thoracic Wall

Expose the lumbar and costal origins of the external abdominal oblique and detach them. Reflect the muscle ventrally to the rectus abdominis. Reflect the mammae if necessary. Free the aponeurotic thoracic attachment of the rectus abdominis close to the sternum and first costal cartilage. Reflect the rectus abdominis caudally, noting and cutting any nerves or vessels that enter the deep face of the muscle from any of the intercostal spaces.

The **cranial epigastric artery** is a terminal branch of the internal thoracic artery that emerges from the thorax in the angle between the costal arch and the sternum. It passes caudally on the deep surface of the rectus abdominis. The cranial epigastric artery gives rise to the **cranial superficial epigastric** (see Figs. 3-7, 4-2, 4-33), which perforates the muscle and runs caudally on its external surface. This artery supplies the skin over the rectus abdominis and the caudal thoracic and cranial abdominal mammae. The cranial epigastric vessels continue on the deep surface of the rectus abdominis. Most of their branches terminate in this muscle.

Make a sagittal incision completely through the thoracic wall, including the costal cartilages, 1 cm from the median plane on each side. These incisions should extend from the thoracic inlet through the ninth costal cartilage. The **transversus thoracis** muscle is a flat, fleshy muscle on the medial surface of the costal cartilages of ribs 2 through 8 (see Figs. 3-4, *A*, *B*, 3-6, 6-36). Its fascicles extend from the costochondral junctions to the sternum. Connect the caudal ends of the right and left sagittal incisions and free the sternum, except for the wide, thin fold of mediastinum that is now its only attachment.

On the right half of the thorax, clean and transect the origin of the latissimus dorsi and reflect it toward the forelimb. Locate and transect the caudal portion of the origin of the serratus ventralis, exposing the ribs. Starting at the costal arch and using bone cutters, *cut only the ribs,* close to their vertebral articulation *within the*

thorax, without damaging the sympathetic trunk. Reflect the thoracic wall *without removing it.* As this is done, cut the attachments of the internal abdominal oblique, transversus abdominis, and diaphragm from the ribs along the costal arch. If this is done carefully, the peritoneal cavity will not be opened. Reflect the left thoracic wall in a similar manner.

On the internal surface of the thoracic wall, notice the intercostal vessels and nerves coursing along the caudal border of the ribs. Ventrally, the vessels bifurcate and anastomose with the ventral intercostal branches of the internal thoracic artery and vein. The intercostal nerves supply the intercostal musculature. Their sensory branches were seen as lateral and ventral cutaneous branches.

The **pleurae** (Figs. 3-8, 3-9) are serous membranes that cover the lungs and line the walls of the thorax. These form right and left sacs that enclose the pleural cavities. Each consists of visceral and parietal parts, depending on their location.

The **pulmonary** or **visceral pleura** closely attaches to the surfaces of the lungs, following all their small irregularities as well as the fissures that separate the lobes.

The **parietal pleura** is attached to the thoracic wall by the endothoracic fascia. This pleura may be divided into costal, diaphragmatic, and mediastinal parts. Each of these is named after the region or surface it covers, and all are continuous, one with another. The **costal pleura** covers the inner surfaces of the ribs and their associated intercostal and transversus thoracis muscles. The **diaphragmatic pleura** covers the cranial surface of the diaphragm. The **mediastinal pleurae** are the layers that cover the sides of the partition between the two pleural cavities. The **mediastinum** includes the two mediastinal pleurae and the space between them. Enclosed in the mediastinum are the thymus, the lymph nodes, the heart, the aorta, the trachea, the esophagus, the vagus nerves, and other nerves and vessels. The **pericardial mediastinal pleura** is that portion covering the heart.

The **mediastinum** can be divided into a cranial part, that lying cranial to the heart; a middle part, that containing the heart; a dorsal portion dorsal to the heart; a ventral portion, ventral to the heart; and a caudal part, lying caudal to the heart. The caudal mediastinum is thin. It attaches to the diaphragm far to the left of the median

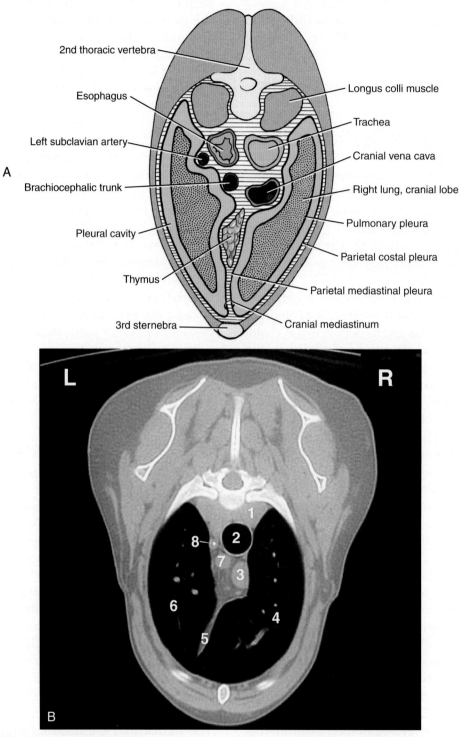

Fig. 3-8   A, Schematic transverse section of thorax through cranial mediastinum, caudal view. **B,** CT image, cranial thorax.

1. Longus colli muscle
2. Trachea
3. Cranial vena cava
4. Right cranial lobe
5. Cranial mediastinum
6. Cranial part of left cranial lobe
7. Brachiocephalic trunk
8. Left subclavian artery

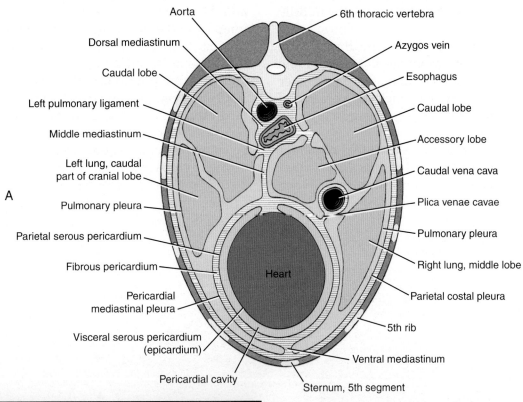

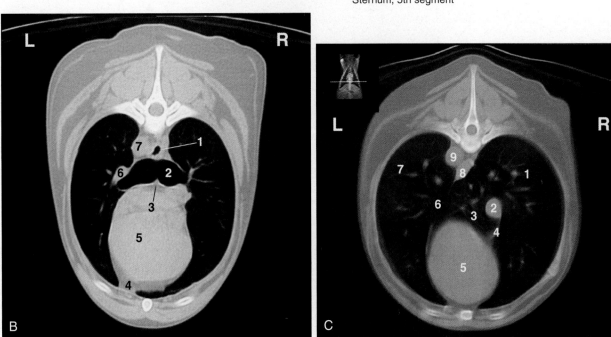

Fig. 3-9 A, Schematic transverse section of thorax through heart, caudal view. **B,** CT image, midthorax. **C,** CT image, caudal thorax.

1. Esophagus
2. Right principal bronchus
3. Carina of trachea
4. Ventral mediastinum-phrenicopericardial ligament
5. Heart
6. Left pulmonary artery
7. Aorta

1. Right caudal lobe
2. Caudal vena cava
3. Accessory lobe
4. Plica venae cavae
5. Heart
6. Caudal mediastinum
7. Left caudal lobe
8. Esophagus
9. Aorta

plane. Cranially, it is continuous with the middle mediastinum.

Note the passage of the esophagus through the mediastinum and the esophageal hiatus of the diaphragm. At the esophageal hiatus, a thin layer of pleura, peritoneum, and enclosed connective tissue attaches the esophagus to the muscle of the diaphragm.

The **plica venae cavae** is a loose fold of pleura derived from the right caudal mediastinal portion of the pleural sac that surrounds the caudal vena cava. The **root** of the lung is composed of pleura

and the bronchi, vessels, and nerves entering the lung. Here the mediastinal parietal pleura is continuous with the pulmonary pleura. Caudal to the hilus this connection forms a free border, known as the **pulmonary ligament** (see Figs. 3-9, 3-10), between the caudal lobe of the lung and the mediastinum at the level of the esophagus. Observe this ligament. In thoracic surgery this must be cut to reflect the caudal lung lobe cranially.

The **thymus** (see Figs. 3-8, 3-11, 3-12, 3-14, 3-16, 3-20) is a bilobed, compressed structure situated in the cranial mediastinum. It is largest in the

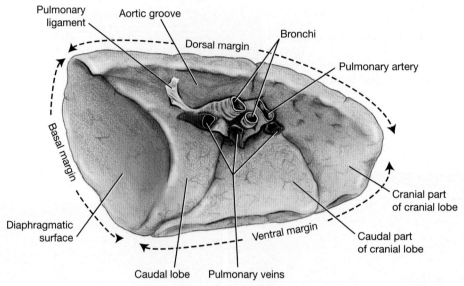

Fig. 3-10   Left lung, medial view.

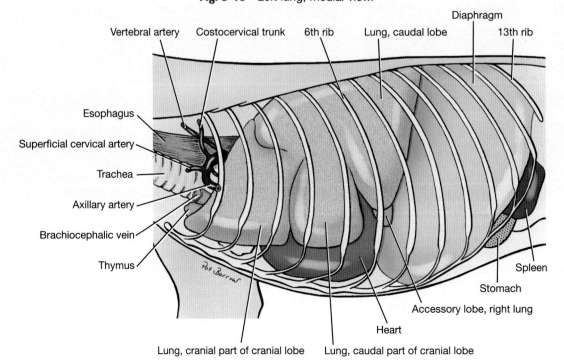

Fig. 3-11   Thoracic viscera, left lateral view.

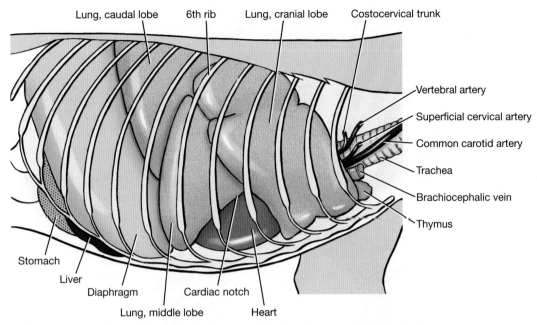

Fig. 3-12 Thoracic viscera within the rib cage, right lateral view.

young dog and usually atrophies with age until only a trace remains. When maximally developed, the caudal part of the thymus is molded on the cranial surface of the pericardium.

The **internal thoracic artery** (see Figs. 3-14, 3-16 through 3-20) leaves the subclavian artery, courses ventrocaudally in the cranial mediastinum, and disappears deep to the cranial border of the transversus thoracis muscle. It supplies many branches to surrounding structures—the phrenic nerve, the thymus, the mediastinal pleurae, and the dorsal intercostal spaces. The perforating branches to the superficial structures of the ventral third of the thorax have been seen. The anastomoses with the dorsal intercostal arteries on the medial side of the thoracic wall have been seen. Near the attachment of the costal arch with the sternum, the internal thoracic artery terminates in the musculophrenic artery and the larger cranial epigastric artery. The latter has been dissected along with its cranial superficial epigastric branch. The **musculophrenic artery** (see Fig. 4-33) runs caudodorsally in the angle formed by the diaphragm and lateral thoracic wall. Dissect its origin. Cut the mediastinum near the sternum and reflect the sternum cranially.

Lungs

Each lung is divided into lobes based on the branching pattern of its principal bronchus into lobar bronchi (Fig. 3-13). The **left lung** (see Figs. 3-10, 3-11) is divided into **cranial** and **caudal lobes** by deep fissures. The cranial lobe is further divided into cranial and caudal parts. The **right lung** (see Fig. 3-12) is divided into **cranial, middle, caudal**, and **accessory lobes**. A part of the accessory lobe can be seen from the left through the caudal mediastinum (see Fig. 3-20) or from the right through the plica venae cavae, where it lies in the space between these two structures. Reflect the caudal lung lobes to observe this.

Examine the **cardiac notch** (see Fig. 3-12) of the right lung at the fourth and fifth intercostal spaces. The apex of the notch is continuous with the fissure between cranial and middle lobes. A larger area of the ventral convexity of the heart is exposed on the right side. The right ventricle occupies this area of the heart and is accessible for cardiac puncture here.

Remove the lungs by transecting all structures that enter the hilus. On the right side, this will involve slipping the accessory lobe over the caudal vena cava. Make the transection far enough from the heart so that the vagal nerves crossing the heart are not severed but close enough so that the lobes are not removed individually.

Examine the structures that attach the lungs. The trachea bifurcates into left and right **principal bronchi**. The **carina** is the partition between them at their origin from the trachea (see Fig. 3-9, *B*). Each principal bronchus divides into **lobar bronchi** that supply the lobes of the lung. Find these on

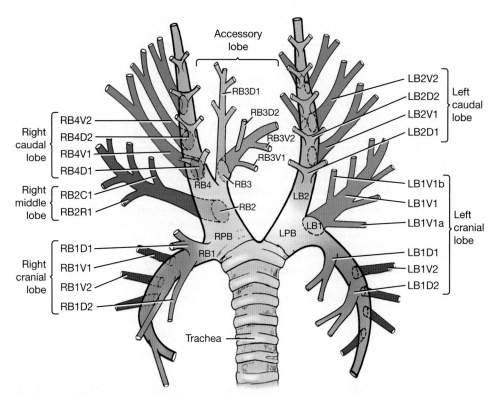

Fig. 3-13 Schematic bronchial tree of the dog, in dorsal view. Letters and numbers identify the principal, lobar, and segmental bronchi by their bronchoscopic order of origin and their anatomical orientation. Lower case *a* and *b* represent subsegmental bronchi. (From Amis TC, McKiernan BC: Systematic identification of endobronchial anatomy during bronchoscopy in the dog, *Am J Vet Res* 47:2649-2657, 1986.)

the lungs that were removed. They can be identified by the cartilage rings within their walls.

At the level of the carina, the right principal bronchus gives off the right cranial bronchus to the right cranial lobe of the lung, directly laterally. This is followed by the right middle bronchus that branches off ventrally. The principal bronchus terminates caudally as the accessory bronchus medially and right caudal bronchus laterally. On the left, the left principal bronchus gives off the left cranial bronchus laterally. This divides into cranial and caudal parts, and the left principal bronchus continues caudally as the left caudal bronchus. Within each lobe segmental bronchi branch off the lobar bronchus dorsally and ventrally except for the right middle lobe, where they are cranial and caudal (see Fig. 3-13).

Notice that there is usually a single pulmonary vein from each lobe that drains directly into the left atrium of the heart. (The pulmonary veins contain red latex because the specimen was prepared by injecting the latex into the common carotid artery. Moving in a retrograde direction, the latex in turn filled the aorta, left ventricle, left atrium, and pulmonary veins. Because latex does not cross capillary beds, there is usually no latex in the pulmonary arteries. Occasionally, the pressure of injection ruptures the interatrial or interventricular septum in the heart, flooding the right chambers with the latex and thus filling the pulmonary arteries as well as the veins.)

The pulmonary trunk supplies each lung with a pulmonary artery. At the root of the lung, the left pulmonary artery usually lies cranial to the left principal bronchus. The right pulmonary artery is ventral to the right principal bronchus. The artery and bronchus are at a more dorsal level than the veins. Using a scissors or scalpel, open a few of the major bronchi to observe the lumen.

Note the **tracheobronchial lymph nodes** (see Fig. 3-20) located at the bifurcation of the trachea and also farther out on the bronchi.

Determine which structures form the various grooves and impressions by replacing the lungs in the thorax. Observe the long **aortic impression** of the left lung. The most marked impressions on the right lung are on the accessory lobe. This lobe is interposed between the caudal vena cava on one side and the esophagus on the other, and both leave impressions on it. Observe the vascular impressions on the cranial lobes of the lungs and the costal impressions on each lung.

Veins Cranial to the Heart

Carefully expose the larger veins cranial to the heart. Reflect the sternum to one side to facilitate this exposure.

The **cranial vena cava** (see Figs. 3-14, 3-15, 3-17, 3-20, 3-22, 3-35) drains into the right atrium after its formation by the union of the right and left brachiocephalic veins at the thoracic inlet. The **brachiocephalic vein** is formed on each side by the **external jugular** and **subclavian veins**. Usually the last branch entering the cranial vena

cava is the **azygos vein** (Fig. 3-14, *A*). Only the right azygos vein develops in the dog. The azygos vein may enter the right atrium directly. It is seen from the right in the mediastinal space winding ventrocranially around the root of the right lung. It originates dorsally in the abdomen and collects all of the dorsal intercostal veins on each side as far cranially as the third or fourth intercostal space.

The **thoracic duct** (Fig. 3-14, *B*) is the chief channel for the return of lymph from lymphatic capillaries and ducts to the venous system. It begins in the sublumbar region between the crura of the diaphragm as a cranial continuation of the **cisterna chyli**. The latter is a dilated structure that receives the lymph drainage from abdominal and pelvic viscera and the pelvic limbs. The thoracic duct runs cranially on the right dorsal border of

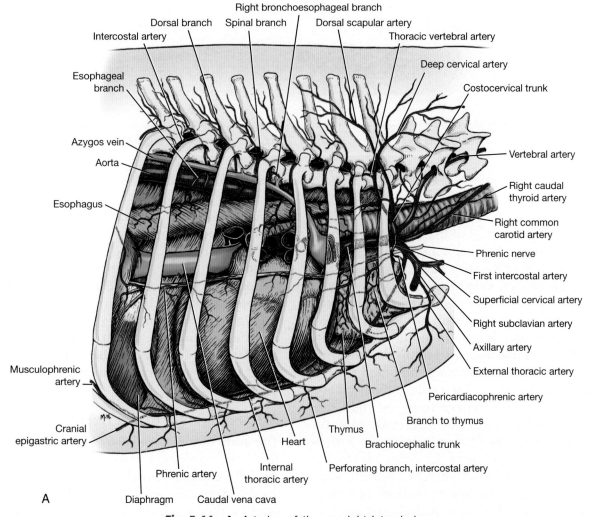

Fig. 3-14 A, Arteries of thorax, right lateral view.

Continued

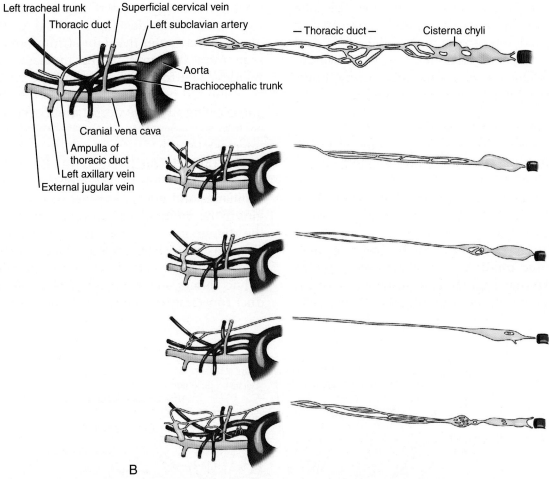

Fig. 3-14, cont'd   B, Variations of the thoracic duct and its entrance into the cranial vena cava. (Part **B** modified from Huber F: *Der ductus thoracicus,* Inaugural Dissertation, Dresden, 1909.)

the thoracic aorta and the ventral border of the azygos vein to the level of the sixth thoracic vertebra. (It may not be visible.) Here it crosses the ventral surface of the fifth thoracic vertebra and courses on the left side of the middle mediastinal pleura. It continues cranioventrally through the cranial mediastinum to the left brachiocephalic vein, where it usually terminates (see Fig. 3-17). The thoracic duct also receives the lymph drainage from the left thoracic limb and the **left tracheal trunk** (from the left side of the head and neck). The lymph drainage from the right thoracic limb and the **right tracheal trunk** (from the right side of the head and neck) form a right lymphatic duct that enters the venous system in the vicinity of the right brachiocephalic vein. There are often multiple terminations of a complicated nature, which may include swellings or anastomoses. All lymphatic channels will be difficult to see unless they are congested with lymph or refluxed blood. They are frequently double.

Look for the thoracic duct. It is not always visible, but it may be identified by the reddish brown or straw color of its contents and the numerous random constrictions in its wall. The tracheal trunks may be found in each carotid sheath or parallel to the sheath and its contents.

Arteries Cranial to the Heart

The **aorta** (see Figs. 3-5, 3-9, 3-15 through 3-20) is the large, unpaired vessel that emerges from the left ventricle medial to the pulmonary trunk. As the **ascending aorta,** it extends cranially, covered by the pericardium; it makes a sharp bend dorsally and to the left as the **aortic arch**; it runs caudally as the **descending aorta** located ventral to the vertebrae. The part cranial to the diaphragm is the thoracic aorta, and the caudal part is the abdominal aorta. Cranial to the heart are several branches of the aorta. Reflect the veins that were dissected cranial to the heart to observe these arteries.

The right and left **coronary arteries** are branches of the ascending aorta that supply the heart muscle. They will be studied with the heart.

The **brachiocephalic trunk** (see Figs. 3-14, 3-16 through 3-20), the first branch from the aortic arch, passes obliquely to the right across the ventral surface of the trachea. It gives rise to the **left common**

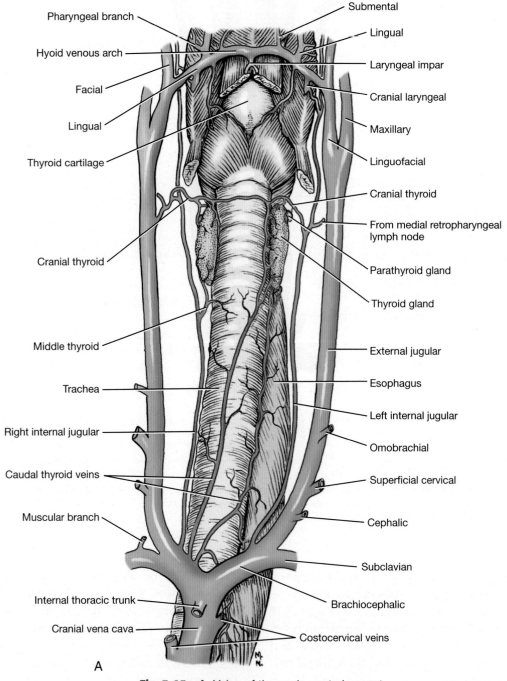

Labels, left: Pharyngeal branch, Hyoid venous arch, Facial, Lingual, Thyroid cartilage, Cranial thyroid, Middle thyroid, Trachea, Right internal jugular, Caudal thyroid veins, Muscular branch, Internal thoracic trunk, Cranial vena cava

Labels, right: Submental, Lingual, Laryngeal impar, Cranial laryngeal, Maxillary, Linguofacial, Cranial thyroid, From medial retropharyngeal lymph node, Parathyroid gland, Thyroid gland, External jugular, Esophagus, Left internal jugular, Omobrachial, Superficial cervical, Cephalic, Subclavian, Brachiocephalic, Costocervical veins

Fig. 3-15 A, Veins of the neck, ventral aspect.

Continued

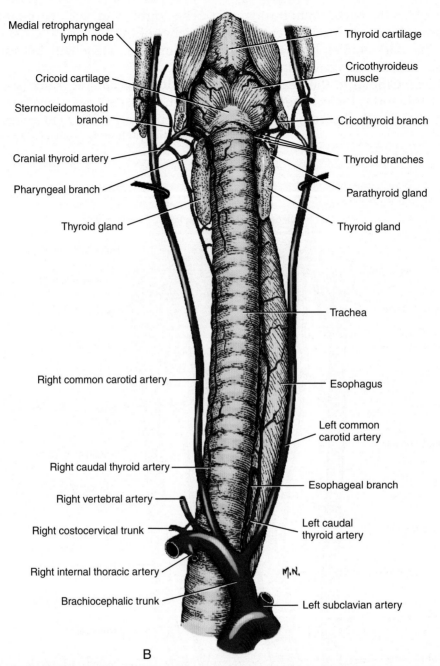

Medial retropharyngeal
lymph node

Cricoid cartilage

Sternocleidomastoid
branch

Cranial thyroid artery

Pharyngeal branch

Thyroid gland

Right common carotid artery

Right caudal thyroid artery

Right vertebral artery

Right costocervical trunk

Right internal thoracic artery

Brachiocephalic trunk

Thyroid cartilage

Cricothyroideus
muscle

Cricothyroid branch

Thyroid branches

Parathyroid gland

Thyroid gland

Trachea

Esophagus

Left common
carotid artery

Esophageal branch

Left caudal
thyroid artery

Left subclavian artery

M.N.

B

Fig. 3-15, cont'd   B, The relation of the common carotid arteries to the larynx, trachea, and related structures, ventral aspect. (Part **B** from Evans HE, de Lahunta A: *Miller's anatomy of the dog,* ed 4, St Louis, 2013, Saunders.)

carotid artery and terminates as the **right common carotid artery** and the **right subclavian artery**.

The **left subclavian artery** (see Figs. 3-16 through 3-20) originates from the aortic arch beyond the level of the brachiocephalic trunk and passes obliquely to the left across the ventral surface of the esophagus.

The branches of the right and left subclavian arteries are similar; only the right subclavian

artery will be described. For each artery described, there is a comparable vein with a similar area of distribution. The terminations of the veins are variable, and they will not be dissected. Remove them when necessary to expose the arteries. The right subclavian artery has four branches that arise medial to the first rib or intercostal space. They are the vertebral artery, the costocervical trunk, the superficial cervical artery, and

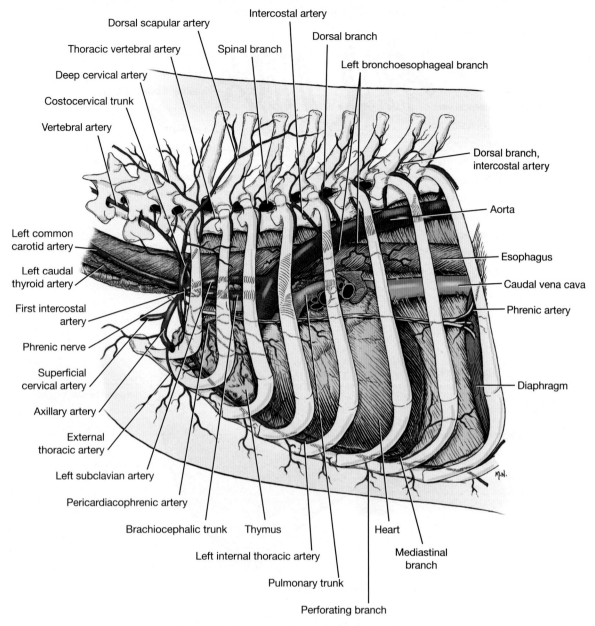

Fig. 3-16 Arteries of thorax, left lateral view.

the internal thoracic artery. Do not sever the nerves or arteries.

The **vertebral artery** (see Figs. 3-14, 3-16 through 3-20) crosses the medial surface of the first rib and disappears dorsally between the longus colli and the scalenus muscles. It enters the transverse foramen of the sixth cervical vertebra and passes through the transverse foramina of the first six cervical vertebrae. It supplies both muscular branches to the cervical muscles and also spinal branches at each intervertebral foramen to the spinal cord and its coverings. At the level of the atlas, it terminates by entering the vertebral canal through the lateral vertebral foramen and contributes to the ventral spinal and basilar arteries. These will be seen later in the dissection of the nervous system.

The **costocervical trunk** (see Figs. 3-14, 3-16 through 3-20) arises distal to the vertebral artery, crosses its lateral side, and extends dorsally as far as the vertebral end of the first rib. By its various branches it supplies the structures of the first, second, and third intercostal spaces; the muscles at the base of the neck; and the muscles dorsal to the first few thoracic vertebrae. These need not be dissected.

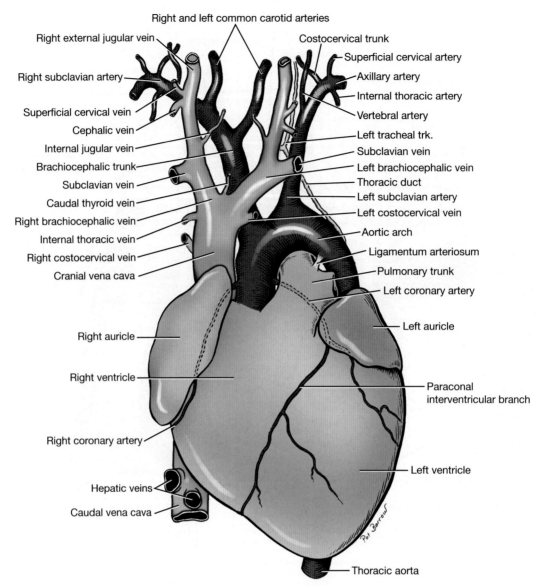

Right and left common carotid arteries

Right external jugular vein

Right subclavian artery

Superficial cervical vein

Cephalic vein

Internal jugular vein

Brachiocephalic trunk

Subclavian vein

Caudal thyroid vein

Right brachiocephalic vein

Internal thoracic vein

Right costocervical vein

Cranial vena cava

Right auricle

Right ventricle

Right coronary artery

Hepatic veins

Caudal vena cava

Costocervical trunk

Superficial cervical artery

Axillary artery

Internal thoracic artery

Vertebral artery

Left tracheal trk.

Subclavian vein

Left brachiocephalic vein

Thoracic duct

Left subclavian artery

Left costocervical vein

Aortic arch

Ligamentum arteriosum

Pulmonary trunk

Left coronary artery

Left auricle

Paraconal interventricular branch

Left ventricle

Thoracic aorta

Fig. 3-17   Heart and great vessels, ventral view.

The **superficial cervical artery** (see Figs. 3-14, 3-16 through 3-20, 3-26) arises from the subclavian opposite the origin of the **internal thoracic artery**, medial to the first rib (see Deep Vessels and Nerves of the Thoracic Wall). It emerges from the thoracic inlet to supply the base of the neck and the adjacent scapular region.

Branches of the Thoracic Aorta

The **esophageal** and **bronchial arteries** vary in number and origin. Usually the small **broncho-esophageal artery** (see Figs. 3-14, 3-16) leaves the right fifth intercostal artery close to its origin and crosses the left face of the esophagus, which it supplies. It terminates shortly afterward in the **bronchial arteries**, which supply the lung.

There are eight to nine pairs of **dorsal intercostal arteries** that leave the aorta (see Figs. 3-4, 3-5, 3-16, 3-19, 3-20). These start with either the fourth or the fifth intercostal artery and continue caudally, there being an artery in each of the remaining intercostal spaces. Each lies close to the caudal border of the rib. The costocervical trunk supplies the first three or four intercostal spaces (see Fig. 3-19). The dorsal costoabdominal artery courses ventrally, caudal to the last rib.

The **phrenic nerves** (see Figs. 3-14, 3-16, 3-20) supply the diaphragm. Find each nerve as it passes through the thoracic inlet. The nerve arises from the ventral branches of the fifth, the sixth, and usually the seventh cervical spinal nerves. Follow the phrenic nerves through the mediastinum to

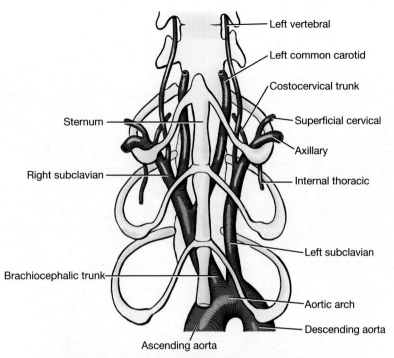

Fig. 3-18 Branches of aortic arch, ventral view.

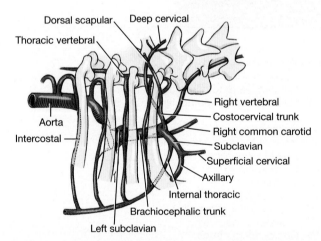

Fig. 3-19 Branches of brachiocephalic trunk, right lateral view.

the diaphragm. Each is both motor and sensory to the corresponding half of the diaphragm except at its periphery. This part of the muscle receives sensory fibers from the caudal intercostal nerves.

INTRODUCTION TO THE AUTONOMIC NERVOUS SYSTEM

The **nervous system** is highly organized both anatomically and functionally. It is composed of a **central nervous system** and a **peripheral**

nervous system. The central nervous system includes the **brain** and the **spinal cord**. The peripheral nervous system comprises the **cranial nerves,** which connect with structures of the head and body, and the **spinal nerves**, which connect the spinal cord to structures of the neck, trunk, tail, and limbs. The peripheral nervous system can be further classified on the basis of anatomy and function. The nerves in this system contain axons myelinated by Schwann cells that conduct impulses *to* the central nervous system—**sensory, afferent axons**—and axons that conduct impulses *from* the central nervous system to muscles and glands of the body—**motor, efferent axons**. Most nerves have both sensory and motor axons. When one speaks of a motor nerve, it is an indication of the primary function of the majority of the neurons, but it is understood that sensory neurons are also present. Likewise, so-called sensory nerves also contain the axons of motor neurons. This duality is the basis of feedback regulation. All the nerves you dissect are bundles of neuronal processes belonging to both sensory and motor neurons.

The **motor portion** of the peripheral nervous system is classified according to the type of tissue being innervated. Motor neurons supplying voluntary, striated, skeletal muscle are **somatic**

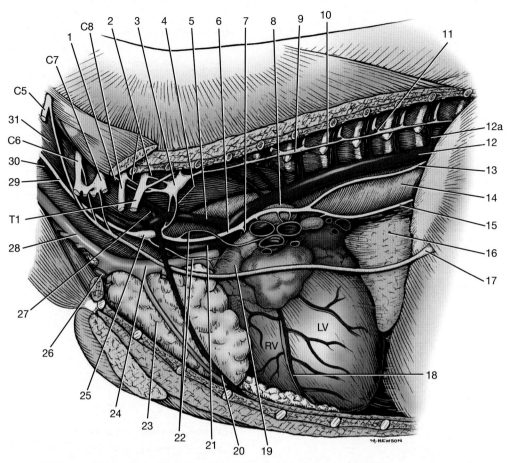

Fig. 3-20   Thoracic autonomic nerves, left lateral view, lung removed.

1. Vertebral artery and nerve
2. Communicating rami from cervico-thoracic ganglion to ventral branches of cervical and thoracic nerves
3. Left cervicothoracic ganglion
4. Ansa subclavia
5. Left subclavian artery
6. Left vagus nerve
7. Left recurrent laryngeal nerve
8. Left tracheobronchial lymph node
9. Sympathetic trunk ganglion
10. Sympathetic trunk
11. Ramus communicans
12. Aorta
12a. Dorsal intercostal artery
13. Dorsal branch of vagus nerve
14. Esophagus
15. Ventral trunk of vagus nerve
16. Accessory lobe of lung
17. Phrenic nerve to diaphragm
18. Paraconal interventricular a., v., and groove
19. Pulmonary trunk
20. Internal thoracic artery and vein
21. Brachiocephalic trunk
22. Cardiac autonomic nerves
23. Thymus
24. Cranial vena cava
25. Middle cervical ganglion
26. Left subclavian vein
27. Costocervical trunk
28. External jugular vein
29. Vagosympathetic trunk
30. Common carotid artery
31. Longus colli muscle

efferent neurons. *Somatic* refers to the body, body wall, or head, neck, trunk, and limbs where these striated skeletal muscles are located. Those supplying involuntary, smooth muscle of viscera, blood vessels, cardiac muscle, and glands are **visceral efferent neurons**.

A **neuron** is composed of a cell body and its processes. A somatic motor neuron of the peripheral nervous system has its cell body located in the gray matter of the spinal cord or brain stem, and its process, or axon, courses through the spinal or cranial nerve to end in the muscle innervated. Thus there is only one neuron spanning the distance from the central nervous system to the innervated structure.

The autonomic nervous system consists of components of the peripheral and central nervous systems. Its function is to control involuntary activity, to maintain homeostasis, and to respond to stress. The visceral efferent system is the peripheral motor part of this **autonomic nervous system**. It differs anatomically from the somatic efferent system in having a second motor neuron interposed between the central nervous system and the innervated structures. One neuron has its cell body located in the gray matter of the central nervous system. Its axon courses in the nerves only part of the way toward the structure to be innervated. Along the course of the nerve is a gross enlargement called a **ganglion**. By definition, a ganglion is a collection of neuronal cell bodies located outside the central nervous system. Some ganglia have a motor function, others a sensory function. Groups of neuronal cell bodies within the central nervous system are called **nuclei**. Autonomic ganglia contain the cell bodies of the second motor neurons in the pathway of the visceral efferent system. Their axons complete the pathway to the structure being innervated. Because of its relationship to the cell bodies in the autonomic ganglia, the first visceral efferent neuron with its cell body in the central nervous system is called the **preganglionic neuron**. The cell body of the second neuron is in an autonomic ganglion. Therefore this neuron is ganglionic and its axon is **postganglionic**.

A synapse occurs between these two neurons where the preganglionic axon meets the cell body of the postganglionic axon.

The visceral efferent system is divided into two subdivisions on the basis of anatomical, pharmacological, and functional characteristics. They are the sympathetic and parasympathetic divisions (Fig. 3-21). (It should be kept in mind that the autonomic nerves we observe also have visceral afferent or sensory axons within them.)

In the **sympathetic division** the preganglionic cell bodies are limited to the segments of the spinal cord from approximately the first thoracic to the fifth lumbar segments—the **thoracolumbar** portion (see Fig. 3-21). The cell bodies of postganglionic axons are located in ganglia that are usually only a short distance from the spinal cord. At most of the postganglionic nerve endings of this portion of the autonomic nervous system, a humoral transmitter substance, norepinephrine, is released, which causes a response in the structures innervated. The overall effect of this system is to help the body withstand unfavorable environmental conditions or conditions of stress.

In the **parasympathetic division** the preganglionic cell bodies are located in specific nuclei in the brain stem associated with cranial nerves III, VII, IX, and X and in the three sacral segments of the spinal cord—the **craniosacral** portion. The cell bodies of the postganglionic axons are often located in terminal ganglia on or in the wall of the structure being innervated. Others are found in specifically named ganglia near the innervated structure. At the postganglionic nerve endings, a humoral transmitter substance, acetylcholine, is released, which causes a response in the structures innervated. This system is associated with the normal homeostatic activity of the visceral body functions—the conservation and restoration of body resources and reserves.

The sensory afferent portion of the peripheral nervous system is also classified as somatic or visceral, depending on the structure innervated. Somatic afferent neurons innervate the cutaneous surface of the body, striated muscle, tendons, joints, and two specialized structures in the head: the eye and the inner ear. Visceral afferent neurons innervate the mucosal surface and wall of all tubular visceral organs, exocrine glands, and specialized vascular structures. *All* of these peripheral sensory neurons are single neurons between the structure innervated and the central nervous system. Their cell bodies are contained in spinal ganglia of all spinal nerves and in cranial nerve ganglia. In these ganglia there is no synapse because the synapse is in the central nervous system.

Each spinal cord segment is connected with its spinal nerve on each side via dorsal and ventral roots. The ventral roots contain the axons of the motor neurons, and the dorsal roots contain the axons of the sensory neurons. These roots leave the spinal cord and merge just distal to the spinal ganglion to form the segmental spinal nerve. Here the axons of the sensory and motor neurons intermingle and form the various peripheral branches of spinal nerves.

The anatomy of the sympathetic division of the visceral efferent system requires further description before it is dissected. The cell bodies of the preganglionic cell bodies are located in the gray matter of the thoracic and first five lumbar spinal cord segments. Their axons leave the spinal cord along with those of other motor neurons in the ventral rootlets of each of these spinal cord segments. Each **ventral root** unites with the

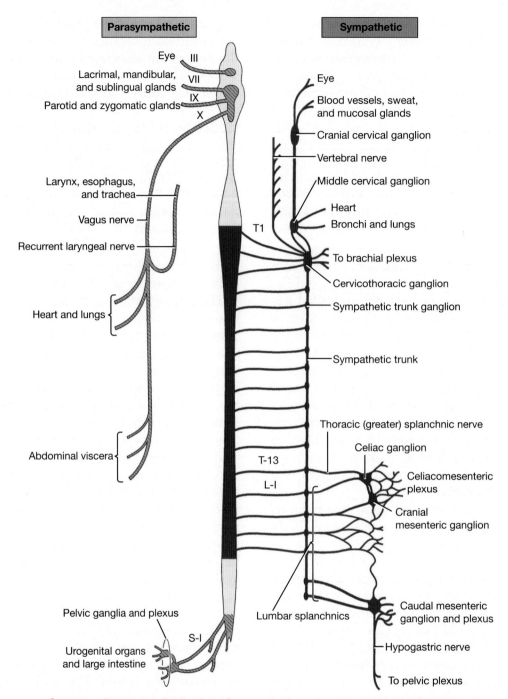

Parasympathetic   **Sympathetic**

Eye III

Lacrimal, mandibular, and sublingual glands VII

Parotid and zygomatic glands IX
X

Eye

Blood vessels, sweat, and mucosal glands

Cranial cervical ganglion

Vertebral nerve

Middle cervical ganglion

Larynx, esophagus, and trachea

Vagus nerve

Recurrent laryngeal nerve

Heart
Bronchi and lungs

To brachial plexus

Cervicothoracic ganglion

Sympathetic trunk ganglion

Sympathetic trunk

Heart and lungs

T1

Abdominal viscera

Thoracic (greater) splanchnic nerve

Celiac ganglion

Celiacomesenteric plexus

Cranial mesenteric ganglion

T-13

L-I

Pelvic ganglia and plexus

Lumbar splanchnics

Caudal mesenteric ganglion and plexus

Hypogastric nerve

S-I

Urogenital organs and large intestine

To pelvic plexus

Fig. 3-21   Peripheral distribution of sympathetic and parasympathetic divisions.

corresponding sensory **dorsal root** at the level of the intervertebral foramen to form the spinal nerve (see Figs. 6-20, 6-21). The dorsal branch of the **spinal nerve** branches off immediately. Just beyond this point, a nerve leaves the ventral branch of the spinal nerve, the **ramus communicans**. It courses a short distance ventrally to join the **sympathetic trunk**, which runs in a craniocaudal direction just lateral to the vertebral column (see Fig. 3-20). A ganglion is usually located

in the trunk at the point where each ramus joins it. This is the **sympathetic trunk ganglion** and contains the cell bodies of postganglionic sympathetic axons (see Figs. 3-20, 4-27).

Leaving the caudal thoracic and lumbar portions of the sympathetic trunk are nerves that course into the abdominal cavity, the **splanchnic nerves** (see Fig. 4-27). These form plexuses around the main blood vessels of the abdominal organs. Additional sympathetic ganglia are located in association with these plexuses and blood vessels. The cell bodies of sympathetic postganglionic axons are located here. These axons follow the terminal branching of the blood vessels of the abdominal organs to reach the organ innervated. These abdominal plexuses and ganglia are named according to the major artery with which they are associated. They will be dissected later.

Each preganglionic sympathetic axon must pass through the ramus communicans of its spinal nerve to reach the sympathetic trunk. Its fate from here is variable and mostly dependent on the structure to be innervated. A few examples will illustrate this.

Smooth muscle of blood vessels, piloerector muscles, and sweat glands are innervated by postganglionic sympathetic axons in spinal nerves. The preganglionic axon enters the sympathetic trunk through the ramus communicans. It may synapse in the ganglion where it entered, or it may pass up or down the sympathetic trunk a few segments and synapse in the ganglion of that segment. The postganglionic axons then return to the segmental spinal nerve via the ramus communicans, usually of the segment in which the synapse occurred. The postganglionic axon then courses with the distribution of the spinal nerve to the smooth muscle and sweat glands. Thus the rami communicantes of spinal cord segments T1 to L5 contain both preganglionic and postganglionic axons.

For the sympathetic innervation of smooth muscle and glands of the head, the preganglionic axons enter the sympathetic trunk in the cranial thoracic region. Some may synapse in ganglia as they enter the sympathetic trunk. Many others continue cranially as preganglionic axons in the sympathetic trunk in the neck. At the cranial end of this trunk, just ventral to the base of the skull, a ganglion is located—the **cranial cervical ganglion**. All remaining preganglionic axons to the head will synapse here. The postganglionic axons are then distributed with the blood vessels to the structures of the head innervated by this sympathetic system.

The sympathetic trunk is located along the full length of the vertebral column on both sides. Throughout the thoracic, lumbar, and sacral levels, it is joined to each segmental spinal nerve by a ramus communicans. Only those from spinal cord segments T1 to L5 contain preganglionic axons.

For smooth muscle and glands in the abdominal and pelvic cavities, the preganglionic sympathetic axon reaches the sympathetic trunk via the ramus communicans. It may synapse with a postganglionic neuron in a trunk ganglion, but more often it continues through the ganglion without synapsing and enters a splanchnic nerve. The preganglionic (or occasionally postganglionic) axon courses through the appropriate splanchnic nerve to the abdominal plexuses and their ganglia. Preganglionic axons synapse in one of these ganglia with a cell body of a postganglionic axon. The postganglionic axons follow the terminal branches of abdominal blood vessels to the organs innervated.

Dissection
Selected portions of the autonomic nervous system will be dissected as they are exposed in the regions being studied.

Examine the dorsal aspect of the interior of the pleural cavities (see Fig. 3-20). Notice the sympathetic trunks coursing longitudinally across the ventral surface of the necks of the ribs. The small enlargements in these trunks at each intercostal space are sympathetic trunk ganglia. Dissect a portion of the trunk and a few ganglia on either side. Notice the fine filaments that run dorsally between the vertebrae to join the spinal nerve of that space. These are the rami communicantes of the sympathetic trunk.

Follow the thoracic portion of the sympathetic trunk cranially. Notice the irregular enlargement of the trunk medial to the dorsal end of the first intercostal space on the lateral side of the longus colli. This is the **cervicothoracic ganglion**. It is formed by a collection of cell bodies from a fusion of the caudal cervical ganglion and the first two or three thoracic ganglia. Locate this ganglion on both sides.

Many branches leave the cervicothoracic ganglion. Rami communicantes connect to the ventral branches of the first and second thoracic spinal nerves and to the ventral branches of the seventh and eighth cervical spinal nerves. These spinal nerves contribute to the formation of the **brachial plexus**, which provides a pathway for postganglionic axons to reach the thoracic limb. A branch or plexus from the cervicothoracic ganglion follows the vertebral artery through the transverse foramina. This is the **vertebral nerve**. This is a source of postganglionic axons for the remaining cervical spinal nerves via branches at each intervertebral space from the vertebral nerve to each cervical spinal nerve. Postganglionic axons may leave the cervicothoracic ganglion and course directly to the heart.

Cranial to the cervicothoracic ganglion, the sympathetic trunk divides to form a loop, the **ansa subclavia,** around the subclavian artery. The two branches of the loop unite at the **middle cervical ganglion**. This ganglion lies at the junction of the ansa and the vagosympathetic trunk and appears as a swelling of the combined structures. Locate these structures on both sides. Numerous branches, **cardiac nerves**, leave the ansa and middle cervical ganglion and course to the heart.

The **vagosympathetic trunk** in the neck lies in the carotid sheath. Its sympathetic portion carries preganglionic and postganglionic sympathetic axons cranially to structures in the head. The **cranial cervical ganglion** is located at its most cranial end. This is at the level of the base of the ear, just caudomedial to the tympanic bulla. It will be dissected later. The tenth cranial or **vagus nerve** contains parasympathetic preganglionic axons that course caudally down the neck to thoracic and abdominal organs.

At the level of the middle cervical ganglion, notice the vagus nerve as it leaves the vagosympathetic trunk to continue its course caudally. Cardiac nerves leave the vagus to innervate the heart. Study the caudal course of the vagus nerve on each side.

On the left side, at the level of the aortic arch, the **left recurrent laryngeal nerve** leaves the vagus, curves medially around the ligamentum arteriosum and the arch of the aorta, and becomes related to the ventrolateral aspect of the trachea and the ventromedial edge of the esophagus. In this position it courses cranially in the neck to reach the larynx. In this course it reaches the dorsolateral aspect of the trachea. On the right side, at the middle cervical ganglion, or slightly caudal to it, the **right recurrent laryngeal nerve** leaves the vagus, curves dorsocranially around the right subclavian artery, reaches the dorsolateral surface of the trachea, and courses cranially to the larynx. It may be found in the angle between the trachea and the longus colli. Each recurrent nerve sends branches to the heart, trachea, and esophagus before terminating in the laryngeal muscles as the **caudal laryngeal nerve**. The laryngeal nerves will be dissected later.

Follow each **vagus nerve** as it courses over the base of the heart (see Fig. 3-20) and supplies cardiac nerves to it. Branches are supplied to the bronchi as the vagus passes over the roots of the lungs. Between the azygos vein and the right bronchus on the right and the area just caudal to the base of the heart on the left, each vagus divides into dorsal and ventral branches. The right and left ventral branches soon unite with each other to form the **ventral vagal trunk** on the esophagus. The dorsal branches of each vagus do not unite until farther caudally near the diaphragm, where they form the **dorsal vagal trunk**, which lies dorsal to the esophagus. The termination of these trunks in the abdomen will be studied later.

HEART AND PERICARDIUM

The **pericardium** (see Fig. 3-9) is the fibroserous covering of the heart. It is a thin but strong layer consisting of three inseparable components: an inner **parietal serous pericardium**, a middle **fibrous pericardium**, and an outer **pericardial mediastinal pleura**. The heart and pericardium are located in the middle part of the mediastinum from the level of the third to the sixth rib. The continuation of the fibrous pericardium to the sternum and diaphragm forms the **phrenicopericardial ligament**. This is located in the ventral mediastinum along with a variable amount of fat. The **serous pericardium** is a closed sac that envelops most of the heart. The **parietal layer** adheres to the fibrous pericardium. At the base of the heart it is continuous with the **visceral layer,** or **epicardium,** which tightly adheres to the heart. Between the parietal and visceral serous pericardium is the **pericardial cavity**, which contains a small amount of pericardial fluid. Incise the combined pericardial mediastinal pleura, fibrous pericardium, and parietal serous pericardium to expose the heart.

The **heart** (Figs. 3-22 through 3-24) consists of a dorsal base, where the great vessels are attached, and an apex that faces ventrally, caudally, and usually to the left, depending on the shape of the thorax. The surface of the heart facing the left thoracic wall is called the **auricular surface** because the tips of the two auricles project on this side. The auricles are small appendages of each atrium. The opposite surface facing the right thoracic wall is the **atrial surface.** The thin-walled

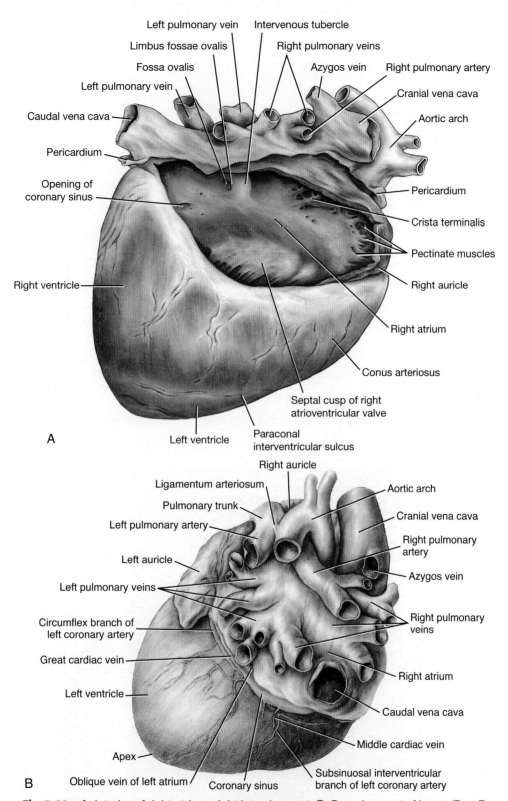

Fig. 3-22 **A,** Interior of right atrium, right lateral aspect. **B,** Dorsal aspect of heart. (Part **B** from Evans HE, de Lahunta A: *Miller's anatomy of the dog,* ed 4, St Louis, 2013, Saunders.)

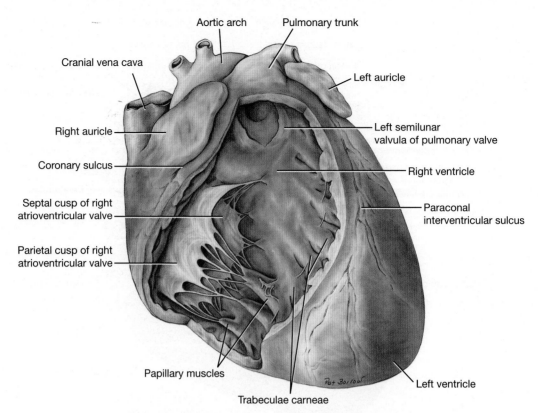

Fig. 3-23   Interior of right ventricle, left lateral aspect.

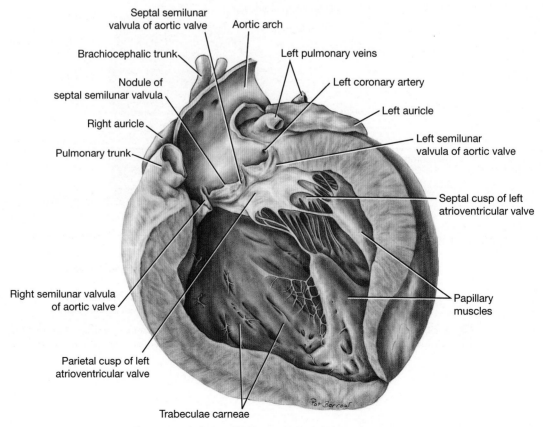

Fig. 3-24   Interior of left ventricle, left lateral aspect.

right ventricle winds across the cranial surface from the **atrial surface** of the heart.

Trace the **coronary sulcus** around the heart. It lies between the atria and ventricles and contains the coronary vessels and fat. The **interventricular sulci** are the superficial separations of the right and left ventricles. They represent the approximate position of the oblique interventricular septum. Obliquely traversing the auricular surface of the heart is the **paraconal interventricular sulcus.** It begins at the base of the pulmonary trunk, where it is covered by the left auricle. It is adjacent to the conus arteriosus (paraconal), which is the outflow tract of the right ventricle. This sulcus contains the paraconal interventricular branch of the left coronary artery. The shorter and less distinct **subsinuosal interventricular sulcus** lies on the caudal aspect of the atrial surface ventral to the level of the coronary sinus (subsinuosal) that enters the right atrium. This sulcus contains the terminal branch of the left coronary artery.

The **right atrium** (see Fig. 3-22) receives the blood from the systemic veins and most of the blood from the heart itself. It lies dorsocranial to the right ventricle. It is divided into a main part, the **sinus venarum**, and a blind cranial part, the **right auricle**.

Open the right atrium by a longitudinal incision through its lateral wall from the cranial vena cava to the caudal vena cava. Extend a cut from the middle of the first incision to the tip of the auricle.

There are four openings into the sinus venarum of the right atrium. The **caudal vena cava** enters the atrium caudally. Ventral to this opening is the **coronary sinus**, the enlarged venous return for most of the blood from the heart. The subsinuosal interventricular groove is ventral to this sinus on the atrial surface of the heart. The **cranial vena cava** enters the atrium dorsally and cranially. Ventral and cranial to the coronary sinus is the large opening from the right atrium to the right ventricle, the **right atrioventricular orifice**. The valve will be described with the right ventricle.

Examine the dorsomedial wall of the sinus venarum, the **interatrial septum**. Between the two caval openings is a transverse ridge of tissue, the **intervenous tubercle**. It diverts the inflowing blood from the two caval veins toward the right atrioventricular orifice. Caudal to the intervenous tubercle is a slitlike depression, the **fossa ovalis**. In the fetus there is an opening at the site of the fossa, the foramen ovale, which allows blood to pass from the right to the left atrium.

The **right auricle** is the blind, ear-shaped pouch of the right atrium that faces cranially and to the left. The internal surface of the wall of the right auricle is strengthened by interlacing muscular bands, the **pectinate muscles** (see Fig. 3-22). These are also found on the lateral wall of the atrium proper. The internal surface of the heart is lined everywhere with a thin, glistening membrane, the **endocardium,** which is continued in the blood vessels as the endothelium-lined tunica intima. The **crista terminalis** is the smooth-surfaced, thick portion of heart muscle shaped like a semilunar crest at the entrance into the auricle. Pectinate muscle bands radiate from this crest into the auricle.

Locate the **pulmonary trunk** leaving the right ventricle at the left craniodorsal angle of the heart. Begin at the cut end of the left pulmonary artery and extend an incision through the wall of this artery, the pulmonary trunk, and the wall of the right ventricle along the paraconal interventricular groove. Continue this cut around the right ventricle following the interventricular septum to the origin of the subsinuosal interventricular groove. Cut through the caudal angle of the right atrioventricular valve and continue the cut through the caudal vena cava. Reflect the ventricular wall.

The greater part of the base of the right ventricle communicates with the right atrium through the atrioventricular orifice. This opening contains the right **atrioventricular valve** (see Figs. 3-23, 3-25).

There are two main parts to the valve in the dog: a wide but short flap that arises from the parietal margin of the orifice, the **parietal cusp**, and a flap from the septal margin, the **septal cusp**, which is nearly as wide as it is long. Subsidiary leaflets are found at each end of the septal flap. The points of the flaps of the valve are continued to the septal wall of the ventricle by the chordae tendineae. The **chordae tendineae** are attached to the septal wall by means of conical muscular projections, the **papillary muscles**, of which there are usually three to four. The **trabeculae carneae** are the muscular irregularities of the interior of the ventricular walls. The **trabecula septomarginalis** is a muscular strand that extends across the lumen of the ventricle from the septal to the parietal wall. The septal attachment is often to a papillary muscle. The right ventricle passes across the cranial surface of the heart and terminates as the funnel-shaped **conus**

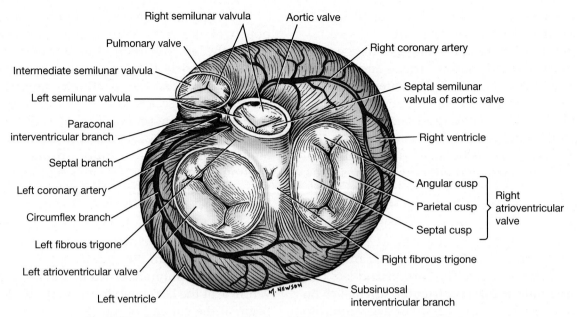

Fig. 3-25 Atrioventricular, aortic, and pulmonary valves, dorsoventral view.

arteriosus, which gives rise to the pulmonary trunk. This is at the left craniodorsal aspect of the heart. The paraconal interventricular groove is adjacent to the caudal border of the conus arteriosus on the auricular surface of the heart.

At the junction between the right ventricle and the pulmonary trunk is the **pulmonary valve**, which consists of three **semilunar cusps** (Figs. 3-23, 3-25). A small fibrous **nodule** is located at the middle of the free edge of each cusp. The pulmonary trunk bifurcates into right and left pulmonary arteries, each going to its respective lung.

Open the left side of the heart with one longitudinal cut through the lateral wall of the left atrium, left atrioventricular valve, and left ventricle midway between the subsinuosal and paraconal interventricular grooves. Extend the incision into the left auricle.

The **left atrium** is situated on the left dorsocaudal part of the base of the heart dorsal to the left ventricle. Five or six openings mark the entrance of the pulmonary veins into the atrium. The inner surface of the atrium is smooth except for pectinate muscles confined to the **left auricle**. A thin concave fold of tissue is present on the cranial part of the interatrial septal wall. This is the **valve of the foramen ovale**, a remnant of the passageway for blood from the right atrium to the left atrium in the fetus.

Notice the thickness of the left ventricular wall as compared with the right. The **left atrioventricular valve** (see Figs. 3-24, 3-25) is composed of two major

cusps, the **septal** and **parietal**, but the division is indistinct. Secondary cusps are present at the ends of the two major ones. Notice the two large papillary muscles and their chordae tendineae attached to the cusps. The trabeculae carneae are not as numerous in the left ventricle as in the right.

Remove the fat, pleura, and pericardium from the aorta. In doing this, isolate the **ligamentum arteriosum**, a fibrous connection between the pulmonary trunk and the aorta just caudal to the left subclavian artery (see Fig. 3-17). In the fetus it was the patent ductus arteriosus and served to shunt the blood destined for the nonfunctional lungs to the aorta. Observe the left recurrent laryngeal nerve as it turns around the caudal surface of the ligamentum arteriosum (see Fig. 3-20). Isolate the origins of the pulmonary trunk and aorta.

From the left ventricle, insert scissors into the aortic valve, located beneath the septal cusp of the left atrioventricular valve, and cut the septal cusp, aortic valve, aortic wall, and left atrium. This exposes the aortic valve and the first centimeter of the ascending aorta. The **aortic valve**, like the pulmonary valve, consists of three semilunar cusps (see Figs. 3-24, 3-25). Notice the nodules of the semilunar cusps in the middle of their free borders. Behind each cusp, the aorta is slightly expanded to form the **sinus of the aorta**.

The **right coronary artery** (see Figs. 3-17, 3-25) leaves the right sinus of the aorta. It encircles the right side of the heart in the coronary groove and often extends to the subsinuosal interventricular groove. It sends many small and one or two large descending branches over the surface of the right ventricle. Remove the epicardium and fat from its surface and follow the artery to its termination.

The **left coronary artery** (see Figs. 3-17, 3-25) is about twice as large as the right. It is a short trunk that leaves the left sinus and immediately terminates in (1) a **circumflex branch,** which extends caudally in the left part of the coronary sulcus and supplies the subsinuosal interventricular branch, and (2) a **paraconal interventricular branch**, which obliquely crosses the auricular surface of the heart in the paraconal interventricular sulcus. Both of these branches send large rami over the surface of the left ventricle. Expose the artery and its large branches by removing the epicardium and fat. A **septal branch** courses into the interventricular septum, which it supplies.

The **coronary sinus** is the dilated terminal end of the great cardiac vein. The **great cardiac vein,** which begins in the paraconal interventricular sulcus, returns blood supplied to the heart by the left coronary artery. Clean the surface of the great cardiac vein and open the coronary sinus. Usually one or two poorly developed valves are present in the coronary sinus.

LIVE DOG

Observe the thorax and watch it expand and contract with each inspiration and expiration, respectively. Place the middle finger of one hand over the dorsal aspect of the ninth or tenth intercostal space. Tap the distal end of this finger just behind the nail with the middle finger of the other hand. Listen for the sound produced by this method of percussion. Compare this with an area over the epaxial muscles or abdomen. A resonating sound will result where normal air-filled lung is beneath the region percussed. This method of physical examination can be used to define the extent of normal lung tissue in the thorax.

Place your hands over the ventral thorax and feel the heartbeat. It should be more evident on the left, where the apex of the heart is directed.

It is important to know the relationship of the cardiac chambers and valve areas for auscultation. A simple hand rule may be helpful. Make a fist with your left hand and extend your thumb at the proximal interphalangeal joint. Your fist represents the left ventricle, and your thumb is the aorta arising from it. The metacarpophalangeal joint of your thumb is at

the position of the left atrioventricular valve. Hold your right hand with the fingers extended. Place the palm of your right hand against the closed fingers of your left fist. Wrap the fingers of your right hand around the front of your left fist and curve the second digit of your right hand around your left thumb. Your right hand is in the position of the right ventricle (right and cranial sides of the heart). Your right second digit represents the pulmonary valve and trunk on the left craniodorsal aspect of the heart to the left of the aortic valve. Your right thumb is in the position of the right atrioventricular valve. The paraconal interventricular groove is between the ends of your right fingers and the metacarpophalangeal joints of your left fist. The subsinuosal interventricular groove is between the base of the palms of your two hands.

VESSELS AND NERVES OF THE THORACIC LIMB
Primary Vessels of the Thoracic Limb

Subclavian
 Vertebral
 Costocervical trunk
 Internal thoracic
 Superficial cervical
Axillary
 Deltoid branch
 External thoracic
 Lateral thoracic
 Subscapular
 Caudal circumflex humeral
 Thoracodorsal
 Circumflex scapula
 Cranial circumflex humeral
Brachial
 Deep brachial
 Bicipital
 Collateral ulnar
 Superficial brachial
 Transverse cubital
Common interosseous
 Ulnar
 Cranial interosseous
 Caudal interosseous
 Deep antebrachial (author's experience)
Median
 Radial
 Deep palmar arch
 Superficial palmar arch

The main arterial blood supply to the thoracic limb arises within the thorax as the subclavian artery, which is a terminal branch of the brachio-cephalic on the right side and a direct branch of the aorta on the left side. The preceding list of arteries shows the various components of this arterial supply. The subclavian artery has four branches: vertebral, superficial cervical, costo-cervical trunk, and internal thoracic. The **superficial cervical artery** (see Figs. 3-11, 3-12, 3-14, 3-16 through 3-19, 3-26) arises from the subclavian just inside the thoracic inlet. It runs dorso-cranially between the scapula and the neck. It supplies the superficial muscles of the base of the neck, the superficial cervical lymph nodes, the muscles of the scapula, and the shoulder.

There are usually two **superficial cervical lymph nodes** (see Fig. 3-26), which lie on the serratus ventralis and scalenus cranial to the supraspinatus, covered by the omotransversarius and the cleidocephalicus. These nodes receive the afferent lymph vessels from the superficial part of the lateral surface of the neck, the caudal surface of the head including the ear and pharynx, and the thoracic limb.

Brachial Plexus

The brachial plexus (see Figs. 3-20, 3-27) is formed by the ventral branches of the sixth, seventh, and eighth cervical and the first and second thoracic spinal nerves. In some dogs there is a small contribution from the ventral branch of the fifth cervical spinal nerve. These branches arise from their spinal nerve just lateral to their respective intervertebral foramen. They emerge along the ventral border of the scalenus and extend across the axillary space to the thoracic limb. In the axilla numerous branches of these nerves communicate to form the brachial plexus. From the plexus arise nerves of mixed origin that supply the structures of the thoracic limb and adjacent muscles and skin (see Fig. 3-27).

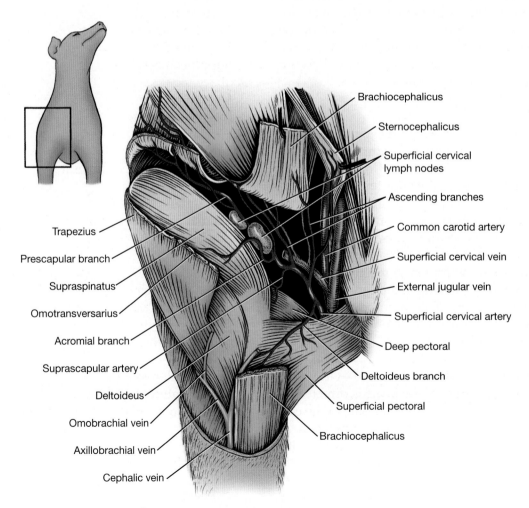

Fig. 3-26 Branches of superficial cervical artery.

The pattern of interchange in the brachial plexus is variable, but the specific spinal nerve composition of the named nerves that continue into the thoracic limb is consistent. These nerves include the suprascapular, subscapular, axillary, musculocutaneous, radial, median, ulnar, thoracodorsal, lateral thoracic, and pectoral nerves. Expose the brachial plexus in the axilla. It will be studied later.

Reflect the superficial and deep pectoral muscles toward their insertions to expose the vessels and nerves on the medial aspect of the arm.

Axillary Artery

The axillary artery (Figs. 3-17, *C*, 3-28, 3-29) is the continuation of the subclavian and extends from the first rib to the conjoined tendons of the teres major and latissimus dorsi. It has four primary branches: the external thoracic, the lateral thoracic, the subscapular, and the cranial circumflex humeral.

In the following dissection some variability may be encountered in the origin of specific blood vessels and nerves. However, although the origin

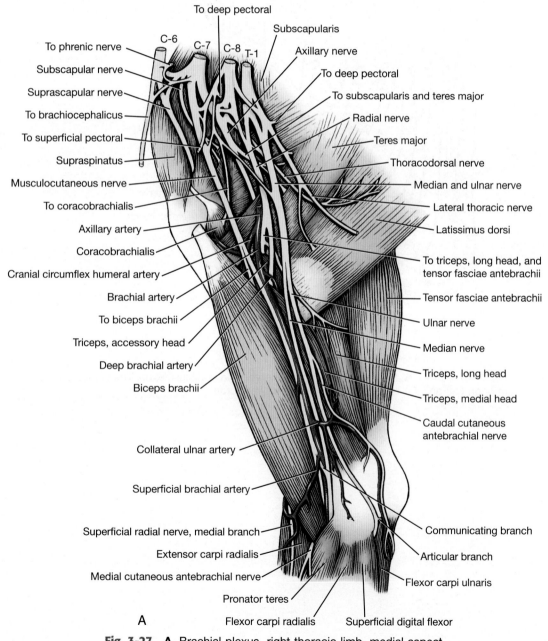

Fig. 3-27 A, Brachial plexus, right thoracic limb, medial aspect.

Continued

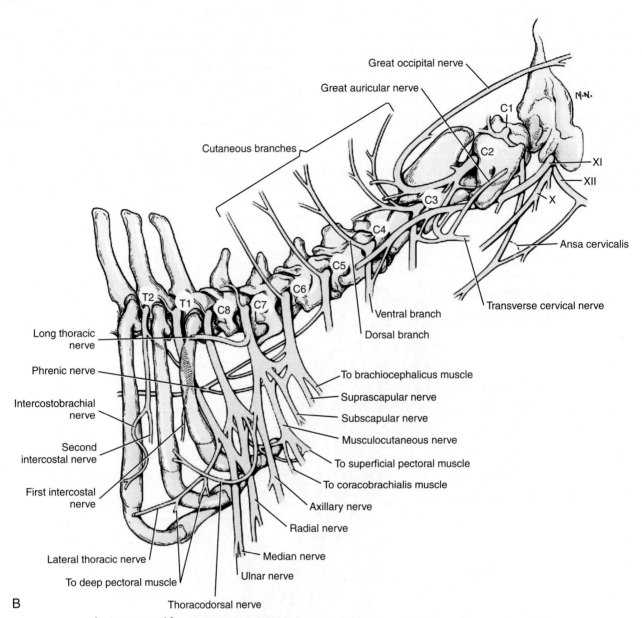

Fig. 3-27, cont'd   B, Schema of the cervical nerves and brachial plexus. The numbers C-1 through C-8 and T-1 refer to spinal nerves, not vertebrae.

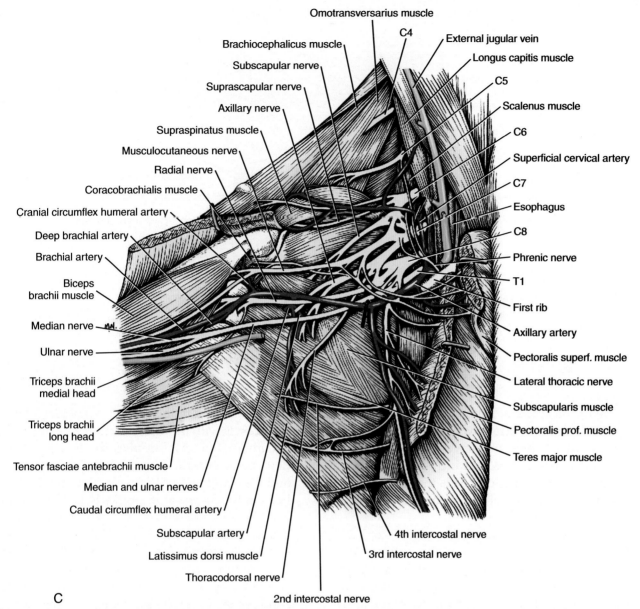

Fig. 3-27, cont'd   C, The right brachial plexus, medial aspect. (Parts **B** and **C** from Evans HE, de Lahunta A: *Miller's anatomy of the dog,* ed 4, St Louis, 2013, Saunders.)

may vary, the area or structures supplied are usually consistent.

1. The **external thoracic artery** (see Figs. 3-14, 3-16, 3-28, 3-29) leaves the axillary near its origin. The external thoracic artery curves around the craniomedial border of the deep pectoral with the nerve to the superficial pectorals and is distributed almost entirely to the superficial pectorals. It may arise from a common trunk with the lateral thoracic artery, or it may arise from the deltoid branch of the superficial cervical artery.

2. The **lateral thoracic artery** (see Figs. 3-7, 3-28, 3-29) runs caudally across the lateral surface

of the axillary lymph node and along the dorsal border of the deep pectoral ventral to the latissimus dorsi. It usually arises from the axillary artery distal to the external thoracic. The vessel may arise distal to the subscapular artery. It supplies parts of the latissimus dorsi, deep pectoral, and cutaneous trunci muscles, and the thoracic mammae.

3. The **subscapular artery** (see Figs. 3-3, 3-7, 3-28, 3-29) is larger than the continuation of the axillary in the arm. Only a short part of the subscapular is now visible. It passes caudodorsally between the subscapularis and the teres major and becomes subcutaneous near the caudal

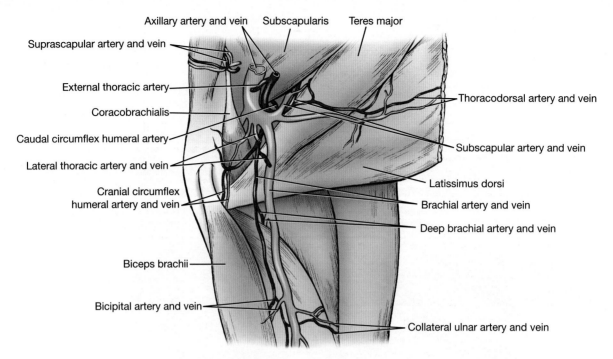

Fig. 3-28 Vessels of right axillary region, medial view.

angle of the scapula. Each bone is supplied by at least one main artery, which enters through a nutrient foramen in the cortex of the bone. The nutrient artery is a branch of an adjacent artery, which for the scapula is the subscapular artery. Dissect the following branches of the subscapular artery:

The **thoracodorsal artery** (see Figs. 3-28, 3-29) leaves the dorsal surface of the subscapular near its origin. It supplies a part of the teres major and latissimus dorsi and ends in the skin. It is readily seen on the deep surface of the latissimus dorsi. Transect the teres major and reflect both ends to expose the subscapular artery.

The **caudal circumflex humeral artery** (see Figs. 3-3, 3-28, 3-29) leaves the subscapular opposite the thoracodorsal and courses laterally between the head of the humerus and the teres major. Pull the subscapular artery medially to see this branch coursing laterally. Expose the caudal circumflex humeral artery from the lateral side, where branches become superficial at the dorsal part of the lateral head of the triceps. Transect the insertion of the deltoideus. Reflect the deltoideus proximally and observe the axillary nerve and caudal circumflex humeral artery entering the deep surface of the muscle. These are located caudal to the shoulder between the adjacent origins of the long and lateral heads of the triceps.

Notice the large branch of the axillobrachial vein that travels with the artery and nerve. The caudal circumflex humeral supplies the triceps, deltoideus, coracobrachialis, and infraspinatus muscles and the shoulder joint capsule. Transect the long head of the triceps at its origin. Reflect it and follow the continuation of the subscapular artery caudodorsally along the caudal surface of the scapula. Numerous branches supply the adjacent musculature and bone. One of these is the **circumflex scapula** artery, which branches off of the subscapular at about the middle of the caudal border of the scapula and supplies the subscapularis and infrapinatus muscles.

4. The **cranial circumflex humeral artery** (see Figs. 3-27 through 3-29) arises from the axillary artery distal or proximal to the subscapular artery. It courses cranially to supply the biceps brachii and the joint capsule of the shoulder.

Brachial Artery

The brachial artery (see Figs. 3-27 through 3-30) is a continuation of the axillary from the conjoined tendons of the teres major and latissimus dorsi. It courses distally across the body of the humerus to reach the craniomedial surface of the elbow, where it gives rise to several branches. The deep brachial and bicipital arteries are muscular branches of the brachial in the arm. Other branches

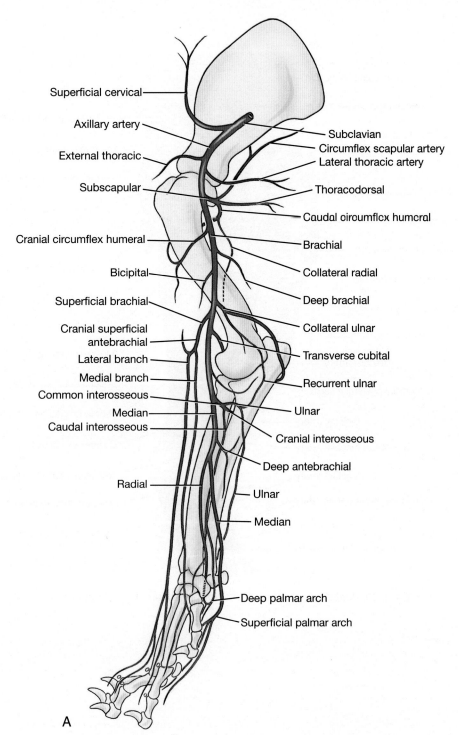

Superficial cervical

Axillary artery

External thoracic

Subscapular

Cranial circumflex humeral

Bicipital

Superficial brachial

Cranial superficial antebrachial

Lateral branch

Medial branch

Common interosseous

Median

Caudal interosseous

Radial

Subclavian

Circumflex scapular artery

Lateral thoracic artery

Thoracodorsal

Caudal circumflex humeral

Brachial

Collateral radial

Deep brachial

Collateral ulnar

Transverse cubital

Recurrent ulnar

Ulnar

Cranial interosseous

Deep antebrachial

Ulnar

Median

Deep palmar arch

Superficial palmar arch

A

Fig. 3-29 A, Arteries of right forelimb, schematic medial view.

Continued

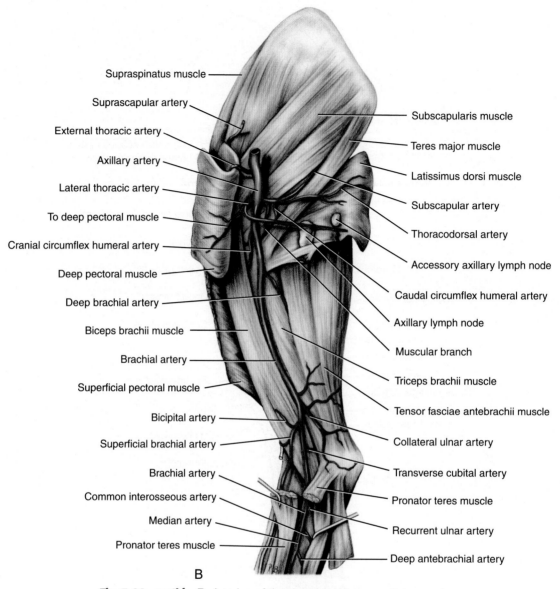

Supraspinatus muscle

Suprascapular artery

External thoracic artery

Axillary artery

Lateral thoracic artery

To deep pectoral muscle

Cranial circumflex humeral artery

Deep pectoral muscle

Deep brachial artery

Biceps brachii muscle

Brachial artery

Superficial pectoral muscle

Bicipital artery

Superficial brachial artery

Brachial artery

Common interosseous artery

Median artery

Pronator teres muscle

Subscapularis muscle

Teres major muscle

Latissimus dorsi muscle

Subscapular artery

Thoracodorsal artery

Accessory axillary lymph node

Caudal circumflex humeral artery

Axillary lymph node

Muscular branch

Triceps brachii muscle

Tensor fasciae antebrachii muscle

Collateral ulnar artery

Transverse cubital artery

Pronator teres muscle

Recurrent ulnar artery

Deep antebrachial artery

B

Fig. 3-29, cont'd   B, Arteries of the right brachium, medial aspect.

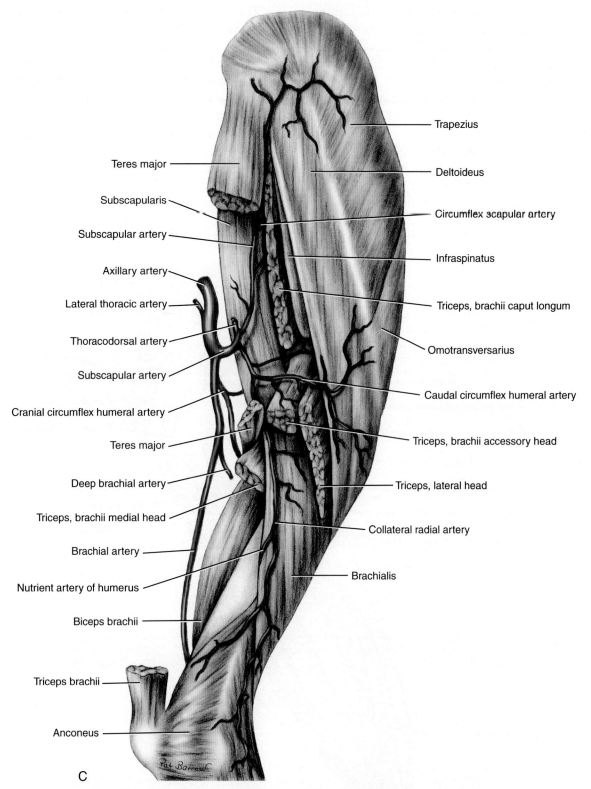

Teres major

Subscapularis

Subscapular artery

Axillary artery

Lateral thoracic artery

Thoracodorsal artery

Subscapular artery

Cranial circumflex humeral artery

Teres major

Deep brachial artery

Triceps, brachii medial head

Brachial artery

Nutrient artery of humerus

Biceps brachii

Triceps brachii

Anconeus

Trapezius

Deltoideus

Circumflex scapular artery

Infraspinatus

Triceps, brachii caput longum

Omotransversarius

Caudal circumflex humeral artery

Triceps, brachii accessory head

Triceps, lateral head

Collateral radial artery

Brachialis

C

Fig. 3-29, cont'd **C,** Arteries of the right brachium, caudolateral aspect. (Parts **B** and **C** from Evans HE, de Lahunta A: *Miller's anatomy of the dog,* ed 4, St Louis, 2013, Saunders.)

are the collateral ulnar, superficial brachial, transverse cubital, and deep antebrachial arteries. The brachial artery continues into the proximal forearm and gives off its largest branch, the common interosseus, followed by a smaller deep antebrachial artery given off by the median artery.

Dissect the following branches of the brachial artery:

1. The **collateral ulnar artery** (see Figs. 3-27 through 3-30) is a caudal branch of the brachial in the distal third of the arm. It supplies the triceps, the ulnar nerve, and the elbow.

2. The **superficial brachial artery** (Figs. 3-27, 3-29 through 3-31) loops around the cranial surface of the distal end of the biceps brachii, deep to the cephalic vein. It continues in the forearm as the **cranial superficial antebrachial artery.** Medial and lateral rami arise from the latter, and both course distally on either side of the cephalic vein accompanied by the medial and lateral branches of the superficial radial nerve. These vessels supply blood to the dorsum of the forepaw (see Fig. 3-37) via the dorsal common digital arteries.

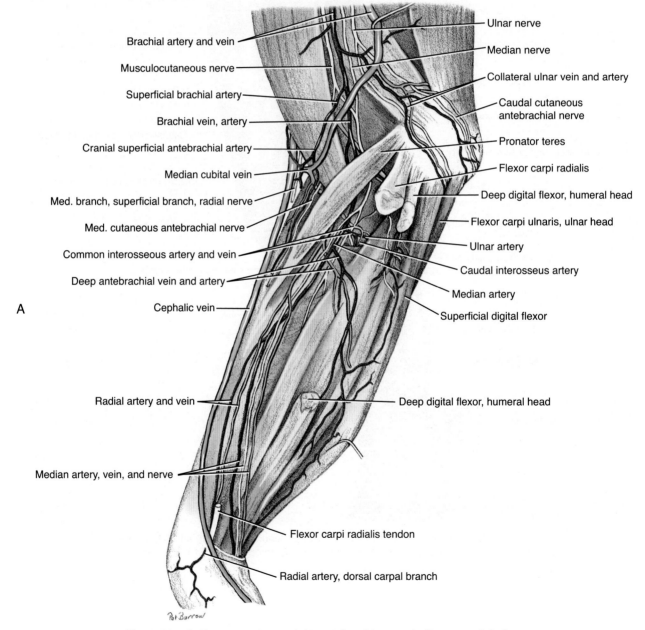

Fig. 3-30   A, Deep structures, right antebrachium and elbow, medial view.

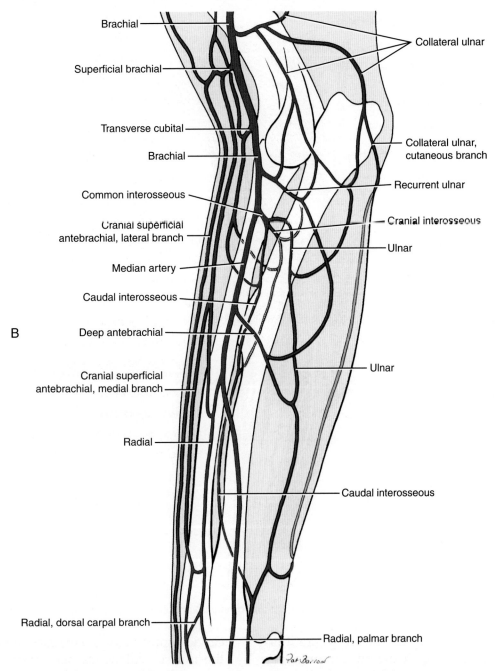

Brachial

Superficial brachial

Transverse cubital

Brachial

Common interosseous

Cranial superficial
antebrachial, lateral branch

Median artery

Caudal interosseous

Deep antebrachial

B

Cranial superficial
antebrachial, medial branch

Radial

Radial, dorsal carpal branch

Collateral ulnar

Collateral ulnar,
cutaneous branch

Recurrent ulnar

Cranial interosseous

Ulnar

Ulnar

Caudal interosseous

Radial, palmar branch

Fig. 3-30, cont'd   B, Arteries of the right antebrachium, medial aspect.

The **transverse cubital artery** (see Fig. 3-30) supplies the elbow and adjacent muscles and need not be dissected. The brachial artery courses deep to the pronator teres and flexor carpi radialis. Its branches in the forearm will be dissected later.

Nerves of the Scapular Region and Arm

All of the following 10 nerves contain somatic efferent neurons to striated muscles and afferent neurons from these muscles. Cutaneous somatic

afferents are found only in the musculocutaneous, axillary, radial, median, and ulnar nerves.

1. **Cranial pectoral nerves** (see Fig. 3-27) are derived from ventral branches of the sixth, seventh, and eighth cervical spinal nerves. They innervate the superficial pectoral muscle. These need not be dissected.
2. The **suprascapular nerve** (see Fig. 3-27) leaves the sixth and seventh cervical spinal nerves and courses between the supraspinatus and subscapularis muscles near the neck of the scapula.

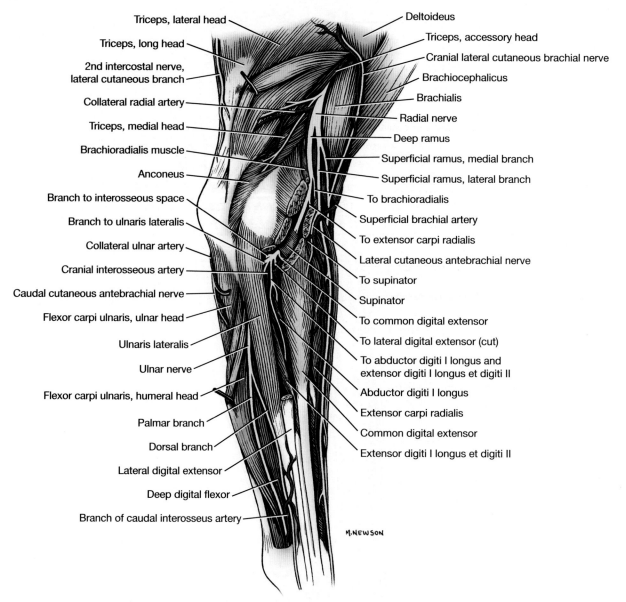

Triceps, lateral head

Triceps, long head

2nd intercostal nerve, lateral cutaneous branch

Collateral radial artery

Triceps, medial head

Brachioradialis muscle

Anconeus

Branch to interosseous space

Branch to ulnaris lateralis

Collateral ulnar artery

Cranial interosseous artery

Caudal cutaneous antebrachial nerve

Flexor carpi ulnaris, ulnar head

Ulnaris lateralis

Ulnar nerve

Flexor carpi ulnaris, humeral head

Palmar branch

Dorsal branch

Lateral digital extensor

Deep digital flexor

Branch of caudal interosseus artery

Deltoideus

Triceps, accessory head

Cranial lateral cutaneous brachial nerve

Brachiocephalicus

Brachialis

Radial nerve

Deep ramus

Superficial ramus, medial branch

Superficial ramus, lateral branch

To brachioradialis

Superficial brachial artery

To extensor carpi radialis

Lateral cutaneous antebrachial nerve

To supinator

Supinator

To common digital extensor

To lateral digital extensor (cut)

To abductor digiti I longus and extensor digiti I longus et digiti II

Abductor digiti I longus

Extensor carpi radialis

Common digital extensor

Extensor digiti I longus et digiti II

M. NEWSON

Fig. 3-31   Deep structures, right antebrachium and elbow, lateral view.

It passes across the scapular notch, where it is subject to injury from external compressive forces. It supplies the supraspinatus and infraspinatus muscles.

Transect the supraspinatus at its insertion and reflect the distal end. Trace the branches of the suprascapular nerve to this muscle. Note the continuation of the nerve distal to the scapular spine, where it enters the infraspinatus muscle.

3. The **subscapular nerve** (see Fig. 3-27) is a branch from the sixth and seventh cervical spinal nerves to the subscapularis. Sometimes two nerves enter the muscle.

4. The **musculocutaneous nerve** (Figs. 3-27, 3-30, 3-32) arises from the sixth, seventh, and eighth

cervical spinal nerves. Throughout the brachium the musculocutaneous nerve lies between the biceps brachii cranially and the brachial vessels caudally. It supplies the coracobrachialis, the biceps brachii, and the brachialis. A branch communicates with the median nerve proximal to the flexor surface of the elbow. The musculocutaneous nerve courses deep to the insertion of the biceps. It supplies the distal end of the brachialis and gives off the **medial cutaneous antebrachial nerve** (see Figs. 3-27, 3-30, 3-32), which is usually removed with the skin. This nerve is sensory to the skin on the medial aspect of the forearm.

5. The **axillary nerve** (see Fig. 3-27) arises as a branch from the combined seventh and eighth

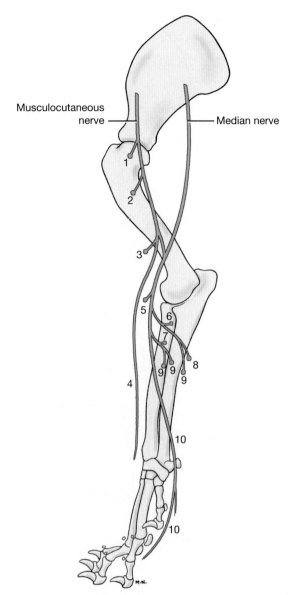

Fig. 3-32 Distribution of musculocutaneous and median nerves, right forelimb, schematic medial view.
Musculocutaneous nerve
1. Coracobrachialis
2. Biceps brachii
3. Brachialis
4. Skin of medial antebrachium
Median nerve
5. Pronator teres
6. Flexor carpi radialis
7. Pronator quadratus
8. Superficial digital flexor
9. Deep digital flexor, humeral, ulnar, and radial heads
10. Skin of caudal antebrachium and palmar paw

terminal branches of the axillary nerve are closely associated with the caudal circumflex humeral vessels and axillobrachial vein

The **cranial lateral cutaneous brachial nerve** (see Figs. 3-3, 3-31) appears subcutaneously on the lateral surface of the brachium just caudal to the deltoideus. It supplies the skin on the lateral surface of the brachium and caudal scapular region. There are cranial cutaneous antebrachial branches of this nerve that supply the skin on the cranial surface of the forearm. The latter overlap with cutaneous antebrachial branches of the superficial branch of the radial nerve laterally and the musculocutaneous nerve medially.

6. The **thoracodorsal nerve** (see Fig. 3-27) arises primarily from the eighth cervical spinal nerve. It supplies the latissimus dorsi muscle. It courses with the thoracodorsal vessels on the medial surface of the muscle.

7. The **radial nerve** (see Figs. 3-3, 3-27, 3-31, 3-33) arises from the last two cervical and first two thoracic spinal nerves, runs a short distance distally with the trunk of the median and ulnar nerves, and enters the triceps distal to the teres major. The radial nerve is motor to all the extensor muscles of the elbow, carpal, and phalangeal joints. The muscles of the arm supplied by the radial nerve are the triceps, the tensor fasciae antebrachii, and the anconeus. Observe the branches to the triceps. The radial nerve spirals around the humerus on the caudal surface and then on the lateral surface of the brachialis muscle. On the lateral side at the distal third of the arm, the radial nerve terminates as a **deep** and a **superficial branch** (see Fig. 3-31). Transect the lateral head of the triceps at its origin and reflect it to expose these terminal branches. The distribution in the antebrachium will be dissected later.

8. The **median** and **ulnar nerves** (see Figs. 3-27, 3-30 through 3-32, 3-34, Table 3-1) arise by a common trunk from the eighth cervical and the first and second thoracic spinal nerves. The common trunk lies on the medial head of the triceps between the brachial vein caudally and the brachial artery cranially. The **median nerve,** the cranial division of the common trunk, runs to the antebrachium in contact with the caudal surface of the brachial artery. It receives a branch from the musculocutaneous nerve at the level of the elbow. The brachial artery and

cervical spinal nerves. It enters the space between the subscapularis and the teres major on a level with the neck of the scapula. The following muscles are supplied by the axillary nerve: the teres major, the teres minor, the deltoideus, and part of the subscapularis. The

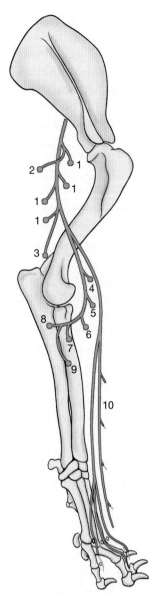

Fig. 3-33 Distribution of radial nerve, right forelimb, schematic lateral view.
1. Triceps brachii
2. Tensor fasciae antebrachii
3. Anconeus
4. Extensor carpi radialis
5. Supinator
6. Common digital extensor
7. Lateral digital extensor
8. Ulnaris lateralis
9. Abductor digiti I longus
10. Skin of cranial and lateral antebrachium and dorsal paw

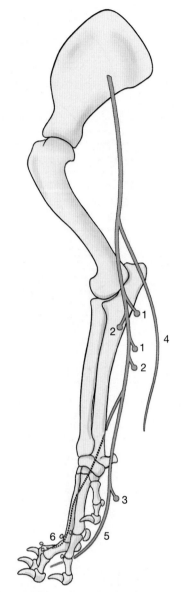

Fig. 3-34 Distribution of ulnar nerve, right forelimb, schematic medial view.
1. Flexor carpi ulnaris, ulnar and humeral heads
2. Deep digital flexor, ulnar and humeral heads
3. Interossei
4. Skin of caudal antebrachium
5. Skin of palmar paw
6. Skin of fifth metacarpal, lateral surface of digit

vein and median nerve pass just cranial to the medial epicondyle to enter the forearm. The median nerve branches to several of the muscles of the forearm and to the skin of the palmar surface of the paw.

The **ulnar nerve,** the caudal division of the common trunk, separates from the median nerve in the distal arm and crosses the elbow caudal to the medial epicondyle of the humerus. Trace it with the collateral ulnar artery to the cut edge of the skin. The **caudal cutaneous antebrachial nerve** (see Figs. 3-3, 3-27, 3-30, 3-31, 3-34) leaves the ulnar near the middle of the arm and runs caudodistally across the medial surface of the triceps and olecranon. This supplies the skin of the distal medial aspect of the brachium and the caudal aspect of the antebrachium.

Table 3-1 | Vessels and Nerves of the Thoracic Limb

Area	Arterial Supply	Nerve Supply
Lateral Muscles of Scapula and Shoulder Stabilizers, flexors, and extensors of shoulder: Supraspinatus, infraspinatus	Superficial cervical	Suprascapular
Caudal Muscles of Scapula and Shoulder Flexors of shoulder: Deltoideus, teres major, teres minor	Subscapular	Axillary
Cranial Muscles of Arm Flexors of elbow, extensor of shoulder: Biceps brachii, brachialis	Superficial cervical, axillary, brachial	Musculocutaneous
Caudal Muscles of Arm Extensor of elbow: Triceps brachii	Axillary, brachial	Radial
Cranial Muscles of Forearm Carpal extensors Digital extensors	Brachial: Common interosseous Median: Deep antebrachial	Radial
Caudal Muscles of Forearm Carpal flexors Digital flexors	Brachial: Common interosseous, deep antebrachial	Median and ulnar
Dorsal Surface of Paw	Superficial brachial, dorsal carpal rete	Radial
Palmar Surface of Paw	Median, caudal interosseous	Median and ulnar

The median and ulnar nerves supply the flexor muscles of the carpus and digits.

9. **Caudal pectoral nerves** are derived from the ventral branches of the eighth cervical and first and second thoracic spinal nerves. They innervate the deep pectoral muscle and are often combined with the lateral thoracic nerve at their origin. They need not be dissected.

10. The **lateral thoracic nerve** (see Fig. 3-27) is derived from the ventral branches of the eighth cervical and first thoracic spinal nerves. It leaves the caudal portion of the brachial plexus and courses caudally between the latissimus dorsi and deep pectoral and is the sole innervation of the cutaneous trunci. The lateral thoracic nerve was dissected previously at its termination in the cutaneous trunci muscle.

Incise the skin from the olecranon to the palmar surface of the third digit. Pass through the carpal, metacarpal, and third digital pads. Remove the skin from the forearm and paw, leaving the vessels and nerves on the specimen wherever possible.

The **cephalic vein** (see Figs. 3-3, 3-15, 3-17, 3-26, 3-30, 3-35 through 3-38) begins on the palmar side of the paw from the superficial palmar venous arch. This need not be dissected. The **accessory cephalic vein** arises from small veins on the dorsum of the paw and joins the cephalic on the cranial surface of the distal third of the forearm.

At the flexor surface of the elbow, the **median cubital vein** forms a connection between the cephalic and brachial veins. From this connection the cephalic continues proximally on the craniolateral surface of the arm in a furrow between the brachiocephalicus cranially and the origin of the lateral head of the triceps caudally. In the middle of the arm, the **axillobrachial vein** leaves the caudal aspect of the cephalic vein. The **cephalic vein** runs deep to the brachiocephalicus and enters the external jugular near the thoracic inlet. The axillobrachial vein continues proximally and passes deep to the caudal border of the deltoideus to join the axillary vein at this site. The **omobrachial vein** arises from the axillobrachial vein and continues subcutaneously across the cranial surface of the arm and shoulder and brachiocephalicus muscle before entering the external jugular vein cranial to the cephalic vein.

Arteries of the Forearm and Paw

Make a longitudinal incision through the medial part of the antebrachial fascia midway between the cranial and caudal borders. Extend this incision to the carpus. Remove the fascia from the forearm. Transect the pronator teres and flexor carpi radialis close to their origins and reflect them to uncover the brachial artery.

The **brachial artery** (see Figs. 3-27, 3-29, 3-30) in the forearm gives rise to the common

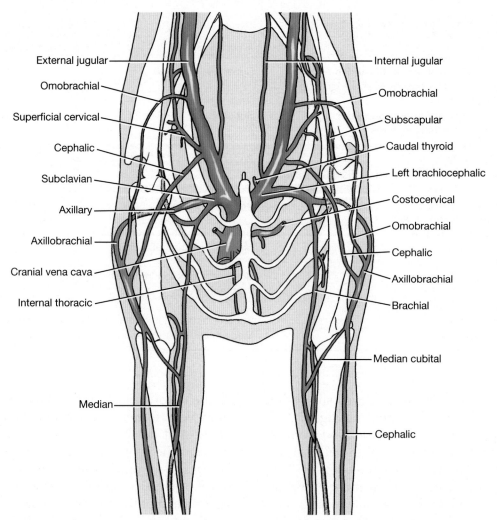

Fig. 3-35 Veins of neck, thoracic inlet, and proximal forelimb, schematic cranial aspect.

interosseous and continues as the **median artery**. The median extends to the superficial palmar arch in the paw.

The **common interosseous artery** (see Figs. 3-29, 3-30) is short and passes to the proximal part of the interosseous space between the radius and ulna before dividing into three branches. Pull the brachial artery medially to see the branches of the common interosseous. The common interosseous and ulnar arteries may arise together from the brachial.

The **ulnar artery** courses caudally. Separate the muscles on the caudomedial side of the forearm to expose its course. A recurrent branch extends proximally between the humeral and ulnar heads of the deep digital flexor. The ulnar artery continues distally with the ulnar nerve between the humeral head of the deep digital flexor and the flexor carpi ulnaris. It supplies the ulnar and humeral heads of the deep digital flexor and the flexor carpi ulnaris.

The **caudal interosseous artery** lies between the apposed surfaces of the radius and ulna. On the medial side of the forearm, expose the pronator quadratus muscle between the radius and ulna. Cut the attachments of this muscle between the two bones and scrape it with the scalpel handle to remove it from the interosseous space. The caudal interosseous artery lies deep in this space. In its course down the forearm, the artery supplies many small branches to adjacent structures. It passes through the lateral side of the carpal canal (see Figs. 2-22, 3-29, 3-38) and in the carpometacarpal region it joins with branches of the radial and median arteries to form arches that supply the palmar surface of the forepaw (see Figs. 3-29, 3-38). These will not be dissected.

The **cranial interosseous artery** (see Figs. 3-29 through 3-31) passes through the proximal part of the interosseous space cranially to supply the muscles lying laterally and cranially in the forearm. This artery will not be dissected.

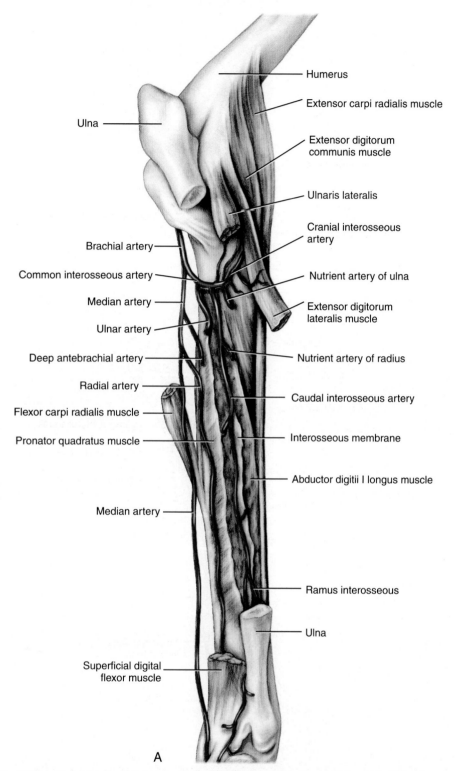

A

Fig. 3-36 A, Arteries of the right antebrachium, caudolateral aspect. (The shaft of the ulna is removed.) (Part **A** from Evans HE, de Lahunta A: *Miller's anatomy of the dog,* ed 4, St Louis, 2013, Saunders.)

Continued

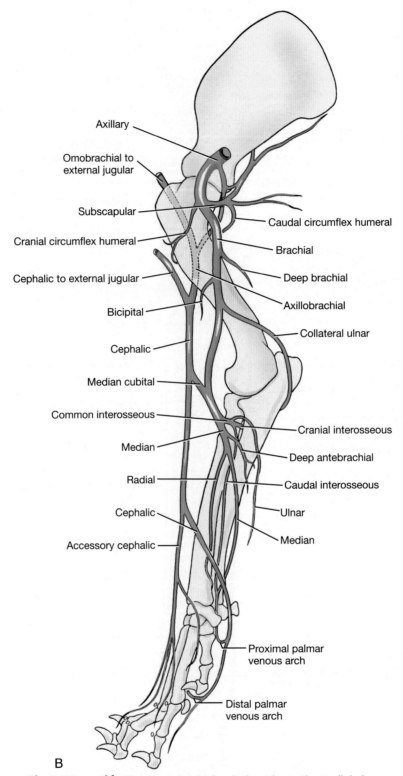

Axillary

Omobrachial to external jugular

Subscapular

Cranial circumflex humeral

Cephalic to external jugular

Bicipital

Cephalic

Median cubital

Common interosseous

Median

Radial

Cephalic

Accessory cephalic

Caudal circumflex humeral

Brachial

Deep brachial

Axillobrachial

Collateral ulnar

Cranial interosseous

Deep antebrachial

Caudal interosseous

Ulnar

Median

Proximal palmar venous arch

Distal palmar venous arch

B

Fig. 3-36, cont'd   B, Veins of right forelimb, schematic medial view.

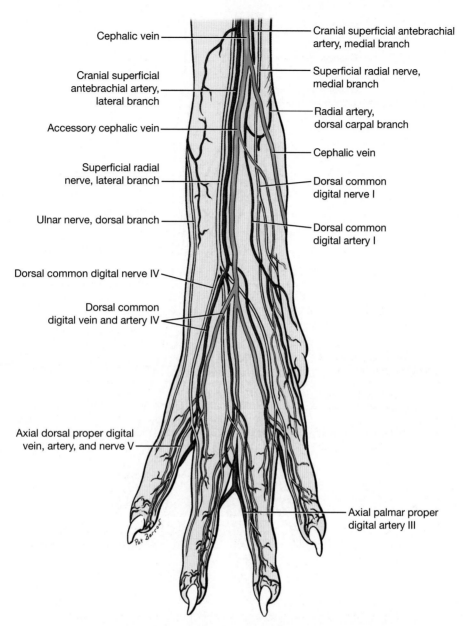

Cephalic vein

Cranial superficial antebrachial artery, lateral branch

Accessory cephalic vein

Superficial radial nerve, lateral branch

Ulnar nerve, dorsal branch

Dorsal common digital nerve IV

Dorsal common digital vein and artery IV

Axial dorsal proper digital vein, artery, and nerve V

Cranial superficial antebrachial artery, medial branch

Superficial radial nerve, medial branch

Radial artery, dorsal carpal branch

Cephalic vein

Dorsal common digital nerve I

Dorsal common digital artery I

Axial palmar proper digital artery III

Fig. 3-37 Arteries, veins, and nerves of right forepaw, dorsal view.

The **median artery** (see Figs. 3-29, 3-30, 3-38) is the continuation of the brachial artery beyond the origin of the common interosseous. It gives off the deep antebrachial and the radial artery in the forearm and continues into the paw deep to the flexor carpi radialis. It is the principal source of blood to the paw. It is accompanied by the median nerve along the humeral head of the deep digital flexor. The median artery and nerve pass through the carpal canal between the superficial and deep digital flexor tendons. Transect the flexor retinaculum and superficial digital flexor tendon. Reflect these and follow this artery through the carpal canal to the proximal end of the metacarpus, where it forms the **superficial palmar arch** with a branch of the caudal interosseous artery. This arch gives rise to the palmar common digital arteries, which course to the palmar surface of the forepaw (these need not be dissected).

The **radial artery** (see Figs. 3-29, 3-30, 3-37, 3-38) arises from the medial side of the median artery in the middle of the forearm. It follows the medial border of the radius. At the carpus it divides into palmar and dorsal carpal branches that supply the deep vessels of the forepaw. These need not be dissected.

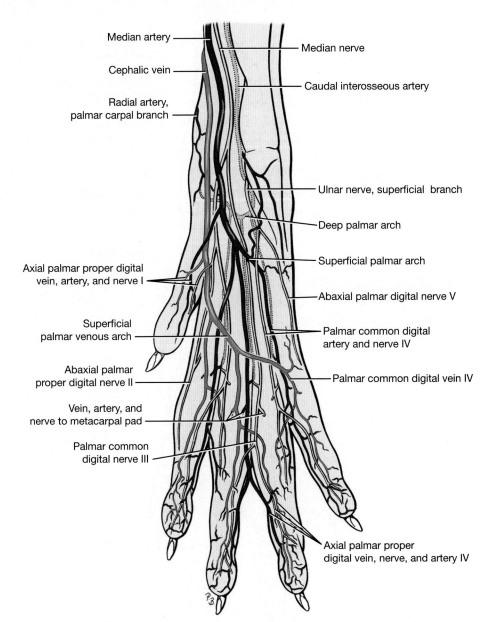

Fig. 3-38 Arteries, veins, and nerves of right forepaw, palmar view.

The **deep antebrachial artery** (see Figs. 3-29, 3-30) is a caudal branch of the median artery. Follow it deep to the flexor carpi radialis and transect the humeral head of the deep digital flexor, which covers the vessel. The deep antebrachial artery supplies the flexor carpi radialis, the deep digital flexor, the flexor carpi ulnaris, and the superficial digital flexor.

Nerves of the Forearm and Paw

The skin of the antebrachium is innervated by four nerves: the cranial surface by the axillary and radial nerves; the lateral surface by the radial nerve; the caudal surface by the ulnar nerve; and

the medial surface by the musculocutaneous nerve. There is considerable overlap in their cutaneous areas of distribution.

1. The **radial nerve** (see Figs. 3-27, 3-31, 3-33) supplies the extensors of the elbow, carpus, and digital joints. Reflect the lateral head of the triceps. Observe the radial nerve near the elbow, where it divides into superficial and deep branches. Transect the extensor carpi radialis and reflect the proximal end. The **deep branch** of the radial nerve crosses the medial surface of the extensor carpi radialis in its course into the forearm with the brachialis muscle. Transect the supinator, which lies over

the radial nerve. The radial nerve innervates the extensor carpi radialis, the common digital extensor, the supinator, the lateral digital extensor, the abductor digiti I longus, and the ulnaris lateralis.

The **superficial branch** divides into a **lateral cutaneous antebrachial nerve** and medial and lateral branches (see Fig. 3-31). The small **medial branch** follows the medial ramus of the cranial superficial antebrachial artery and continues distally in the forearm on the medial side of the cephalic vein. The **lateral branch** becomes associated with the lateral side of the cephalic vein and enters the forearm with the lateral branches of the cranial superficial antebrachial artery. These branches continue to the paw on either side of the accessory cephalic vein (see Fig. 2-22). These medial and lateral branches are sensory to the skin on the cranial and lateral surface of the forearm and the dorsal surface of the carpus, metacarpus, and digits (Fig. 3-39). They terminate in dorsal common digital nerves in the paw (Fig. 3-37).

2. The **median nerve** (see Figs. 3-27, 3-30, 3-32, 3-38) runs distally into the antebrachium with the brachial artery. It innervates the pronator teres, the pronator quadratus, the flexor carpi radialis, the superficial digital flexor, and the radial head and parts of the humeral and ulnar heads of the deep digital flexor.

Transect and reflect the pronator teres and reflect the flexor carpi radialis and the humeral head of the deep digital flexor to observe the course of the nerve. The median nerve passes through the carpal canal with the median artery and branches to supply sensory innervation to the palmar surface of the forepaw. Note the course of the nerve through the carpal canal (Figs. 2-22, 3-38).

3. The **ulnar nerve** (see Figs. 3-27, 3-30, 3-31, 3-34, 3-38) diverges caudally from the median nerve at the distal third of the arm. At this point the caudal cutaneous antebrachial nerve arises from the ulnar. The ulnar nerve enters the antebrachial muscles caudal to the medial epicondyle of the humerus and is distributed to the flexor carpi ulnaris and parts of the ulnar and humeral heads of the deep digital flexor. In the middle of the antebrachium the **dorsal branch** of the ulnar nerve arises and becomes subcutaneous on the lateral surface. It is distributed to

the lateral surface of the metacarpus and the fifth digit (see Fig. 3-37).

Transect and reflect the ulnar and humeral heads of the flexor carpi ulnaris. The ulnar nerve lies on the caudal surface of the deep digital flexor deep to the humeral head of the flexor carpi ulnaris.

Trace the **palmar branch** of the ulnar nerve into the forepaw. The nerve lies on the deep surface of the flexor carpi ulnaris, just above the carpus. It then enters the lateral side of the carpal canal (see Fig. 3-22), where it divides into a superficial and a deep branch (see Fig. 3-38). Reflect the flexor carpi ulnaris and flexor retinaculum to expose the nerve in the carpal canal. In the metacarpus the superficial and deep branches further divide to supply sensory innervation to the palmar surface of the forepaw and motor innervation to the intrinsic muscles of the forepaw. Although the terminal cutaneous distribution of nerves in the forelimb is difficult to dissect, it is important to know both the cutaneous areas and the autonomous zones of these nerves for local anesthetic procedures and for the diagnosis of nerve lesions. The **cutaneous area** is the entire area of skin innervated by a nerve. The **autonomous zone** is that area of skin innervated solely by a specific peripheral nerve with no overlap from adjacent nerves. Fig. 3-39 shows the autonomous zones for the nerves of the forelimb and adjacent neck and trunk regions.

The distribution of vessels and nerves to the digits will not be dissected, but you should understand the pertinent terminology (see Fig. 3-40). These are more important clinically in large animals that walk on one (horse) or two (most farm animals) digits. In the metacarpus there are superficial and deep branches on both the dorsal and palmar sides, but there are no deep nerves dorsally. Superficial branches are called **dorsal** or **palmar common digital** vessels or nerves and deep branches are called **dorsal** or **palmar metacarpal** vessels and nerves. These four branches are oriented in a sagittal plane between the metacarpal bones. At the metacarpophalangeal joint, the common digital and metacarpal branches unite to form a common trunk on the dorsal and palmar surfaces. Each common trunk then divides into medial and lateral branches to the digits. These digital branches are called axial or abaxial dorsal or palmar proper digital vessels or nerves. *Axial* or *abaxial* refers to whether they are

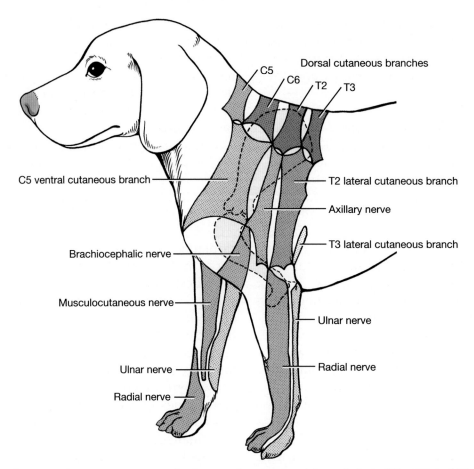

Fig. 3-39   Autonomous zones of cutaneous innervation of thoracic limb. (After Kitchell RL et al: Electrophysiologic studies of cutaneous nerves of the thoracic limb of the dog, *Am J Vet Res* 41:61–76, 1980.)

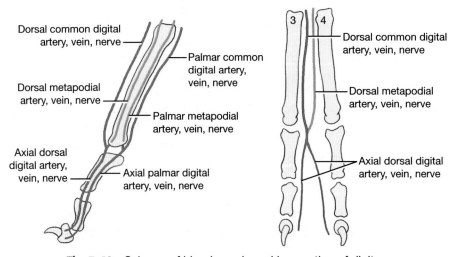

Fig. 3-40   Schema of blood supply and innervation of digits.

Table 3-2	Blood Supply and Innervation of the Digits of the Thoracic Limb		
Dorsal Surface			
Arteries			
Superficial	Superficial brachial a.: Lateral br. of cranial superficial antebrachial	Dorsal common digital a.	
	Medial br. of cranial superficial antebrachial		Axial or abaxial dorsal digital a.
Deep	Dorsal carpal rete: Radial a., dorsal carpal br. Caudal interosseous a.	Dorsal metacarpal a.	
Nerves			
Superficial only	Superficial br. radial n.: Medial and lateral br. Ulnar n., dorsal br.	Dorsal common digital n.	Axial or abaxial dorsal digital n. Abaxial dorsal digital n. V
Palmar Surface			
Arteries			
Superficial	Superficial palmar arch: Median a., br. caudal Interosseous a.	Palmar common digital a.	Axial or abaxial palmar proper digital a.
Deep	Deep palmar arch: Caudal interosseous a. Radial a., palmar carpal br.	Palmar metacarpal a.	
Nerves			
Superficial	Median n. Ulnar n., superficial br.	Palmar common digital nn.	Axial or abaxial palmar proper digital n.
Deep	Ulnar n., deep br.	Palmar metacarpal nn. I–IV	

on the surface of the digit that faces toward the axis (axial) or away from the axis (abaxial) of the paw. The axis of the paw passes between digits III and IV. As a rule, the largest digital vessels are the palmar axial proper digitals. (Table 3-2 shows the arrangement of these vessels and nerves in the forepaw.)

LIVE DOG

On the medial side of the arm, feel the vessels and nerves coursing distally between the biceps brachii cranially and the medial head of the triceps brachii caudally. Palpate a pulse in the brachial artery. Arterial injections can be made into this artery.

Palpate the medial epicondyle of the humerus. The brachial vessels and median nerve course just cranial to this and pass beneath the pronator teres. These cannot be felt here. The ulnar nerve courses caudal to the medial epicondyle and can be palpated by stroking the skin in a caudal to cranial direction toward the epicondyle. The ulnar nerve will be felt when it slips beneath your fingers.

On the lateral side of the distal arm, the radial nerve can be felt where it emerges from under the distal border of the lateral head of the triceps on the brachialis muscle and divides into superficial and deep branches. Press firmly on the skin over the brachialis muscle here and stroke from proximal to distal. The superficial branch will be felt as it slips out from under your fingers.

Place your fingers across the flexor surface of the elbow and compress this area. This will distend the cephalic vein in the forearm, which is commonly used for venipuncture. Remember that a small artery and sensory nerve accompany this vein on both sides. Repeated needle punctures may injure them and contribute to subcutaneous hemorrhage, as well as being a painful experience for the patient. In some short-haired breeds, the cephalic, axillobrachial, and omobrachial veins may be visible in the arm and shoulder region.

Place your fingers on the distal medial side of the forearm and extend the carpus. Feel the tendon of the flexor carpi radialis as it becomes taut. Palpation here may detect a pulse in the median artery where it passes deep to this tendon.

Review the location of the autonomous zones of the nerves in the forelimb of the dog.

4

CHAPTER

The Abdomen, Pelvis, and Pelvic Limb

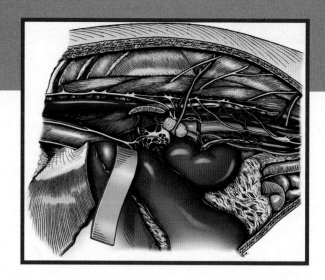

CHAPTER OUTLINE

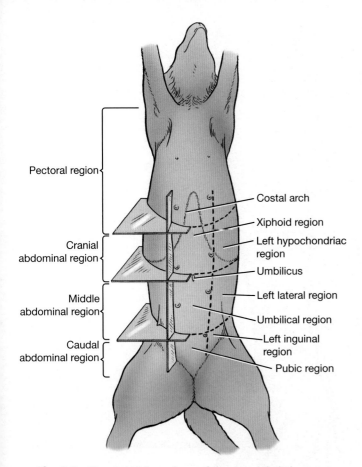

Pectoral region

Cranial
abdominal region

Middle
abdominal region

Caudal
abdominal region

Costal arch
Xiphoid region
Left hypochondriac
region
Umbilicus
Left lateral region
Umbilical region
Left inguinal
region
Pubic region

Fig. 4-1 Topographic regions of thorax and abdomen.

The surface anatomy of the abdomen is divided into cranial, middle, and caudal regions (Fig. 4-1). Reflect the skin from the right abdominal wall, leaving the mammary papillae in the female, the prepuce in the male, and the cutaneous trunci. Extend a perpendicular incision from the ventral midline to the middle of the medial surface of the right thigh and then to its cranial border. Continue this incision dorsally along the cranial edge of the thigh past the crest of the ilium to the mid-dorsal line. Starting on the medial surface of the thigh, reflect or remove the skin of the right side of the abdomen.

VESSELS AND NERVES OF THE VENTRAL AND LATERAL PARTS OF THE ABDOMINAL WALL

The arteries that supply the superficial part of the ventral abdominal wall are branches of the superficial epigastric arteries (Fig. 4-2). The origin of the cranial superficial epigastric artery is from the cranial epigastric (see Fig. 4-33).

The subcutaneous tissue of the ventral abdominal wall contains the abdominal and inguinal mammae and the vessels and nerves that supply them. In

the female, the cranial superficial epigastric vessels are seen subcutaneously near the cranial abdominal papilla. By blunt dissection, separate the right row of mammae from the fascia and turn them laterally.

Dissect the **external pudendal artery** (see Figs. 2-79, 4-2, 4-33, 4-40), which emerges from the superficial inguinal ring. Its origin from the pudendoepigastric trunk, a branch from the deep femoral artery, will be seen later. The external pudendal artery courses caudoventrally to the cranial border of the gracilis. The caudal superficial epigastric artery is large and appears as a direct continuation of the external pudendal artery dorsal to the superficial inguinal lymph node. The **caudal superficial epigastric artery** (see Fig. 4-2) runs cranially to the deep surface of the inguinal mamma and supplies the mammary branches. The artery continues to supply the caudal abdominal mamma and anastomose with branches of the cranial superficial epigastric artery. In the male it supplies the prepuce. A small branch of the external pudendal artery courses caudally to supply the labia in the female and the scrotum in the male.

Expose the **superficial inguinal lymph nodes** (see Fig. 4-40), which lie adjacent to the caudal superficial epigastric vessels and cranial to their origin from the external pudendal vessels. The afferent lymphatics of these nodes drain the mammae, the prepuce, the scrotum, and the ventral abdominal wall as far cranially as the umbilicus. Their efferent lymphatics course through the inguinal canal to reach lymph nodes in the sublumbar region.

The abdominal wall receives its vascular supply primarily from four vessels (see Fig. 4-33): cranial abdominal artery (craniodorsal), cranial epigastric artery (cranioventral), caudal epigastric artery (caudoventral), and deep circumflex iliac artery (caudodorsal).

Reflect the superficial fascia from the lateral abdominal wall. Emerging from the dorsolateral abdominal wall, caudal to the last rib, are superficial branches of the **cranial abdominal artery** (see Fig. 4-33). The latter arises from a common origin with the caudal phrenic artery off the aorta and perforates the abdominal musculature, which it supplies, to reach the skin.

The **cutaneous nerves** of the abdomen differ somewhat from those of the thorax. The lateral cutaneous branches from the last five thoracic nerves do not follow the convexity of the costal arch but run in a caudoventral direction and supply the ventral and ventrolateral parts of the abdominal wall (Fig. 4-3). The cutaneous branches of

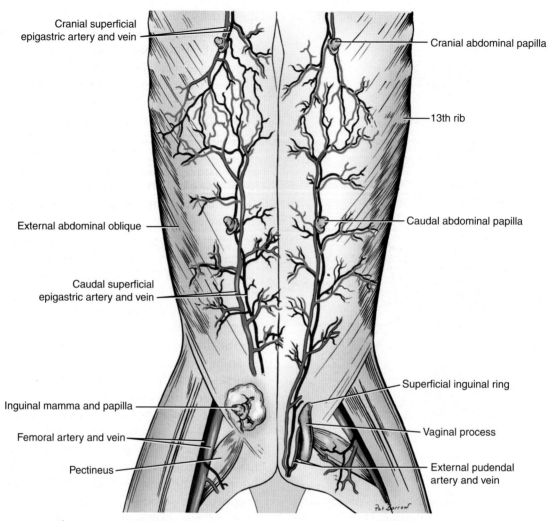

Cranial superficial epigastric artery and vein

Cranial abdominal papilla

13th rib

External abdominal oblique

Caudal abdominal papilla

Caudal superficial epigastric artery and vein

Superficial inguinal ring

Inguinal mamma and papilla

Vaginal process

Femoral artery and vein

Pectineus

External pudendal artery and vein

Fig. 4-2   Superficial veins and arteries of abdomen. Left vaginal process exposed.

the first three lumbar nerves perforate the lateral part of the abdominal wall and, as small nerves, run caudoventrally. They supply the skin of the caudolateral and caudoventral abdominal wall and the thigh in the region of the stifle. Do not dissect these cutaneous nerves. Cranial to the cranioventral iliac spine, the **lateral cutaneous femoral nerve** (see Fig. 4-3) and the **deep circumflex iliac artery** and vein (see Fig. 4-33) perforate the internal abdominal oblique and appear superficially. The nerve arises from the fourth lumbar spinal nerve and is cutaneous to the cranial and lateral surfaces of the thigh. The artery arises from the aorta and supplies the caudodorsal abdominal wall. Dissect these vessels and trace the nerve as far as the present skin reflection will allow.

Transect the lumbar origin of the external abdominal oblique and reflect it ventrally.

Transect the internal abdominal oblique at the origin of the muscle fibers from the thoracolumbar

fascia. Extend the transection caudally to the level of the deep circumflex iliac vessels and lateral cutaneous femoral nerve. Separate the internal abdominal oblique muscle from the underlying transverse muscle and reflect it ventrally to expose the ventral branches of the last few thoracic spinal nerves and the first four lumbar spinal nerves. These are parallel to each other and supply the ventral and lateral parts of the thoracic and abdominal wall. The ventral branches of the first four lumbar nerves form the **cranial iliohypogastric, caudal iliohypogastric, ilioinguinal,** and **lateral cutaneous femoral nerves,** respectively. It may be difficult to differentiate between the ventral branches of T13 and L1 without tracing them to the intervertebral foramina, which is not necessary. Usually the ventral branch of T13 courses along the caudal aspect of the thirteenth rib.

The cranial and caudal iliohypogastric and ilioinguinal nerves (see Fig. 4-3) pass through the

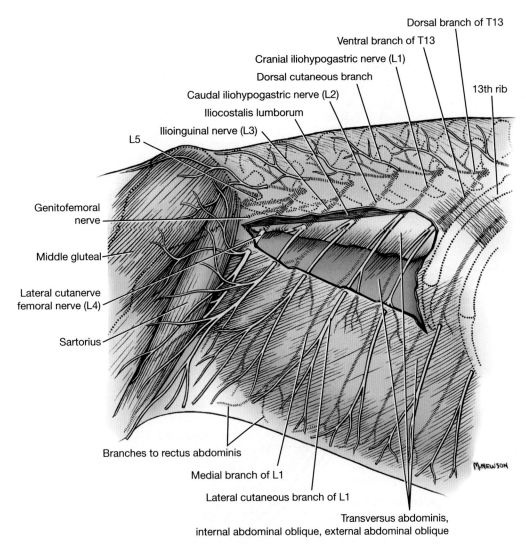

Dorsal branch of T13

Ventral branch of T13

Cranial iliohypogastric nerve (L1)

Dorsal cutaneous branch

13th rib

Caudal iliohypogastric nerve (L2)

Iliocostalis lumborum

Ilioinguinal nerve (L3)

L5

Genitofemoral nerve

Middle gluteal

Lateral cutanerve femoral nerve (L4)

Sartorius

Branches to rectus abdominis

Medial branch of L1

Lateral cutaneous branch of L1

Transversus abdominis, internal abdominal oblique, external abdominal oblique

Fig. 4-3   Lateral view of the first four lumbar nerves.

aponeurosis of origin of the transversus abdominis. Each has a medial branch that descends between the transversus abdominis and the internal abdominal oblique to the rectus abdominis. The medial branches supply these muscles and the underlying peritoneum. The lateral branches of these nerves perforate the internal abdominal oblique and descend between the oblique muscles. They may be seen on the deep surface of the external abdominal oblique. Each lateral branch supplies these muscles, perforates the external abdominal oblique, and terminates subcutaneously as the lateral cutaneous branch to the abdominal wall in that region.

Inguinal Structures

Dissect the structures in the male that pass through the inguinal canal and the superficial inguinal ring (see Figs. 2-79, 2-80, 4-5 through 4-7). Review Figs. 2-79 and 2-80.

Male

The **external pudendal artery** and **vein** leave the superficial inguinal ring caudal and medial to the structures that extend to the testis. Their branches have been dissected.

The **genitofemoral nerve** (see Figs. 4-3, 4-60, 4-65, 4-66, 4-69) arises from the ventral branches of the third and fourth lumbar nerves. It is bound by fascia to the external pudendal vein medial to the spermatic cord. It passes through the inguinal canal with the spermatic cord and innervates the cremaster muscle and the skin covering the inguinal region and proximal medial thigh of both sexes and part of the prepuce in the male.

The **spermatic fascia**, a continuation of abdominal and transversalis fascia, surrounds the structures emerging from the superficial inguinal ring. This includes the vaginal tunic (spermatic cord) and cremaster muscle (Figs. 4-4 through 4-7).

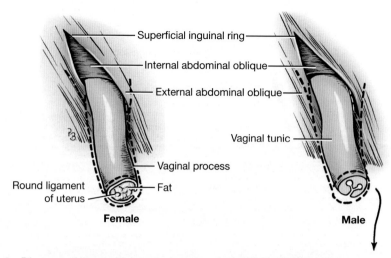

Fig. 4-4 Diagram of transected vaginal process in female and vaginal tunic in male. (*Dotted lines* indicate spermatic fascia. In the male the contents of the vaginal tunic are not shown. See Fig. 4-5.)

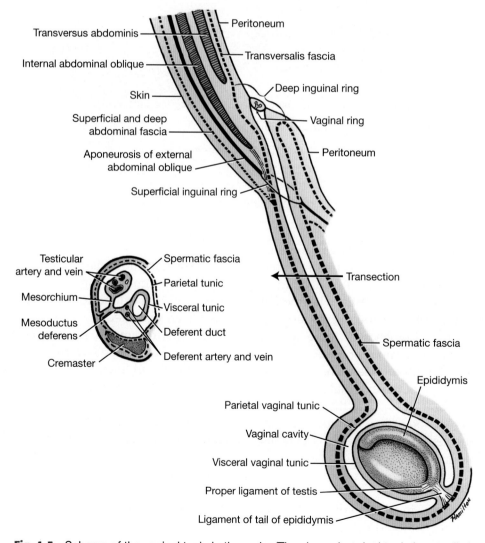

Fig. 4-5 Schema of the vaginal tunic in the male. (The visceral vaginal tunic is actually in contact with the surface of the testis.)

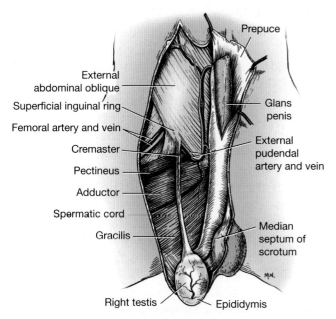

External
abdominal oblique

Superficial inguinal ring

Femoral artery and vein

Cremaster

Pectineus

Adductor

Spermatic cord

Gracilis

Right testis

Prepuce

Glans
penis

External
pudendal
artery and vein

Median
septum of
scrotum

Epididymis

Fig. 4-6 Male genitalia, ventral view. As the vaginal tunic with the spermatic cord leaves the superficial inguinal ring, it is joined by muscle fibers of the internal abdominal oblique, which form the cremaster muscle.

The cremaster muscle is surrounded by this spermatic fascia as it courses along the caudal part of the vaginal tunic. The cremaster muscle arises from the caudal free border of the internal abdominal oblique and attaches to the vaginal tunic near the testis (Figs. 2-80, 4-40). Reflect the spermatic fascia to expose the vaginal tunic, which can be seen extending from its emergence through the superficial inguinal ring to the testis.

The **vaginal process** (see Figs. 4-4 through 4-7) is a diverticulum of the peritoneum present in both sexes. In the male it envelops the testis and structures of the spermatic cord and is referred to as the *vaginal tunic*. It consists of the parietal, visceral, and connecting parts. In the female it surrounds fat and the round ligament of the uterus. It is usually short and ends in the inguinal region.

The **parietal vaginal tunic**, the outer layer of this diverticulum in the male, extends from the deep inguinal ring to the bottom of the scrotum. Incise this parietal tunic along the most ventral part of the testis and along the cranial border of the vaginal tunic to the superficial inguinal ring

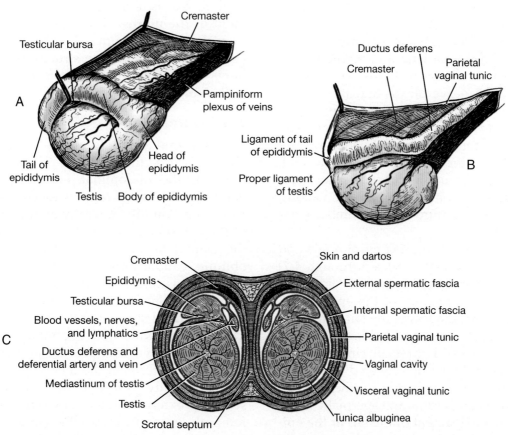

Cremaster

Testicular bursa

A

Tail of
epididymis

Testis   Body of epididymis

Head of
epididymis

Pampiniform
plexus of veins

Ductus deferens

Cremaster

Parietal
vaginal tunic

Ligament of tail
of epididymis

Proper ligament
of testis

B

Cremaster

Epididymis

Testicular bursa

Blood vessels, nerves,
and lymphatics

C

Ductus deferens and
deferential artery and vein

Mediastinum of testis

Testis

Scrotal septum

Skin and dartos

External spermatic fascia

Internal spermatic fascia

Parietal vaginal tunic

Vaginal cavity

Visceral vaginal tunic

Tunica albuginea

Fig. 4-7 Structures of testes and scrotum. **A,** Right testis, lateral aspect. **B,** Left testis, medial aspect. **C,** Schematic cross section through scrotum and testes.

to expose the visceral vaginal tunic. The cavity entered is a continuation of the peritoneal cavity.

The **visceral vaginal tunic** is closely fused to the testis and epididymis and surrounds the ductus deferens. The **mesorchium** is the connecting mesentery of the testis that contains the vessels and nerves of the testis. The **mesoductus deferens** is the connecting mesentery that attaches the ductus deferens to the body wall proximally and the mesorchium distally. It contains the artery, vein, and nerve of the ductus deferens (see Figs. 4-5 through 4-7).

The **spermatic cord** (see Figs. 2-80, 4-4 through 4-7) is carried through the inguinal canal by the descent of the testis and is composed of two distinct parts: the ductus deferens and the testicular artery and vein.

The **ductus deferens** carries the spermatozoa from the epididymis to the urethra. It arises from the tail of the epididymis at the caudal end of the testis and is attached to the mesorchium by the **mesoductus deferens**. The small **deferent artery** and **vein** accompany the deferent duct.

The **testicular artery** and **vein**, as well as the testicular lymph vessels and the testicular plexus of autonomic nerves, are closely associated with each other. These vessels and nerves are covered by a fold of peritoneum, the **mesorchium**, that is continuous with the parietal and visceral vaginal tunics. The artery is tortuous, and woven around it are the nerve plexus and the venous plexus. The venous plexus is the **pampiniform plexus**. The testicular artery and vein are branches of the aorta and caudal vena cava, respectively. They enter the testis at its cranial end. The nerve plexus is autonomic and sensory and contains postganglionic sympathetic axons, which arise from the third to fifth lumbar sympathetic ganglia.

The **testis** and the associated **epididymis** and **ductus deferens** (see Figs. 2-80, 4-5 through 4-7) are intimately covered by the visceral vaginal tunic. At the caudal extremity of the epididymis, the visceral peritoneum leaves the tail of the epididymis at an acute angle and becomes the parietal layer. Thus there is a small circumscribed area on the epididymis not covered by peritoneum. The connective tissue that attaches the epididymis to the vaginal tunic and spermatic fascia at this point is the **ligament of the tail of the epididymis**. Reflect the skin of the scrotum caudally to observe it.

The **epididymis** (see Figs. 2-80, 4-5 through 4-7) lies more on the lateral side of the testis than on its dorsal border. For descriptive purposes it is divided into a cranial extremity, or **head,** where the epididymis communicates with the testis; a middle part, or **body;** and a caudal extremity, or **tail,** which is continuous with the ductus deferens. The tail is attached to the testis by the **proper ligament of the testis** and to the vaginal tunic and spermatic fascia by the **ligament of the tail of the epididymis**. The ductus deferens passes cranially over the testis medial to the epididymis.

Lay the previously reflected skin back over the inguinal region and examine the scrotum. The **scrotum** is a pouch divided by an external raphe and an internal median septum into two cavities, each of which is occupied by a testis, an epididymis, and the distal part of the spermatic cord.

Female

In the female locate the external pudendal blood vessels and the genitofemoral nerve emerging from the superficial inguinal ring. The **vaginal process** (see Figs. 4-2, 4-4) is the peritoneal diverticulum that is accompanied by the **round ligament of the uterus**. (The origin of this ligament from the mesometrium within the abdomen will be seen later.) These two structures, enclosed in fascia and surrounded by fat, may extend as far as the vulva.

The Inguinal Canal

The **inguinal canal** (see Figs. 2-80, 4-5) is a short fissure filled with connective tissue between the abdominal muscles. It extends between the deep and superficial inguinal rings. It is bounded laterally by the aponeurosis of the external abdominal oblique; cranially by the caudal border of the internal abdominal oblique; caudally by the caudal border of the aponeurosis of the external abdominal oblique (inguinal ligament); and medially, in part, by the superficial surface of the rectus abdominis. The vaginal tunic and spermatic cord in the male and the vaginal process and round ligament of the uterus in the female pass obliquely caudoventrally through the canal. In both sexes the external pudendal vessels and genitofemoral nerve traverse the canal. Notice as many of these boundaries as possible before opening the abdomen.

Abdominal and Peritoneal Cavities

The **abdominal cavity** is formed by the muscles of the abdominal wall, the ribs, and the diaphragm. It is lined by peritoneum, which encloses the peritoneal cavity.

The **peritoneal cavity,** like the pleural and pericardial cavities, is a closed space. It is lined by a serous membrane. Serous membranes are thin layers of loose connective tissue covered by a layer of mesothelium. The peritoneum is derived from the somatic and splanchnic mesodermal layers lining the embryonic coelom.

The **parietal peritoneum** is the layer that lines the body wall and has to be incised to open the peritoneal cavity. The **visceral peritoneum** surrounds all organs of the abdominal cavity. Therefore there are no organs "within" the peritoneal cavity because they are all covered by visceral peritoneum. (Only an oocyte when it ovulates is within the peritoneal cavity before it enters the uterine tube.) The **connecting peritoneum** extends between the parietal and visceral peritoneums and forms a mesentery that suspends the organs of the abdominal cavity and contains their blood vessels and nerves (Fig. 4-8).

The transversalis fascia reinforces the parietal peritoneum and attaches it to the abdominal muscles and diaphragm. Make a sagittal incision through the abdominal wall on each side dorsal to the rectus abdominis from the costal arch to the level of the inguinal canal. Connect the cranial ends of these incisions and reflect the ventral abdominal wall. Observe the following structures:

The **falciform ligament** is a fold of peritoneum that passes from the umbilicus to the diaphragm. It is also attached to the liver between the left medial and quadrate lobes. In obese specimens a large accumulation of fat is found in this remnant of the embryonic ventral mesentery. In young animals the **round ligament of the liver** may still be visible in the free border of the falciform ligament. Caudal to the umbilicus, the fold of peritoneum is the **median ligament of the bladder.** In the fetus the umbilical vein courses cranially in the free border of the falciform ligament to enter the liver, whereas the urachus and umbilical arteries are in the free border of the median ligament of the bladder.

Examine the caudoventral aspect of the inside of the peritoneal cavity at the level of the inguinal canal and observe the vaginal ring.

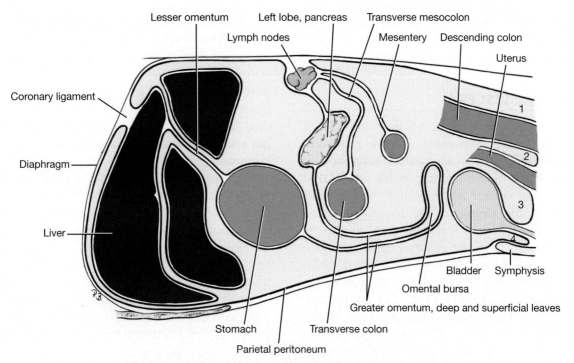

Fig. 4-8 Diagram of peritoneal reflections, sagittal section.
1. Pararectal fossa
2. Rectogenital pouch
3. Vesicogenital pouch
4. Pubovesical pouch

The **vaginal ring** (see Figs. 4-5, 4-11, 4-43) is the opening formed by the parietal peritoneum as it leaves the abdomen and enters the inguinal canal to form the vaginal process or tunic. It marks the position of the **deep inguinal ring,** which is formed by the reflection of the transversalis fascia outside the vaginal ring (see Fig. 4-5). A deposit of fat is usually present in the transversalis fascia around the vaginal ring.

In the male the **ductus deferens** is attached to the abdominal and pelvic walls by a fold of peritoneum, the mesoductus deferens. At the vaginal ring, this fold joins the mesorchium, which contains the testicular artery and vein and the testicular nerve plexuses (see Figs. 4-5, 4-11, 4-43). The ductus deferens courses from the vaginal ring dorsally over the edge of the lateral ligament of the bladder and caudally to the urethra just beyond the neck of the bladder. In the female a fold of peritoneum from the mesometrium, which suspends the uterus, passes into the vaginal ring (see Fig. 4-12). This contains the round ligament of the uterus, which is the remnant of the caudal part of the fetal gubernaculum. In the male this becomes the ligament of the tail of the epididymis.

The **caudal epigastric artery** and **vein** course cranially on the deep face of the caudal part of the rectus abdominis. The origin of the artery from the pudendoepigastric trunk of the deep femoral artery will be dissected later (see Fig. 4-33).

ABDOMINAL VISCERA

The **greater omentum** (Figs. 4-8 through 4-11) is the first structure seen after reflecting the abdominal wall. It is a caudoventral extension of the two layers of connecting peritoneum that pass from the dorsal body wall to the greater curvature of the stomach, the dorsal mesogastrium. As the stomach forms and rotates to its definitive position in the embryo, this mesogastrium grows extensively and forms a double-layered sac that extends caudoventrally beneath many of the abdominal organs. The space contained within the folded mesogastrium is the omental bursa. The fold adjacent to the ventral body wall is the **superficial leaf**. The **deep leaf** is adjacent to the abdominal organs. The greater omentum is lacelike, with depositions of fat along the vessels. The greater omentum covers the jejunum and ileum, leaving the descending colon exposed on the left, the bladder exposed caudally, and the descending duodenum exposed on the right. Reflect the omentum and, using your fingers on opposite sides, separate its superficial and deep walls to expose its cavity, the **omental bursa**. Follow the greater omentum from its ventral attachment on the greater curvature of the stomach to its dorsal attachment to the dorsal body wall. The spleen is enclosed in the superficial leaf of the greater omentum on the left side, and the left lobe of the pancreas is enclosed in the deep leaf dorsally.

Three organs in the abdomen that are capable of considerable variation in size are the stomach, the urinary bladder, and the uterus. If one or more of these are distended, the relations of the organs will be altered.

The **urinary bladder** (see Figs. 4-8, 4-9, 4-11, 4-12, 4-24, 4-37 through 4-39, 4-41 through 4-43), when empty, is contracted and lies on the floor of the pelvic inlet. When distended, it lies on the floor of the abdomen and conforms in shape to the caudal part of the abdominal cavity because it displaces all freely movable viscera. It frequently reaches a transverse plane through the umbilicus.

The nonpregnant **uterus** (see Figs. 4-8, 4-9, *B*, 4-12, 4-24, 4-37, 4-38) is remarkably small even in a bitch that has had several litters. The uterus consists of a short **cervix** and **body** and two long **horns**. The gravid uterus lies on the floor of the abdomen during the second month or last half of pregnancy. As the uterus enlarges, the middle parts of the horns gravitate cranially and ventrally and come to lie medial to the costal arches; thus the uterus bends on itself because the ovarian and vaginal ends move very little during enlargement.

The **spleen** (see Figs. 4-9 through 4-11, 4-13, 4-14, 4-20, 4-26, 4-27, 4-29, 4-30, 4-34) lies in the superficial leaf of the greater omentum to the left of the median plane along the greater curvature of the stomach. Its position, shape, and degree of distention are variable. Its lateral surface lies against the parietal peritoneum of the left lateral abdominal wall and the liver. Its caudal part may reach to a transverse plane through the midlumbar region. Its cranial limit is usually marked by a plane passing between the twelfth and thirteenth thoracic vertebrae. It may reach the floor of the abdomen. The part of the greater omentum that attaches the spleen to the stomach is the gastrosplenic ligament. If your specimen was anesthetized with

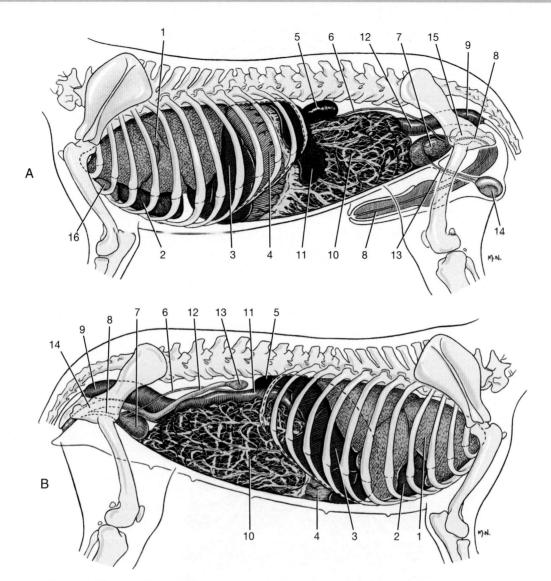

Fig. 4-9 Viscera of the dog.
A, Male dog, left lateral view.

1. Left lung
2. Heart
3. Liver
4. Stomach
5. Left kidney
6. Ureter
7. Bladder
8. Urethra
9. Rectum
10. Greater omentum covering small intestine
11. Spleen
12. Descending colon
13. Ductus deferens
14. Left testis
15. Prostate
16. Thymus

B, Female dog, right lateral view.

1. Right lung
2. Heart
3. Liver
4. Stomach
5. Right kidney
6. Ureter
7. Bladder
8. Urethra
9. Rectum
10. Greater omentum covering small intestine
11. Descending duodenum
12. Right uterine horn
13. Right ovary
14. Vagina

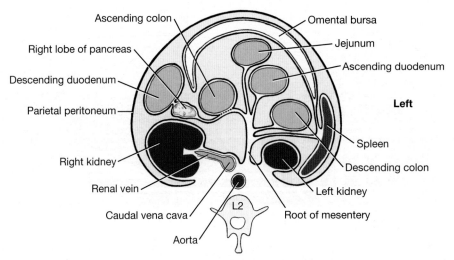

Fig. 4-10   Abdominal mesenteries. Schematic transverse section at the level of the spleen.

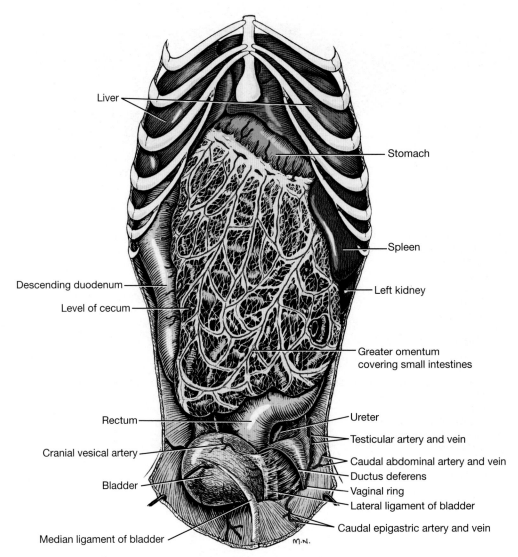

Fig. 4-11   Abdominal viscera of the male dog, ventral aspect.

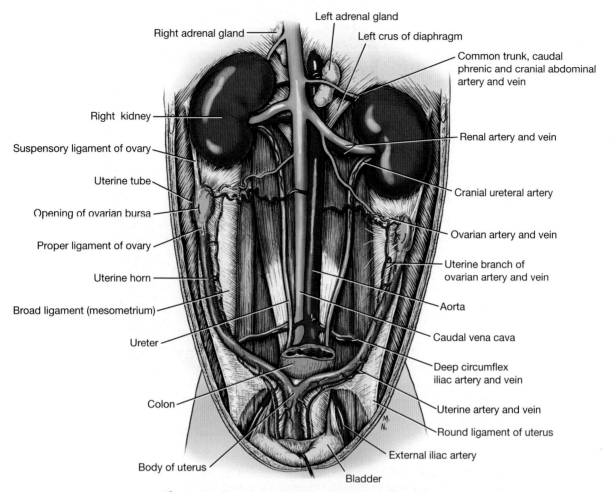

Right adrenal gland
Left adrenal gland
Left crus of diaphragm
Common trunk, caudal phrenic and cranial abdominal artery and vein
Right kidney
Renal artery and vein
Suspensory ligament of ovary
Uterine tube
Cranial ureteral artery
Opening of ovarian bursa
Ovarian artery and vein
Proper ligament of ovary
Uterine branch of ovarian artery and vein
Uterine horn
Broad ligament (mesometrium)
Aorta
Ureter
Caudal vena cava
Deep circumflex iliac artery and vein
Colon
Uterine artery and vein
Round ligament of uterus
Body of uterus
External iliac artery
Bladder

Fig. 4-12 Female urogenital system, ventral aspect.

a barbiturate, the spleen may be abnormally enlarged.

The **diaphragm** (Fig. 4-15), the muscular partition between the thoracic and the abdominal cavities, is a muscle of inspiration. It has an extensive muscular periphery and a small, V-shaped tendinous center. The muscular part of the diaphragm is divided into three parts according to its attachments: lumbar, costal, and sternal. The lumbar part forms the left and right crura that attach to the bodies of the third and fourth lumbar vertebrae by large tendons. The right crus is larger than the left. The costal part of the diaphragm arises from the medial surfaces of the eighth to thirteenth ribs. It interdigitates with the transversus abdominis muscle. The sternal part is narrow and arises from the dorsal surface of the sternum cranial to the xiphoid cartilage. The cupula is the most cranial extent of the dome-shaped diaphragm that bulges into the thorax. The extensions of the V-shaped tendinous center run dorsally between the lumbar

and costal parts of each side. The caudal mediastinum may be severed to expose the tendinous part of the muscle.

The **aortic hiatus** is a dorsal passageway between the crura for the aorta, the azygos vein, and the thoracic duct. The more centrally located **esophageal hiatus** is in the muscular part of the right crus and transmits the esophagus, vagal nerve trunks, and esophageal vessels. The **caval foramen** is located at the junction of the tendinous and muscular parts of the right side of the diaphragm. The caudal vena cava passes through it.

The **liver** (see Figs. 4-8, 4-9, 4-11, 4-14, 4-16, 4-17, 4-20) has six lobes, and its parietal surface conforms to the abdominal surface of the diaphragm. The visceral surface of the liver is related on the left to the stomach and sometimes to the spleen; on the right to the pancreas, right kidney, and duodenum; and ventrally to the greater omentum and through this to the small intestine. Its most caudal part covers the cranial extremity

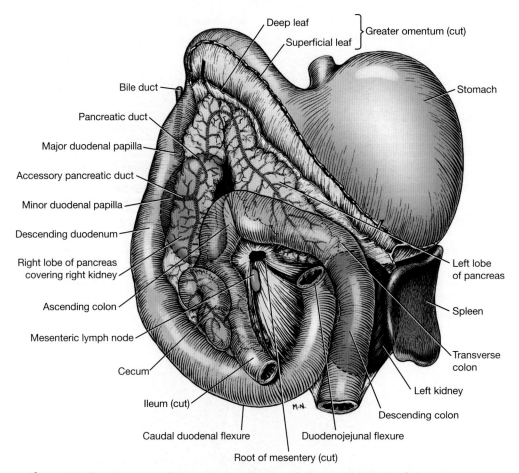

Fig. 4-13 Duodenum and transverse colon in relation to the root of the mesentery. Pancreas in situ and position of kidneys indicated by *dotted line.* Ventral aspect.

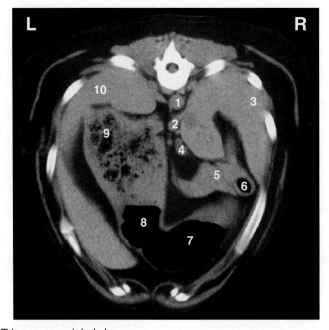

Fig. 4-14 CT image, cranial abdomen.
1. Aorta
2. Caudal vena cava
3. Right lateral lobe—liver
4. Portal vein
5. Right lobe of pancreas
6. Descending duodenum
7. Pyloric antrum
8. Body—stomach
9. Fundus of stomach
10. Spleen

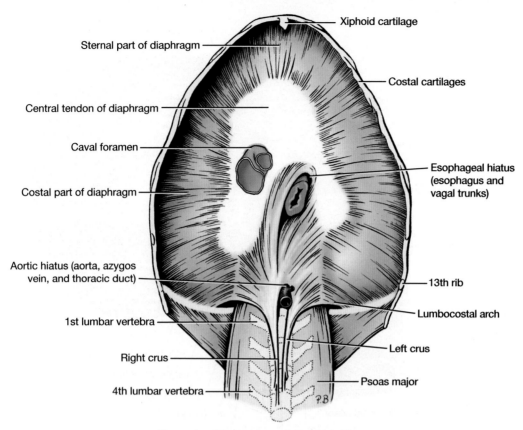

Xiphoid cartilage

Sternal part of diaphragm

Costal cartilages

Central tendon of diaphragm

Caval foramen

Esophageal hiatus (esophagus and vagal trunks)

Costal part of diaphragm

Aortic hiatus (aorta, azygos vein, and thoracic duct)

13th rib

Lumbocostal arch

1st lumbar vertebra

Left crus

Right crus

Psoas major

4th lumbar vertebra

Fig. 4-15   Diaphragm, abdominal view.

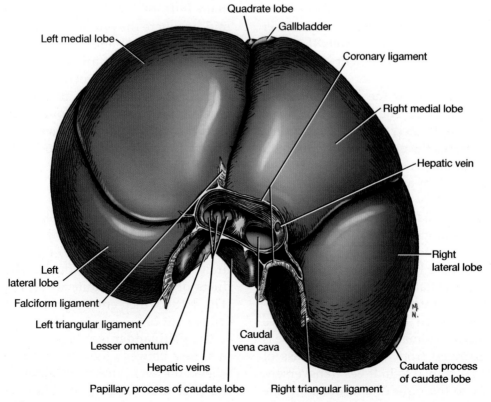

Quadrate lobe

Gallbladder

Left medial lobe

Coronary ligament

Right medial lobe

Hepatic vein

Left lateral lobe

Right lateral lobe

Falciform ligament

Left triangular ligament

Lesser omentum

Caudal vena cava

Hepatic veins

Caudate process of caudate lobe

Papillary process of caudate lobe

Right triangular ligament

Fig. 4-16   Liver, diaphragmatic aspect. Dog in dorsal recumbency: cranial to caudal view.

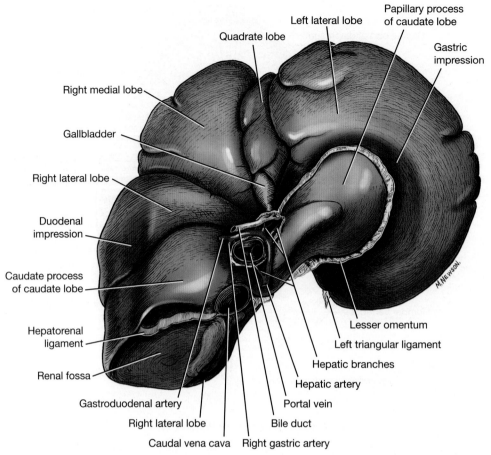

Right medial lobe
Gallbladder
Right lateral lobe
Duodenal impression
Caudate process of caudate lobe
Hepatorenal ligament
Renal fossa
Gastroduodenal artery
Right lateral lobe
Caudal vena cava
Quadrate lobe
Left lateral lobe
Papillary process of caudate lobe
Gastric impression
Lesser omentum
Left triangular ligament
Hepatic branches
Hepatic artery
Portal vein
Bile duct
Right gastric artery

Fig. 4-17   Liver, visceral aspect. Dog in dorsal recumbency: caudal to cranial view.

of the right kidney and reaches a transverse plane through the thirteenth thoracic vertebra. The liver rarely projects caudal to the costal arch. It undergoes slight longitudinal movement with each respiration.

The right medial lobe of the liver contains a fossa for the gallbladder. The right lateral lobe, which is smaller, is located next to the caudate lobe, which embraces the cranial end of the right kidney. The quadrate lobe is narrow and is located between the right and left medial lobes. It forms the left boundary of the fossa of the gallbladder. The left medial lobe is separated by a fissure from the right medial and quadrate lobes. The umbilical vein enters the liver through this fissure. The left lateral lobe is separated by a fissure from the left medial lobe. The free margin of the left lateral lobe is frequently notched. The visceral surface of the left lateral lobe is concave where it contacts the stomach. The caudate lobe is indistinctly separated from the central mass of the liver, which is cranial to it. It lies transversely, but it is mainly to the right of and dorsal to the

main bulk of the organ. It is constricted in its middle where the portal vein enters the liver ventral to it and the caudal vena cava crosses dorsal to it. Its extremities are in the form of two processes. The caudate process caps the cranial end of the right kidney and thus contains the deep renal impression. The papillary process can be seen through the lesser omentum if the liver is tipped forward. It lies in the lesser curvature of the stomach.

Biliary Passages

Much of the biliary duct system within the liver is microscopic. The bile, which is secreted by the liver cells, is collected into the canaliculi, which drain into interlobular ducts. The interlobular ducts of each lobe unite to form **hepatic ducts** (Fig. 4-18), which emerge from each lobe. The arrangement of the hepatic ducts is variable.

The **gallbladder** (see Figs. 4-17, 4-18) is located in a fossa between the quadrate and right medial lobes of the liver. A full gallbladder extends through the liver and contacts the diaphragm (which is

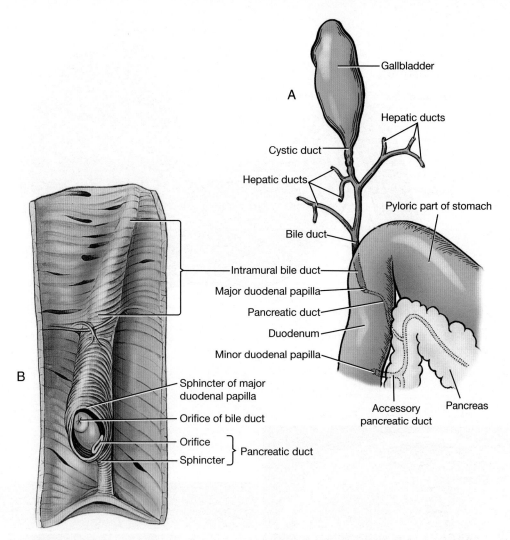

Fig. 4-18 Biliary and pancreatic ducts. **A,** Topographic relations, ventral view. **B,** Interior of the duodenum with the tunica mucosa removed to show musculus proprius in relation to the ducts and major duodenal papilla. (After Eichorn E, Boyden E: The choledochoduodenal junction in the dog: a restudy of Oddi's sphincter, *Am J Anat* 97:431, 1955. Copyright 1955 Wiley-Liss. Reprinted by permission of Wiley-Liss, Inc., a subsidiary of John Wiley & Sons, Inc.)

often stained green in preserved specimens). The neck of the gallbladder is continued as the cystic duct.

The main duct formed by the union of the hepatic ducts and the cystic duct from the gallbladder is the **bile duct (ductus choledochus).** It courses through the wall of the descending duodenum and terminates on the major duodenal papilla alongside the pancreatic duct. There are no valves in the biliary ducts, and bile may flow in either direction. Observe the duct system in your specimen.

The **stomach** (Figs. 4-8, 4-9, 4-11, 4-13, 4-14, 4-19, 4-20) is divided into parts that blend imperceptibly

with one another. The **cardiac part** is the smallest part of the stomach and is situated nearest the esophagus. The **fundus** is dome-shaped and lies to the left of and dorsal to the cardia. The **body** of the stomach is the large middle portion. It extends from the fundus on the left to the pyloric part on the right. The body joins the **pyloric part** at the angular incisure, which is the relatively sharp bend on the lesser curvature. The pyloric part is the distal third of the stomach as measured along the lesser curvature. The initial thin-walled portion is the **pyloric antrum,** which narrows to a **pyloric canal** before joining the duodenum at the sphincter, the **pylorus.**

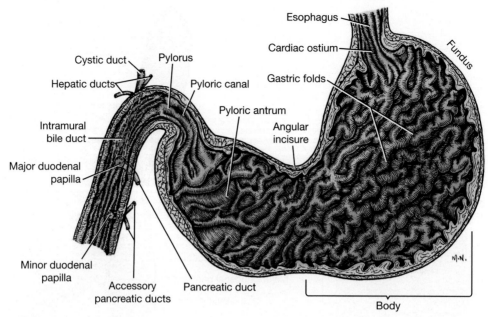

Fig. 4-19   Longitudinal section of stomach and proximal duodenum. Dog in dorsal recumbency: caudal to cranial view.

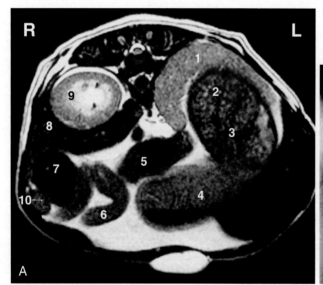

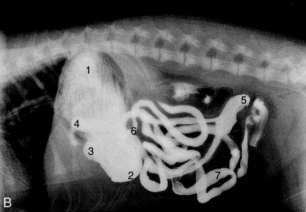

Fig. 4-20   A, MRI of cranial abdomen.
1. Spleen
2. Fundus of stomach
3. Body of stomach
4. Pyloric antrum
5. Transverse colon
6. Jejunum
7. Ascending colon
8. Caudate lobe—liver
9. Right kidney
10. Descending duodenum

B, Lateral radiograph of the abdomen with barium. (Part **B** from Evans HE, de Lahunta A: *Miller's anatomy of the dog,* ed 4, St Louis, 2013, Saunders.)
1. Fundus of stomach
2. Body of stomach
3. Pylorus of stomach
4. Cranial duodenum
5. Caudal duodenal flexure
6. Duodenojejunal flexure
7. Jejunum

The stomach is bent so that its greater curvature faces mainly to the left and its lesser curvature faces mainly to the right; its parietal surface faces cranioventrally toward the liver, and its visceral surface caudodorsally faces the intestinal mass. Its position changes depending on its fullness.

The **empty stomach** is completely hidden from palpation and observation by the liver and diaphragm cranioventrally and the intestinal mass caudally. It lies to the left of the median plane. The empty stomach is cranial to the costal arch and sharply curved, so that it is more V-shaped than C-shaped. The greater curvature faces ventrally, caudally, and to the left. This curvature lies above and to the left of the mass of the small intestine. The lesser curvature is strongly curved around the papillary process of the liver and faces craniodorsally and to the right. The left lobe of the pancreas and transverse colon are dorsocaudal to it.

The **full stomach** lies in contact with the ventral abdominal wall and protrudes beyond the costal arches. It displaces the intestinal mass. Open the stomach along its parietal surface, remove the contents, and observe the longitudinal folds of mucosa—the rugae.

The **duodenum** (see Figs. 4-9 through 4-11, 4-13, 4-14, 4-19, 4-20, 4-26) is the most fixed part of the small intestine. It is suspended by the mesoduodenum, which will be studied later. Reflect the greater omentum cranially and the jejunum to either side to expose the duodenum. The duodenum begins at the pylorus to the right of the median plane. After a short dorsocranial course, it turns as the **cranial duodenal flexure**. It continues caudally on the right as the **descending part**, where it is in contact with the parietal peritoneum. Farther caudally the duodenum turns, forming the **caudal duodenal flexure,** and continues cranially as the **ascending part**. The ascending part is short and lies to the left of the root of the mesentery, where it terminates at the **duodenojejunal flexure** (Fig. 4-20, *B*).

The **jejunum** forms the coils of the small intestine (Figs. 4-9 through 4-11), which occupy the ventrocaudal part of the abdominal cavity. They receive their nutrition from the cranial mesenteric artery, which is in the root of the mesentery. The root of the mesentery attaches the jejunum and ileum to the dorsal body wall. The **mesenteric lymph nodes** lie along the vessels in the mesentery. The jejunum begins at the left of the root of the mesentery and is the longest portion of the small intestine. Trace it from the duodenojejunal flexure on the left to its termination at the ileum on the right side of the abdomen. The **ileum** is the terminal portion of the small intestine (see Figs. 4-13, 4-21, 4-29, 4-31, 4-32, 4-34). It is short and passes cranially on the right side of the root of the mesentery and joins the ascending colon at the **ileocolic orifice**. This narrow orifice is surrounded by a sphincter. There is no clear demarcation between jejunum and ileum. Note the vessel that courses on the antimesenteric side of the ileum from the cecum toward the jejunum. This approximates the length of the ileum (10 cm).

The **cecum** (see Figs. 4-13, 4-21, 4-29, 4-31, 4-32, 4-34), a part of the large intestine, is an S-shaped, blind tube located to the right of the median plane at the junction of the ileum and colon. It is ventral to the caudal extremity of the right kidney, dorsal to the small intestine, and medial to the descending part of the duodenum. The cecum communicates with the ascending colon at the **cecocolic orifice**. Open the cecum, terminal ileum, and adjacent ascending colon and observe the ileocolic and cecocolic orifices.

The **colon** (see Figs. 4-8 through 4-10, 4-13, 4-20, 4-21, 4-29, 4-31, 4-32, 4-34) is located dorsally in the abdomen, suspended by a mesocolon. It is divided into a short **ascending colon,** which lies on the right of the root of the mesentery; a **transverse colon,** which lies cranial to the root of the mesentery; and a long **descending colon,** which lies at its beginning on the left of the root of the mesentery. The bend between the ascending and transverse colons is known as the **right colic flexure,** and that between the transverse and descending colons is

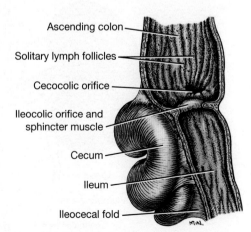

Fig. 4-21 Longitudinal section through ileocolic junction showing cecocolic orifice.

Ascending colon

Solitary lymph follicles

Cecocolic orifice

Ileocolic orifice and sphincter muscle

Cecum

Ileum

Ileocecal fold

known as the **left colic flexure.** The descending colon terminates at a transverse plane through the pelvic inlet. It is continued by the rectum.

The **pancreas** (see Figs. 4-8, 4-13, 4-14, 4-18, 4-26, 4-29, 4-34) is lobulated and is composed of a body and two lobes. The **body** lies at the pylorus. The **right lobe** lies dorsomedial to the descending part of the duodenum enclosed by the mesoduodenum. It is ventral to the right kidney. Pull the descending duodenum ventrally and to the left to expose this right lobe of the pancreas in the mesoduodenum. The **left lobe** of the pancreas lies between the peritoneal layers that form the deep leaf of the greater omentum. It is caudal to the stomach and liver and cranial to the transverse colon. Reflect the greater omentum cranially and the small intestine and transverse colon caudally to observe the pancreas.

The pancreatic duct system (see Figs. 4-13, 4-18, 4-19) is variable. Most dogs have two ducts; these open separately in the duodenum but communicate in the gland. The **pancreatic duct** is the smaller of the two ducts and is sometimes absent. It opens close to the bile duct on the **major duodenal papilla.** Make an incision through the free border of the cranial part of the descending duodenum. Scrape away the mucosa with the scalpel handle and identify the major duodenal papilla. This is on the side where the mesoduodenum attaches. The larger **accessory pancreatic duct** opens into the duodenum on the **minor duodenal papilla** 2 or 3 cm caudal to the major papilla.

Locate the accessory duct by blunt dissection in the mesoduodenum between the right lobe of the pancreas and the descending duodenum.

The **adrenal glands** (see Figs. 4-12, 4-22, 4-27) are light-colored and are located at the cranial aspect of each kidney. Each gland is crossed ventrally by the common trunk of the caudal phrenic and cranial abdominal veins, which leaves a deep groove on its ventral surface.

The right adrenal gland lies between the caudal vena cava and the caudate lobe of the liver ventrally and the sublumbar muscles dorsally. Expose the gland by dissection between the caudal vena cava and the kidney cranial to the renal vein. The left adrenal gland lies between the aorta and the left kidney. Transect each adrenal and note the lighter-colored cortex and darker medulla.

The **kidneys** (see Figs. 4-9 through 4-13, 4-20, 4-22, 4-23, 4-27) are dark brown. They are partly surrounded by fat and are covered only on their ventral surface by peritoneum. For this reason they are considered to be retroperitoneal organs. The lateral border is strongly convex, and the medial, nearly straight. At the middle of the medial border is an indentation, the **hilus** of the kidney, where the renal vessels and nerves and the ureter communicate with the organ.

The **right kidney** lies opposite the first three lumbar vertebrae. It is farther cranial than the left kidney by the length of half a kidney. The right kidney is more extensively related to the liver

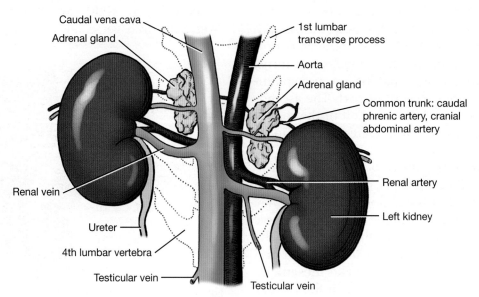

Caudal vena cava
Adrenal gland
1st lumbar transverse process
Aorta
Adrenal gland
Common trunk: caudal phrenic artery, cranial abdominal artery
Renal artery
Left kidney
Renal vein
Ureter
4th lumbar vertebra
Testicular vein
Testicular vein

Fig. 4-22 Kidneys and adrenal glands, ventral view.

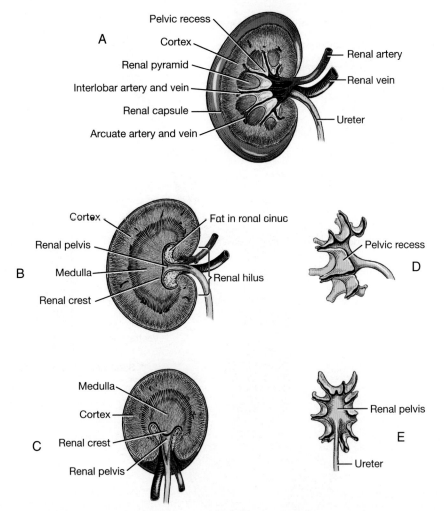

Fig. 4-23 Details of kidney structure. **A,** Sectioned in dorsal plane, off center. **B,** Sectioned in mid-dorsal plane. **C,** Transverse section. **D,** Cast of renal pelvis, dorsal view. **E,** Cast of renal pelvis, medial view.

than to any other organ. Its cranial third is covered by the caudate process of the caudate lobe of the liver. The remaining ventral surface is related to the descending duodenum, the right lobe of the pancreas, the cecum, and the ascending colon. The caudal vena cava is on the medial border of the right kidney.

The **left kidney** lies opposite the second, third, and fourth lumbar vertebrae. It is related ventrally to the descending colon and the small intestine. The spleen is related to the cranial extremity of the kidney. The medial border is close to the aorta.

The expanded part of the **ureter** within the kidney is the **renal pelvis.** The ureter courses caudally in the sublumbar region. It opens into the dorsal part of the neck of the urinary bladder. Throughout this course it is enveloped by a fold of peritoneum from the dorsal body wall. Follow

the course of the ureter. The **renal sinus** is the fat-filled space that contains the renal vessels and surrounds the renal pelvis.

Free the left kidney from its covering peritoneum and fascia. Do not cut its vascular attachment. Make a dorsal plane longitudinal section of the left kidney from its lateral border to the hilus, dividing it into dorsal and ventral halves. Note the granular appearance of the peripheral portion of the renal parenchyma. This is the **renal cortex,** which contains primarily the renal corpuscles and convoluted portions of the tubules. The more centrally positioned parenchyma is the **medulla.** It has a striated appearance owing to numerous collecting ducts. The vessels that are apparent at the corticomedullary junction are the **arcuate branches** of the renal vessels. The longitudinal ridge projecting into the renal pelvis is the **renal crest,** through which collecting

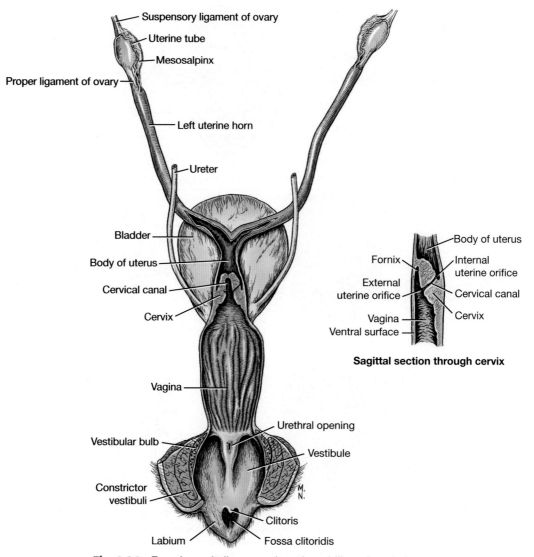

Fig. 4-24   Female genitalia opened on the midline, dorsal view.

tubules of the kidney excrete urine into the renal pelvis. Make a second longitudinal section parallel to the first and note the **renal pyramids** formed by the medulla. The **pelvic recesses** of the renal pelvis project outward between the renal pyramids.

Free the right kidney from its peritoneum and fascia and make a transverse section through it. Note the renal cortex, medulla, crest, and pelvis.

The **ovaries** (see Figs. 4-9, 4-12, 4-24, 4-25) are located near the caudal pole of the kidneys. The right ovary lies cranial to the left ovary and is dorsal to the descending duodenum. The left ovary is between the descending colon and the abdominal wall. Each ovary is enclosed in a thin-walled peritoneal sac, the **ovarian bursa** (see

Fig. 4-25), formed by the mesovarium and mesosalpinx. The **ovarian bursa** is open to the peritoneal cavity by means of a slitlike orifice on the medial surface.

The uterine tube courses cranially and then caudally through the lateral wall of the bursa on its way to the uterine horn. Examine the surface of the bursa and observe the small cordlike thickening within its wall. This is the uterine tube. Open the bursa by a lateral incision dorsal to the uterine tube and examine the ovary and the infundibulum. The infundibulum is the dilated ovarian end of the uterine tube. It has a fimbriated margin and functions to engulf the oocyte after ovulation. Note that several of the fimbriae protrude into the peritoneal cavity from the opening of the ovarian

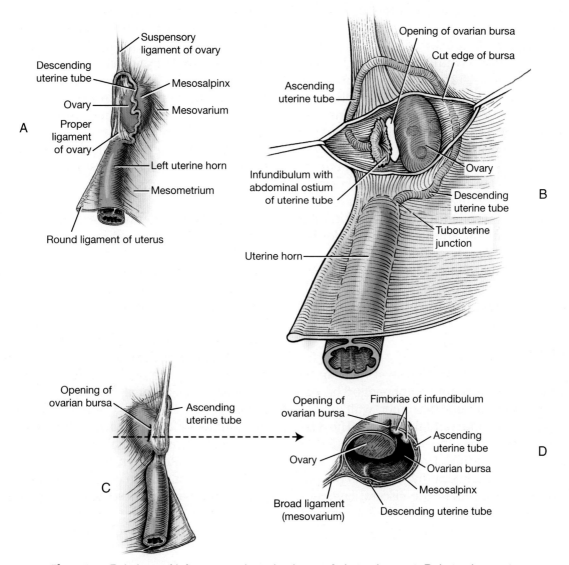

Fig. 4-25   Relations of left ovary and ovarian bursa. **A,** Lateral aspect. **B,** Lateral aspect, bursa opened. **C,** Medial aspect. **D,** Section through ovary and bursa.

bursa. In life, these fimbriae function to close the opening into the peritoneal cavity at the time of ovulation and thus prevent transperitoneal migration of oocytes. The entrance of the infundibulum into the uterine tube is often described as the abdominal ostium, and it is in this region that fertilization takes place. The uterine tube is short and slender. It opens into the much wider uterine horn at the tubouterine junction. This region is of physiological importance because it is here that sperm and ova are regulated in their transit.

The **broad ligaments** of the uterus (see Figs. 4-12, 4-25) are the peritoneal folds on each side that attach to the lateral sublumbar region. They suspend all the internal genitalia except the caudal part of the vagina, which is not covered by peritoneum. Each ligament is divided into three parts: The **mesometrium** arises from the lateral wall of the pelvis and the lateral part of the sublumbar region and attaches to the lateral part of the cranial end of the vagina, uterine cervix, and uterine body, and the corresponding uterine horn. The **mesovarium,** a continuation of the mesometrium, is the cranial part of the broad ligament. It begins at a transverse plane through the cranial end of the uterine horn and attaches the ovary and the ligaments associated with the ovary to the lateral part of the sublumbar region. The **mesosalpinx** is the peritoneum that attaches the uterine tube to the mesovarium and forms with the mesovarium the wall of the ovarian bursa.

The **suspensory ligament of the ovary** joins the transversalis fascia medial to the dorsal end of the last rib (see Figs. 4-12, 4-24, 4-25). It functions to hold the ovary in a relatively fixed position. In ovariohysterectomy this ligament is freed from its attachment to the body wall to facilitate removal of the ovary. The **proper ligament of the ovary** is short and attaches the ovary to the cranial end of the uterine horn. From this point caudolaterally to the inguinal canal, there is a fold from the lateral layer of the mesometrium that contains the **round ligament of the uterus** in its free border (see Figs. 4-12, 4-25). The round ligament, a homologue of the embryonic gubernaculum, has no function in the adult. It passes through the inguinal canal and is wrapped by the vaginal process and adipose tissue.

Peritoneum

The peritoneum is a mesothelial layer that can be divided into three regional components. The **parietal peritoneum** covers the inner wall of the abdominal, pelvic, and scrotal cavities. The **visceral peritoneum** covers the organs suspended in these cavities. The **connecting peritoneum** is a double sheet of peritoneum that connects the parietal and visceral layers or the visceral layers of adjacent organs, forming peritoneal folds referred to as *mesenteries, omenta,* or *ligaments.*

In the embryo the dorsal common mesentery is a double layer of peritoneum that passes from the dorsal abdominal wall to the digestive tube. It serves as a route by which the nerves and vessels reach the organs. In the embryo, the dorsal common mesentery persists from cranial to caudal as the greater omentum, mesoduodenum, mesentery, and mesocolon.

An **omentum** (epiploon) is the connecting peritoneum that attaches the stomach to the body wall or other organs. It is an extended mesogastrium.

The **greater omentum** (see Figs. 4-8 through 4-11, 4-13, 4-26), an extended fold of dorsal mesogastrium, attaches the greater curvature of the stomach to the dorsal body wall. From the greater curvature of the stomach, it extends caudally within the peritoneal cavity as the superficial leaf between the jejunum and the ventral abdominal wall. It turns dorsally on itself near the pelvic inlet and returns as the deep leaf dorsal to the stomach, where it contains the left lobe of the pancreas between its peritoneal layers. It attaches to the dorsal abdominal wall. Caudal and to the left of the fundus of the stomach is the spleen, which lies largely in an outpocketing of the superficial leaf of the greater omentum.

The lesser omentum (see Figs. 4-8, 4-16, 4-17), a part of the ventral mesogastrium, loosely spans the distance from the lesser curvature of the stomach to the porta of the liver. Between the

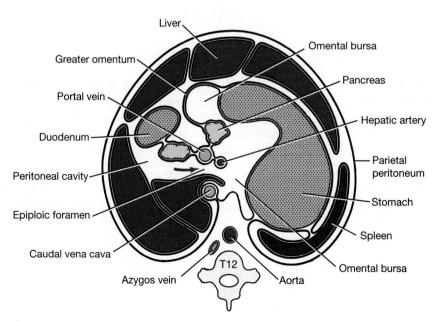

Fig. 4-26 Peritoneal schema. Transverse section through the epiploic foramen.

liver and the cardia of the stomach, it attaches for a short distance to the diaphragm. The papillary process of the liver is loosely enveloped by the lesser omentum. On the right the free edge of the lesser omentum is the hepatoduodenal ligament, which attaches the liver to the duodenum. It contains the portal vein, the hepatic artery, and the bile duct.

The **omental bursa** (see Figs. 4-8, 4-10, 4-26) is formed by the omenta and the adjacent organs. It has an **epiploic foramen** opening into the main peritoneal cavity. This opening lies dorsally to the right of the median plane at the level of the cranial duodenal flexure, caudomedial to the caudate lobe of the liver. It is bounded dorsally by the caudal vena cava, ventrally by the portal vein, caudally by the hepatic artery in the mesoduodenum, and cranially by the liver. Find this foramen and insert a finger through it.

The **mesoduodenum** originates at the dorsal abdominal wall and the root of the mesentery and extends to the duodenum. On the right side it passes to the descending duodenum and encloses the right lobe of the pancreas between its layers. Cranially, it is continuous with the greater omentum across the ventral surface of the portal vein. Caudally, the mesoduodenum passes from the root of the mesentery to the caudal flexure of the duodenum. On the left, it is attached to the ascending duodenum, and at the duodenojejunal flexure, it is continuous with the mesentery of the jejunum. The ascending duodenum is secondarily attached to the mesocolon of the descending colon by the **duodenocolic fold.**

The **mesentery** (mesojejunoileum) attaches to the abdominal wall opposite the second lumbar vertebra by a short peritoneal attachment known as the **root of the mesentery.** Vessels and nerves pass in the mesentery to supply the large and small intestines. The peripheral border of the mesentery attaches to the jejunum and the ileum. At the ileocolic junction, the mesentery is continuous with the ascending mesocolon. The **ascending, transverse,** and **descending mesocolons** respectively connect the ascending, transverse, and descending colons to the dorsal body wall. They are continuous with each other from right to left.

There are a few short peritoneal folds that serve more to fix organs in position than as channels for blood vessels. These are called *ligaments:* The **right triangular ligament** extends from the right crus of the diaphragm above the central tendinous part to the right lateral lobe of the liver. The **left triangular ligament** extends from the left crus of the diaphragm to the left lateral lobe of the liver.

The **coronary ligament** is a sheet of peritoneum that passes between the diaphragm and the liver around the caudal vena cava and hepatic veins. On the right it is continuous with the right triangular ligament, and on the left it is continuous with the left triangular ligament. Ventrally, right and left parts of the coronary ligament converge to form the falciform ligament.

The **falciform ligament** (see Fig. 4-16) extends from the liver to the diaphragm and ventral abdominal wall to the umbilicus. The round ligament of the liver, which is the remnant of the **umbilical vein** of the fetus, may be found in the young animal as a small fibrous cord lying in the free edge of the falciform ligament. It enters the fissure for the round ligament of the liver between the quadrate and left medial lobes. In adult dogs the falciform ligament is filled with fat, and it persists only from the diaphragm to the umbilicus.

Vessels and Nerves of the Abdominal Viscera

Vagal Nerves

The **vagus nerve**, or tenth cranial nerve (see Figs. 3-20, 4-27, 5-50), carries both sensory and motor axons from and to the viscera. About 20% are visceral motor (preganglionic parasympathetic efferent fibers), and about 80% are visceral sensory (afferents from all of the thoracic and most of the abdominal organs). The vagus nerve leaves the cranial cavity via the tympano-occipital fissure and traverses the neck in the carotid sheath with the sympathetic trunk. At the thoracic inlet, the vagus separates from the sympathetic trunk and continues over the base of the heart where the recurrent laryngeal nerve branches from it. Right and left vagus nerves divide caudal to the root of the lung into **dorsal** and **ventral branches**. The dorsal branches unite near the diaphragm to form the **dorsal vagal trunk**. The ventral branches unite caudal to the root of the lung to form the **ventral vagal trunk**. These trunks lie on the dorsal and ventral surfaces of the terminal part of the esophagus. From the trunks, as well as from the dorsal and ventral branches of the vagi, nerves arise to supply the esophagus. The vagal trunks pass through the esophageal hiatus of the diaphragm and course along the lesser curvature of the stomach.

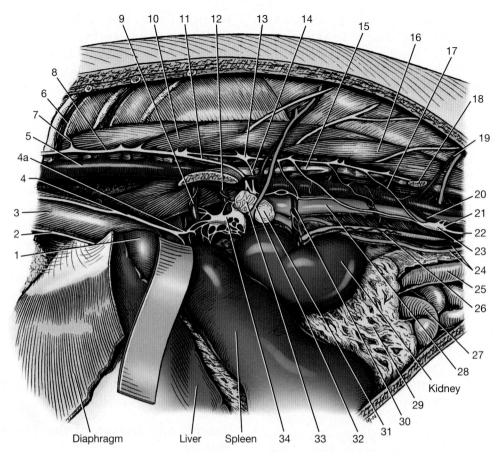

Fig. 4-27   Exposure of abdominal autonomic nervous system on left side.

1. Stomach
2. Ventral trunk of vagus n.
3. Esophagus
4. Dorsal trunk of vagus n.
4a. Celiac br. of dorsal vagal trunk
5. Aorta
6. Intercostal a. and n.
7. Ramus communicans
8. Sympathetic trunk
9. Celiac a.
10. Quadratus lumborum
11. Major splanchnic n.
12. Cranial mesenteric a.
13. Lumbar sympathetic ganglion at L2
14. Minor splanchnic n.
15. Tendon of left crus of diaphragm
16. Psoas major
17. Lumbar splanchnic n.
18. Transected psoas minor

19. Deep circumflex iliac a.
20. Caudal mesenteric a.
21. Left hypogastric n.
22. Caudal mesenteric plexus
23. Caudal mesenteric ganglion
24. Testicular a. and v.
25. Descending colon
26. Cranial ureteral a.
27. Jejunum
28. Caudal vena cava
29. Greater omentum
30. Renal a. and plexus
31. Adrenal gland
32. Common trunk for caudal phrenic and
    cranial abdominal v.
33. Adrenal plexus
34. Celiac and cranial mesenteric ganglia
    and plexus

Transect the left crus of the diaphragm at the esophageal hiatus and reflect it to expose the vagal trunks. Observe the ventral vagal trunk. It supplies the liver, the parietal surface of the stomach, and the pylorus. The terminal branches need not be dissected.

The **dorsal vagal trunk** (see Fig. 4-27) gives off a **celiac branch** that passes dorsocaudally and contributes to the formation of the celiac and cranial

mesenteric plexuses. These abdominal aortic plexuses are nerve networks lying on, lying around, and passing along abdominal vessels for which they are named. Parasympathetic axons in these plexuses follow the terminal branching of the respective blood vessels to the intestines at least as far caudally as the left colic flexure. The dorsal vagal trunk continues along the lesser curvature of the stomach to supply the visceral surface of the stomach, including the pylorus. All of these parasympathetic preganglionic axons will synapse with a second neuron within the wall of the organ where they terminate. The abdominal aortic plexuses are named for the branch of the aorta with which they are associated or, in some instances, for the adjacent organ. They include the celiac, cranial mesenteric, caudal mesenteric, adrenal, and aorticorenal plexuses. The first three will be dissected.

In addition to the parasympathetic preganglionic axons described earlier, these plexuses contain sympathetic visceral efferent processes and numerous visceral afferent processes. Associated with many of these plexuses are abdominal sympathetic ganglia that contain cell bodies of sympathetic postganglionic axons. Within these ganglia are synapses with preganglionic sympathetic neurons that are destined to innervate the abdominal viscera.

Sympathetic Trunk

To expose the caudal thoracic and lumbar parts of the sympathetic trunk on the left side, reflect the abdominal and caudal thoracic walls so that the kidney and the crura of the diaphragm are freely accessible. Reflect the left kidney toward the median plane. The deep circumflex iliac artery and vein arise from the aorta and caudal vena cava in the caudal part of the lumbar region and may be transected and turned aside. These vessels will be described later with the branches of the abdominal aorta and caudal vena cava.

The psoas minor arises from the fascia of the muscle dorsal to it, the quadratus lumborum, and from the last thoracic and the first five lumbar vertebral bodies. It is ventral and medial to the quadratus lumborum and psoas major (see Figs. 2-51, 4-27, 4-65). It inserts on the arcuate line of the ilium dorsal to the iliopubic eminence. Transect the tendon of the psoas minor caudal to the deep circumflex iliac vessels. Remove the muscle from its vertebral origins. Examine the psoas major and its union with the iliacus to form the iliopsoas muscle.

Identify the thoracic and lumbar parts of the sympathetic trunk as it passes along the vertebral bodies. Because most of the preganglionic axons in the sympathetic trunk at levels T10 to T13 pass into the major splanchnic nerve rather than into the lumbar region of the trunk, there is a distinct narrowing of the trunk caudal to the major splanchnic nerve. The trunk widens again as lumbar rami communicantes and splanchnic components enter it (see Fig. 4-27).

Splanchnic Nerves

The **splanchnic nerves** contain sympathetic axons that run between the sympathetic trunk and the abdominal autonomic ganglia as well as axons of visceral afferents coursing to the spinal cord.

The **major splanchnic nerve** (see Fig. 4-27) leaves the sympathetic trunk at the level of the twelfth or thirteenth thoracic sympathetic ganglion. It passes dorsal to the crus of the diaphragm, enters the abdominal cavity, and courses to the adrenal and celiacomesenteric ganglia and plexuses.

The **minor splanchnic nerves** (see Fig. 4-27), generally two, usually leave the last thoracic and first lumbar sympathetic ganglia. They supply nerves to the adrenal gland, ganglion, and plexus, and they terminate in the celiacomesenteric ganglia and plexus. Dissect the origin of these nerves and their course to the adrenal gland.

The **lumbar splanchnic nerves** (see Fig. 4-27) arise from the second to the fifth lumbar sympathetic ganglia. In general, they are distributed to the aorticorenal, cranial mesenteric, and caudal mesenteric ganglia and plexuses. Observe the origin of these nerves.

Abdominal Aortic Nerve Plexuses and Ganglia

As noted previously, branches of the vagus and splanchnic sympathetic nerves intermingle around the major abdominal arteries to form nerve plexuses in the abdomen. The plexuses supply the musculature of the artery and arterioles, and the viscera supplied by the branches of that artery.

Several sympathetic ganglia are located in the abdomen in close association with the plexuses. These ganglia are collections of cell bodies of postganglionic axons. Preganglionic axons of sympathetic splanchnic nerves must synapse in one of these ganglia. Preganglionic vagal axons (parasympathetic) do not synapse here but pass through the ganglia and plexuses to the wall of the organ innervated, where they synapse on a cell body of a postganglionic axon.

The **celiac ganglia** (see Fig. 4-27) lie on the right and left surfaces of the celiac artery close to its origin. They are often interconnected, and numerous nerves from the ganglia follow the terminal branches of the celiac artery as a plexus.

The **cranial mesenteric ganglion** (see Fig. 4-27) is located caudal to the celiac ganglion on the sides and caudal surface of the cranial mesenteric artery, which it partly encircles. Most of its nerves continue distally on the cranial mesenteric artery as the cranial mesenteric plexus. Because of the close relationship of the celiac and cranial mesenteric plexuses and ganglia, they are referred to as the **celiacomesenteric ganglion and plexus.**

The **caudal mesenteric ganglion** (see Fig. 4-27) is located ventral to the aorta around the caudal mesenteric artery, which is an unpaired branch of the aorta caudal to the kidneys that supplies a portion of the colon. Lumbar splanchnic nerves enter the ganglion on each side. Branches may also come from the aortic and celiacomesenteric plexuses. Some of the nerves leaving the ganglion continue along the artery as the **caudal mesenteric plexus.**

The **right** and **left hypogastric nerves** leave the caudal mesenteric ganglion and course caudally near the ureters. They run in the mesocolon, incline laterally, and enter the pelvic canal. Their connections with the pelvic plexuses will be described later.

Branches of the Abdominal Aorta

Lumbar aa.
Celiac a.
  Hepatic a.
    Hepatic branches
      Cystic a.
    Right gastric a.
    Gastroduodenal a.
      Right gastroepiploic a.
      Cranial pancreaticoduodenal a.
  Left gastric a.
    Esophageal branches
  Splenic a.
    Pancreatic branches
    Short gastric aa.
    Left gastroepiploic a.
Cranial mesenteric a.
  Common trunk
    Middle colic a.
    Right colic a.
    Ileocolic a.
      Colic br.
      Mesenteric ileal br.
      Cecal a.
        Antimesenteric ileal br.

    Caudal pancreaticoduodenal a.
    Jejunal aa.
    Ileal aa.
Common trunk (Phrenicoabdominal a.)
  Caudal phrenic a.
  Cranial abdominal a.
Renal aa.
Testicular and ovarian aa.
Caudal mesenteric a.
  Left colic a.
  Cranial rectal a.
Deep circumflex iliac aa.

1. The paired **lumbar arteries** (see Figs. 4-27, 4-28, 4-33) leave the dorsal surface of the aorta. Each extends dorsally and terminates in a spinal and a dorsal branch. The spinal branches pass through the intervertebral foramina into the vertebral canal, where they penetrate the dura and arachnoid that surround the spinal cord. Here they anastomose with the ventral spinal artery that is within the subarachnoid space and supply part of the spinal cord. The dorsal branches supply the muscles and skin above the lumbar vertebrae.

2. The **celiac artery** (see Figs. 4-27 through 4-29) is short and arises from the aorta between the crura of the diaphragm. It has three branches: the hepatic artery, the left gastric artery, and the splenic artery. The celiac plexus of nerves covers the artery in its course through the mesentery.

   The **hepatic artery** (see Figs. 4-28, 4-29) is the first branch to leave the celiac artery. Find its origin. It courses cranially in the cranial border of the mesoduodenum, which is the caudal boundary of the epiploic foramen. It passes to the liver in the hepatoduodenal ligament. Follow this vessel dorsal to the pylorus between the lesser curvature of the stomach and the liver. One to five **hepatic branches** leave the hepatic artery and enter the liver. (These branches are covered with nerves and are closely associated with the hepatic lymph nodes.) The **cystic artery** leaves the last hepatic branch and supplies the gallbladder. It need not be dissected. After giving off branches to the liver, the hepatic artery terminates as the right gastric and the gastroduodenal arteries. This occurs in the lesser omentum.

   The **right gastric artery** is a small artery that extends from the pylorus toward the cardia to supply the lesser curvature of the stomach. It anastomoses with the left gastric artery. It need not be dissected.

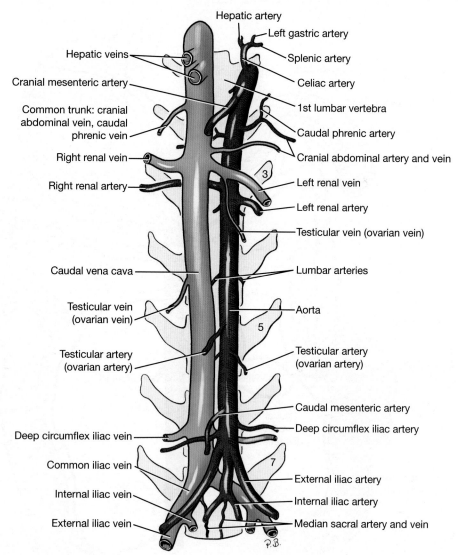

Fig. 4-28 Branches of abdominal aorta and tributaries of the caudal vena cava, ventral view.

The **gastroduodenal artery** supplies the pylorus and terminates as the right gastroepiploic and cranial pancreaticoduodenal arteries. This occurs at the junction of the greater omentum and the mesoduodenum.

The **right gastroepiploic artery** enters and runs in the greater omentum along the greater curvature of the stomach. It supplies the stomach and the greater omentum. The right gastroepiploic artery anastomoses with the left gastroepiploic, a branch of the splenic artery.

The **cranial pancreaticoduodenal artery** follows the mesenteric border of the descending duodenum, where it supplies the duodenum and adjacent right lobe of the pancreas. It anastomoses with the caudal pancreaticoduodenal

artery, which is a branch of the cranial mesenteric artery.

The **left gastric artery** (see Figs. 4-28, 4-29) branches from the celiac and runs in the greater omentum to the lesser curvature of the stomach near the cardia and supplies both surfaces of the stomach. One or more esophageal rami pass cranially on the esophagus. It extends toward the pylorus, where it anastomoses with the right gastric artery.

The **splenic artery** (see Figs. 4-28 through 4-30) crosses the dorsal surface of the left lobe of the pancreas in the deep leaf of the greater omentum—to which it may supply branches—before dividing into dorsal and ventral splenic branches that enter the hilus of the spleen on its

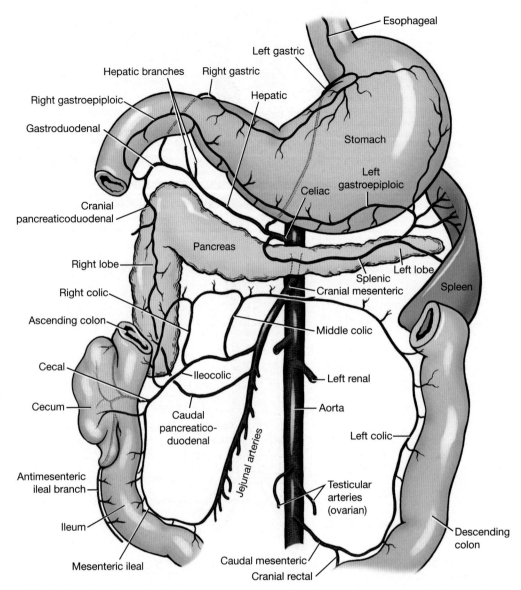

Fig. 4-29 Branches of celiac and cranial mesenteric arteries with principal anastomoses.

visceral surface. The dorsal branch gives rise to several arteries that enter the dorsal end of the spleen and a few **short gastric arteries** that course in the gastrosplenic ligament to the greater curvature of the stomach on the left side. The dorsal splenic branch continues as the **left gastroepiploic artery** on the greater curvature of the stomach. At the pyloric end of the stomach, the left gastroepiploic artery anastomoses with the right gastroepiploic artery, a branch of the hepatic artery. The ventral splenic branch supplies the rest of the spleen by numerous branches that enter at the hilus. Variations in this pattern exist, and you may find that the ventral branch of the splenic, rather than the

dorsal branch, gives rise to the left gastroepiploic artery.

3. The **cranial mesenteric artery** (see Figs. 4-28, 4-29, 4-31) leaves the aorta caudal to the celiac artery. It is surrounded proximally by the cranial mesenteric plexus of nerves and partly by the cranial mesenteric ganglion. Peripheral to the ganglion are the mesenteric lymph nodes and branches of the portal vein. Reflect these from the vessel. Observe the branches of the cranial mesenteric artery.

The middle, right, and ileocolic arteries arise from a common trunk from the cranial mesenteric artery and course through the mesocolon. Reflect the small intestine caudally and expose

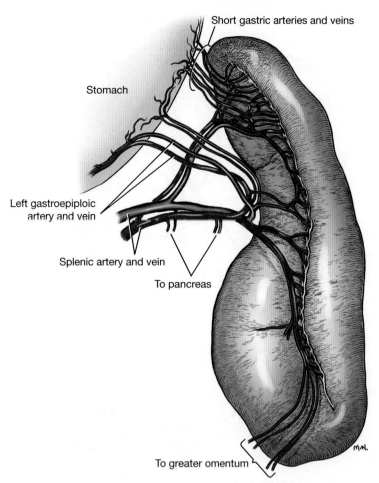

Short gastric arteries and veins

Stomach

Left gastroepiploic
artery and vein

Splenic artery and vein

To pancreas

To greater omentum

M.N.

Fig. 4-30 Blood supply of the spleen.

the colon cranial to the root of the mesentery. Dissect its blood supply within the mesocolon.

The **middle colic artery,** the first branch from the **common trunk,** runs cranially in the mesocolon to the mesenteric border of the left colic flexure and descending part of the colon. It bifurcates near the left colic flexure. One branch runs distally in the descending mesocolon, supplies the descending colon, and then anastomoses with the left colic artery, a branch of the caudal mesenteric artery. The other branch passes to the right and forms an arcade with the smaller right colic artery and supplies the transverse colon.

The **right colic artery** runs in the right mesocolon toward the right colic flexure, giving off branches to the distal part of the ascending colon and the adjacent transverse colon. It forms arcades with the middle colic artery and the colic branch of the ileocolic artery.

The **ileocolic artery** (see Figs. 4-29, 4-31, 4-32) supplies the ileum, cecum, and ascending colon. It is closely associated with the right colic lymph node. The ascending colon is supplied by the **colic branch.** The **cecal** artery crosses the dorsal surface of the ileocolic junction and supplies the cecum and antimesenteric side of the ileum. The ileocolic artery continues as the **mesenteric ileal branch** to anastomose with ileal arteries of the cranial mesenteric artery.

The caudal pancreaticoduodenal artery (see Figs. 4-29, 4-31) arises from the cranial mesenteric artery close to the common trunk for the colon. It runs to the right in the mesoduodenum to the descending portion of the duodenum near the caudal flexure. It supplies the descending duodenum and the right lobe of the pancreas and anastomoses with the cranial pancreaticoduodenal artery.

The **jejunal arteries** arise from the caudal side of the cranial mesenteric artery. They form arcades in the mesentery close to the jejunum.

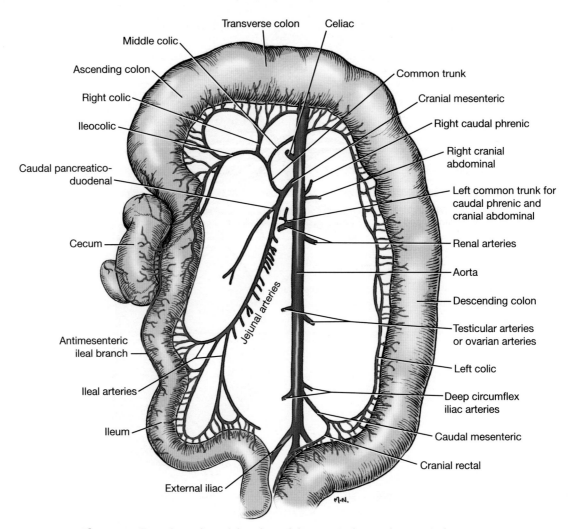

Fig. 4-31   Branches of cranial and caudal mesenteric arteries, ventral aspect.

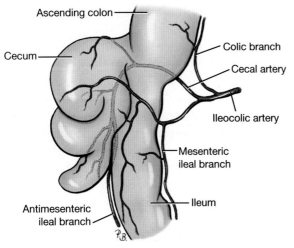

Fig. 4-32   Terminations of ileocolic artery.

The cranial mesenteric artery is terminated by **ileal arteries,** the last of which anastomoses with a branch of the ileocolic artery.

4. The **common trunk** of the caudal phrenic and cranial abdominal arteries (see Figs. 4-12, 4-22, 4-28, 4-31, 4-33) is paired and arises from the aorta between the cranial mesenteric and renal arteries. This common trunk crosses the ventral surface of the psoas muscles dorsal to the adrenal gland. The **caudal phrenic artery** runs cranially to supply the diaphragm. The **cranial abdominal artery** continues into the abdominal wall and ramifies between the transversus abdominis and the internal abdominal oblique, where it was previously dissected.

The adrenal gland may receive branches from the aorta or caudal phrenic, renal, or lumbar arteries.

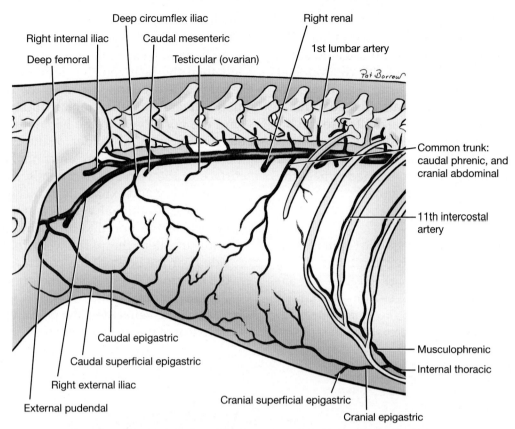

Fig. 4-33 Abdominal aorta in relation to epigastric arteries, lateral view.

5. The **renal arteries** (see Figs. 4-12, 4-22, 4-27, 4-28, 4-31, 4-33) leave the aorta at different levels. The right one arises cranial to the left, in conformity with the more cranial position of the right kidney. It is longer than the left and lies dorsal to the caudal vena cava.

6. The **ovarian artery** (see Figs. 4-12, 4-28, 4-31, 4-33) of the female is homologous to the testicular artery of the male. This paired vessel arises from the aorta about halfway between the renal and external iliac arteries. The ovarian artery varies in size, position, and tortuosity, depending on the degree of development of the uterus. Each ovarian artery divides into two or more branches in the mesovarium just medial to the ovaries. Branches supply the ovary and its bursa and the uterine tube and horn. The branch to the uterine horn anastomoses with the uterine artery, a branch of the vaginal artery that runs cranially in the mesometrium.

   The **testicular artery** (see Figs. 4-27 through 4-29, 4-31, 4-33) leaves the aorta in the midlumbar region and crosses the ventral surface of the ureter. The testicular artery, vein, and nerve

plexus lie in a peritoneal fold, the **mesorchium,** which can be followed to the level of the vaginal ring. Their course in the spermatic cord has been dissected.

The right testicular and ovarian veins enter the caudal vena cava near the origin of the artery from the aorta. However, the left testicular and ovarian veins usually enter the left renal vein. This is important surgically.

7. The **caudal mesenteric artery** (see Figs. 4-27 through 4-29, 4-31) is unpaired and arises near the termination of the aorta. It enters the descending mesocolon and runs caudoventrally to the mesenteric border of the descending colon, where it terminates in two branches of similar size. The **left colic artery** follows the mesenteric border of the descending colon cranially to anastomose with the middle colic artery. The **cranial rectal artery** descends along the rectum and anastomoses with the middle rectal artery from the prostatic or vaginal artery.

8. The **deep circumflex iliac artery** (see Figs. 4-12, 4-27, 4-28, 4-33) is paired and arises from the

aorta close to the origin of the external iliac artery. It crosses the sublumbar muscles laterally, and at the lateral border of the psoas major it supplies the musculature of the caudodorsal portion of the abdominal wall. The deep circumflex iliac artery perforates the abdominal wall and becomes superficial ventral to the tuber coxae. It supplies the skin of the caudal abdominal area, the flank, and the cranial thigh. This vessel was transected when the psoas minor muscle was removed.

Portal Venous System

A venous portal system consists of a capillary bed interposed between veins returning blood to the heart. The **portal vein** (see Figs. 4-17, 4-34, 4-35) carries venous blood to the liver from abdominal viscera such as the stomach, the small intestine, the cecum, the colon, the pancreas, and the spleen.

The liver has a capillary bed of sinusoids through which the blood passes before it exits through large hepatic veins to enter the caudal vena cava and then the heart on the right side (Fig. 4-16). Separate the caudate process of the caudate lobe of the liver from the cranial duodenal flexure. Find the portal vein in the hepatoduodenal ligament at the ventral border of the epiploic foramen. Reflect the peritoneum and fat from the surface of the vein as far caudally as the root of the mesentery and expose its branches.

1. The **gastroduodenal vein** is a small, proximal branch of the portal vein in the mesoduodenum. It enters the portal vein from the right side near the body of the pancreas and drains the pancreas, the stomach, the duodenum, and the greater omentum.
2. The **splenic vein** enters the portal vein from the deep leaf of the greater omentum on the left side

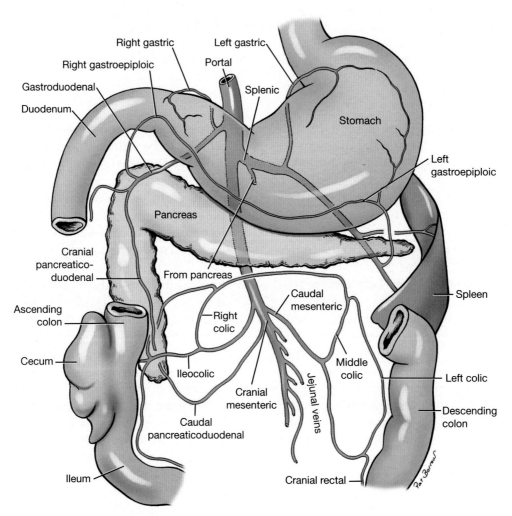

Fig. 4-34   Tributaries of portal vein, ventral view.

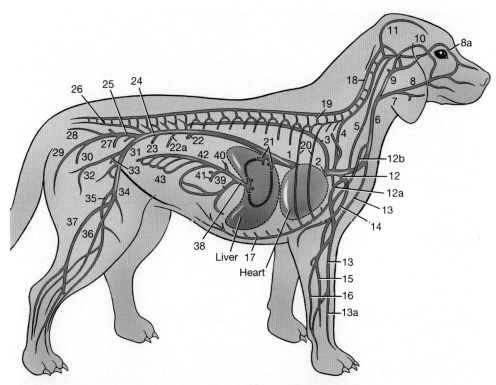

Fig. 4-35 Schema of the venous system, right lateral view.

1. Caudal vena cava
2. Cranial vena cava
3. Azygos
4. Vertebral
5. Internal jugular
6. External jugular
7. Linguofacial
8. Facial
8a. Angularis oculi
9. Maxillary
10. Superficial temporal
11. Dorsal sagittal sinus
12. Axillary
12a. Axillobrachial
12b. Omobrachial
13. Cephalic
13a. Accessory cephalic
14. Brachial
15. Median
16. Ulnar
17. Internal thoracic
18. Right internal ventral vertebral
    venous plexus
19. Intervertebral
20. Intercostal
21. Hepatic
22. Renal
22a. Testicular or ovarian
23. Deep circumflex iliac
24. Common iliac
25. Right internal iliac
26. Median sacral
27. Vaginal or prostatic
28. Lateral caudal
29. Caudal gluteal
30. Internal pudendal
31. Right external iliac
32. Deep femoral
33. Pudendoepigastric trunk
34. Femoral
35. Medial saphenous
36. Cranial tibial
37. Lateral saphenous
38. Portal
39. Gastroduodenal
40. Splenic
41. Caudal mesenteric
42. Cranial mesenteric
43. Jejunal

just caudal to the gastroduodenal branch. It is a large branch that receives blood from the spleen, the stomach, the pancreas, and the greater omentum. It receives the **left gastric vein,** which drains the lesser curvature of the stomach.

3. The **cranial** and **caudal mesenteric veins** are the distal terminal branches of the portal vein. The cranial mesenteric vein arborizes in the mesentery and collects blood from the jejunum, the ileum, the caudal duodenum, and the right lobe of the pancreas. The caudal mesenteric vein in the mesocolon drains the cecum and the colon.

As the portal vein enters the liver in the hepatoduodenal ligament, it divides into a short

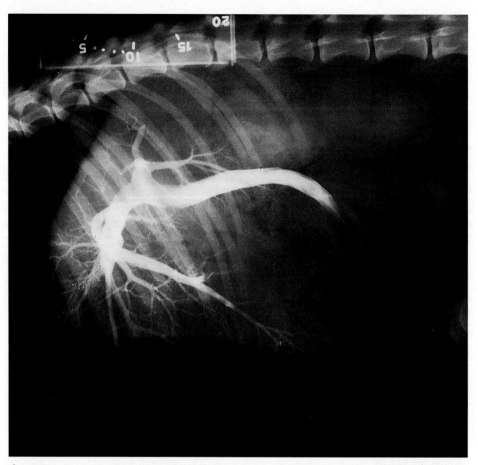

Fig. 4-36   Normal portogram after catheterization of a jejunal vein. In this lateral view the intrahepatic right branch of the portal vein courses dorsally and the left branch courses ventrally.

right and a long left branch. The right branch supplies the right lateral lobe and caudate process of the caudate lobe. The left branch supplies the other lobes. Within these lobes the portal venous branches give rise to a large array of hepatic sinusoids (Fig. 4-36) that form an extensive capillary bed. These are drained by larger branches that give rise to a variable number of hepatic veins that enter the caudal vena cava as it traverses the dorsal aspect of the liver (see Fig. 4-16). Open this part of the caudal vena cava and observe the entrance of these hepatic veins.

PELVIC VISCERA, VESSELS, AND NERVES

To reflect the left pelvic limb, first reflect the penis and scrotum to the right. Cut through the pelvic symphysis with a cartilage knife, saw, or bone cutters. Locate the wing of the left ilium and sever all muscles that attach to its medial and ventral surfaces. Apply even but constant lateral pressure to the left os coxae by abducting the limb and at

the same time cut through the cranioventral aspect of the sacroiliac joint. Cut the attachment of the penis to the left ischiatic tuberosity. Leave the limb attached. All structures more easily traced from the left should be dissected from this side.

The **levator ani** muscle (see Figs. 4-37, 4-45 through 4-47, 4-54, 4-65) lies medial to the **coccygeus muscle**. It is a broad, thin muscle originating on the medial edge of the body of the ilium and the dorsal surface of the pubis and the pelvic symphysis. It covers the cranial part of the internal obturator. The muscle appears caudal to the coccygeus, where it inserts on caudal vertebrae 3 to 7. Transect this muscle on the left side near its origin and reflect it.

The coccygeus muscle (see Figs. 4-37, 4-45 through 4-47, 4-54, 4-65) lies lateral to the levator ani muscle. It is shorter and thicker and arises from the ischiatic spine and inserts on the transverse processes of caudal vertebrae 2 to 4. Transect the muscle at its origin. The levator ani and coccygeus muscles of each side form a pelvic

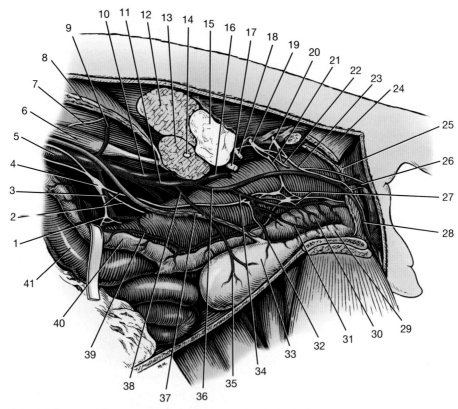

Fig. 4-37 Autonomic nerves and vessels of pelvic region, left lateral view.

1. Caudal mesenteric plexus
2. Right and left hypogastric nerves
3. Caudal mesenteric artery
4. Caudal mesenteric ganglion
5. Aorta
6. Psoas minor
7. Lateral cutaneous femoral nerve
8. Abdominal oblique muscles
9. Deep circumflex iliac artery
10. External iliac artery
11. Internal iliac artery
12. Quadratus lumborum
13. Iliopsoas
14. Femoral nerve
15. Sacroiliac articulation
16. Caudal gluteal artery
17. Lumbar nerves 6 and 7
18. First sacral nerve
19. Second sacral nerve
20. Third sacral nerve
21. Pelvic nerve
22. Caudal cutaneous femoral nerve
23. Pudendal nerve
24. Coccygeus
25. Levator ani
26. Perineal nerve and artery
27. Pelvic plexus
28. Artery and nerve to clitoris
29. Urethra
30. Vagina
31. Urethral branch of vaginal artery
32. Caudal vesical artery
33. Bladder
34. Vaginal artery
35. Cranial vesical artery
36. Internal pudendal artery
37. Ureter and ureteral branch of vaginal artery
38. Umbilical artery
39. Uterine artery
40. Uterine horn
41. Descending colon

diaphragm through which the genitourinary and digestive tracts open to the outside.

The **pelvic plexus** (see Fig. 4-37) lies caudal to a transverse plane passing through the pelvic inlet and dorsal to the prostate. It is closely applied to the surface of the rectum and the vaginal/prostatic artery. It can be identified by tracing the left hypogastric nerve to it. Occasionally, ganglia are large enough to be recognized in the plexus. The pelvic plexus contains

sympathetic fibers from the hypogastric nerve and parasympathetic fibers from the pelvic nerve.

The **pelvic nerve** (see Figs. 4-37, 4-58, 4-65, 4-66) is formed by parasympathetic preganglionic axons that leave the ventral branches of the three sacral spinal nerves. Find the left pelvic nerve on the lateral wall of the caudal portion of the rectum. It is a very small nerve. Attempt to trace it proximally to its origin. It supplies branches to the urogenital organs, the rectum, and the descending colon. The branches to the urogenital organs join the pelvic plexus and follow the vaginal/prostatic vessels to these organs.

The extension of the peritoneal cavity dorsal to the rectum on either side of the mesorectum is the **pararectal fossa** (see Figs. 4-8, 4-41, 4-53). Caudally, it extends approximately to the plane of the second caudal vertebra (see Fig. 4-41). The pararectal fossa is continuous ventrally with the common peritoneal space between the rectum and uterus or prostate. This is the **rectogenital pouch**. In the female the rectogenital pouch communicates ventrally on either side of the uterus with the **vesicogenital pouch** between the uterus and bladder. The vesicogenital pouch in the female and the rectogenital in the male communicate with the short **pubovesical pouch** between the bladder and ventral body wall and pubis. This is divided by the median ligament of the bladder.

Iliac Arteries

Iliac arteries
    External iliac
    Internal iliac
        Umbilical a.
        Internal pudendal a.
            Vaginal a.
                Uterine a.
                    Caudal vesical a.
                Middle rectal a.
            Prostatic a.
                Artery of ductus deferens
                    Caudal vesical a.
                Middle rectal a.
        Urethral a.
        Ventral perineal a.
            Caudal rectal a.
            Dorsal scrotal or labial a.
        Artery of penis or artery of clitoris
            Artery of bulb of penis/vestibule
            Deep artery of penis/clitoris
            Dorsal artery of penis/clitoris
    Caudal gluteal a.

The paired **iliac arteries** (see Figs. 4-28, 4-33, 4-37 through 4-39, 4-55, 4-58) supply the pelvis and pelvic limb. The external iliac runs ventrocaudally and becomes the femoral artery as it leaves the abdomen through the **vascular lacuna**. The **internal iliac** arises caudal to the external iliac and passes caudolaterally into the pelvis.

The internal iliac arteries and the smaller, unpaired median sacral artery terminate the aorta.

Find the origin of these vessels. The internal iliac artery gives off the rudimentary umbilical artery and terminates cranial to the sacroiliac joint as the caudal gluteal and internal pudendal arteries. The caudal gluteal primarily supplies muscles on the outside of the pelvis and in the caudal thigh. The internal pudendal is distributed to the pelvic viscera and external genitalia at the ischial arch. Dissect the following vessels on the left side.

In the fetus the **umbilical artery** is a large, paired vessel that carries blood from the aorta to the placenta through the umbilicus. Find the remnant of this vessel, the **round ligament of the bladder**. It arises near the origin of the internal iliac artery and courses to the apex of the bladder in its lateral ligament. In some specimens it remains patent this far and supplies the bladder with cranial vesical arteries. Distal to the bladder the vessel is obliterated. There are no visible remnants in the median ligament of the bladder.

Find the origin of the **internal pudendal artery** (see Figs. 4-37 through 4-39, 4-55, 4-58) from the internal iliac and dissect its branches. It is the smaller, more ventral branch that runs caudally on the terminal tendon of the psoas minor. At the level of the sacroiliac joint, the internal pudendal gives rise to the vaginal or prostatic artery.

The **vaginal** or **prostatic artery** forms an angle of about 45 degrees with the internal pudendal. It passes ventrally in an arch and terminates in cranial and caudal branches. In the female (see Fig. 4-38) the cranial branch is the **uterine artery.** The uterine artery supplies a **caudal vesical artery** to the bladder and has ureteral and urethral branches. The uterine artery courses cranially along the body and horn of the uterus in the broad ligament and anastomoses with the uterine branch of the ovarian artery in the mesometrium. (This artery must be located on each side and ligated in an ovariohysterectomy procedure.) The caudal branch of the vaginal artery is the **middle rectal artery,** which supplies branches to the rectum and vagina. In the male (see Fig. 4-39) the prostatic artery passes caudoventrally from the internal pudendal toward the prostate gland. Its cranial branch is the **artery of the ductus deferens,** which gives off a **caudal vesical artery** to the bladder, with ureteral and urethral branches. It then continues along the ductus deferens, which it supplies. The caudal branch is the middle rectal artery, which supplies the rectum, prostate, and urethra.

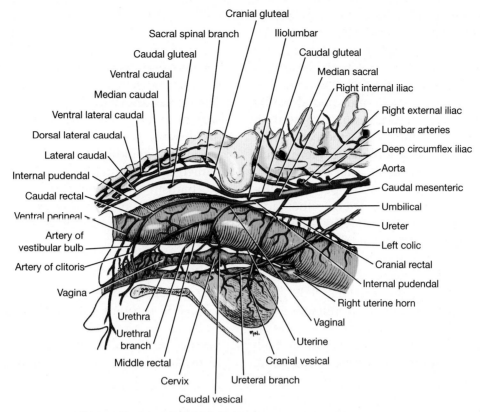

Fig. 4-38 Arteries of female pelvic viscera, right lateral view.

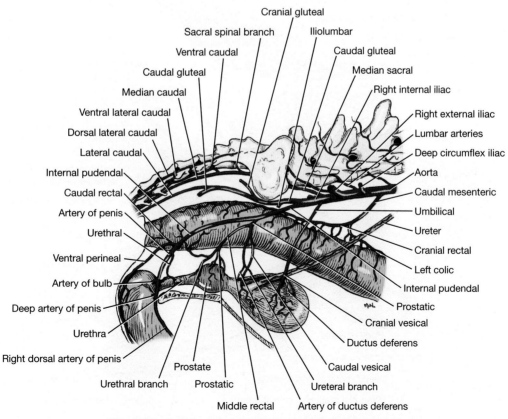

Fig. 4-39 Arteries of male pelvic viscera, right lateral view.

Reflect the skin and fat from the right ischiorectal fossa. The internal pudendal artery (see Figs. 4-37 through 4-40, 4-68) passes obliquely across the greater ischiatic notch. It continues along the dorsal border of the ischiatic spine lateral to the coccygeus muscle and medial to the gluteal muscles and sacrotuberous ligament. It then courses medially into the ischiorectal fossa accompanied by the pudendal nerve. Here it terminates as a ventral perineal artery, a variable urethral artery, and an artery of the penis or clitoris. These vessels may be dissected on either side.

The ventral perineal artery may be seen passing caudally. It supplies a caudal rectal artery to the rectum and anus and terminates in the skin of the perineum and the scrotum or vulva.

The **artery of the penis** (see Figs. 4-39, 4-40, 4-48) courses caudoventrally and terminates at the level of the ischial arch as three branches. The **artery of the bulb of the penis** arborizes in the bulb and continues to supply the corpus spongiosum

penis and penile urethra. Observe this artery as it enters the bulb. The **deep artery of the penis** arises close to the artery of the bulb and enters the corpus cavernosum penis at the crus. This is at the level of the ischial arch lateral to the penile bulb. The **dorsal artery of the penis** runs on the dorsal surface to the level of the bulbus glandis, where it divides and sends branches to the prepuce and pars longa glandis. The penile arteries are accompanied by veins that have an important role in the mechanism of erection (see Fig. 4-40).

In the female the **artery of the clitoris** courses caudoventrally to supply the clitoris and vestibular bulb.

Pelvic Viscera

The **urinary bladder** (see Figs. 4-8, 4-9, 4-11, 4-12, 4-24, 4-37 through 4-39, 4-41 through 4-43, 4-52, 4-53) has an apex, a body, and a neck. Three connecting peritoneal folds (ligaments) are reflected from the bladder on the pelvic and abdominal

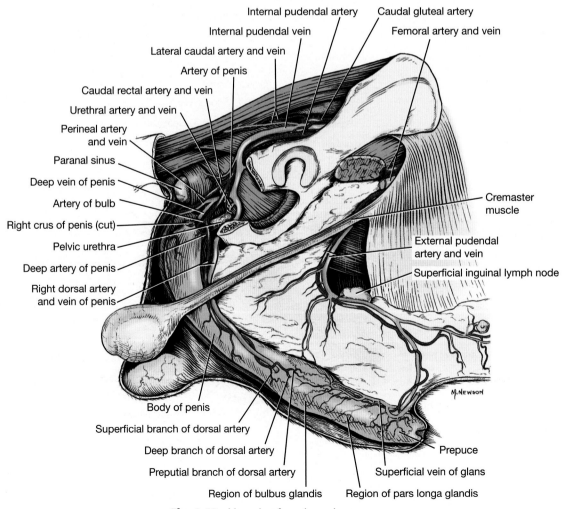

Fig. 4-40 Vessels of penis and prepuce.

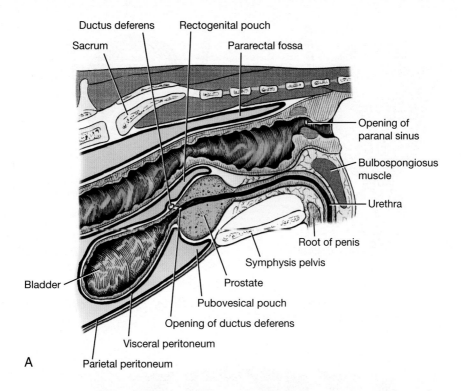

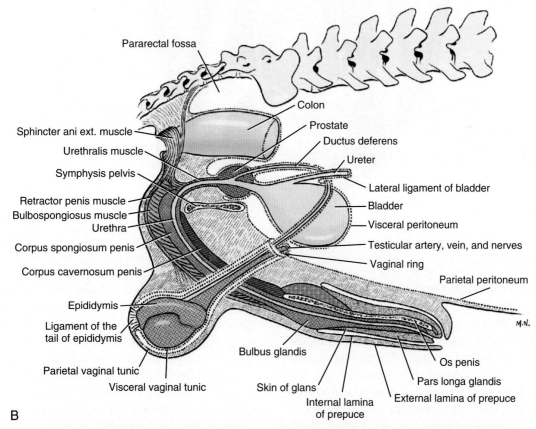

Fig. 4-41   A, Median section through male pelvic region. **B,** Diagram of peritoneal reflections and the male genitalia. (Part **B** from Evans HE, de Lahunta A: *Miller's anatomy of the dog,* ed 4, St Louis, 2013, Saunders.)

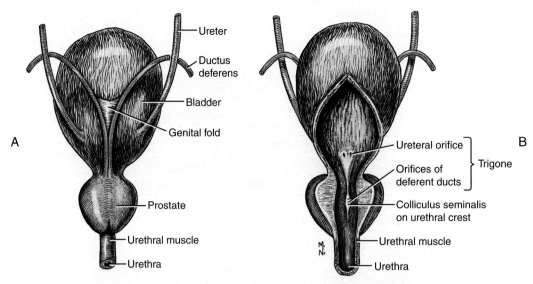

Fig. 4-42   Bladder, prostate, and associated structures. **A,** Dorsal view. **B,** Ventral view with bladder and urethra opened on the midline.

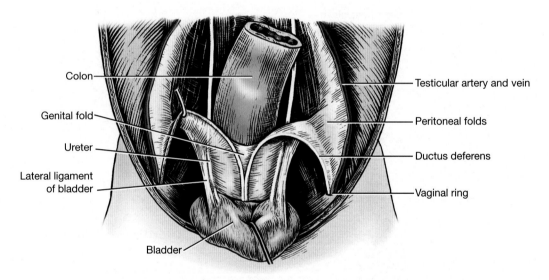

Fig. 4-43   Ligaments and folds associated with the bladder in the male.

walls. The **median ligament of the bladder** (see Figs. 4-11, 4-53) leaves the ventral surface of the bladder and attaches to the abdominal wall as far cranial as the umbilicus. In the fetus it contains the urachus and umbilical arteries. These degenerate and leave no ligamentous remnant in the adult. The **lateral ligament of the bladder** (see Figs. 4-11, 4-43, 4-53) passes to the pelvic wall and often contains an accumulation of fat along with the ureter and umbilical artery.

Observe the pattern of the bundles of smooth muscle on the surface of the bladder. These smooth muscle bundles pass obliquely across the neck of the bladder and the origin of the urethra. The

muscle is innervated by the pelvic nerve (sacral parasympathetic neurons). No gross anatomical sphincter is present in the neck of the bladder, but a physiological sphincter of smooth muscle is maintained by sympathetic visceral efferent innervation.

The **urethral muscle** is striated and is confined to the pelvis, where it surrounds the pelvic urethra and serves as a voluntary sphincter to retain the urine. It is innervated by the pudendal nerve (sacral somatic efferent neurons). Make a midventral incision through the bladder wall and the urethra. In the male this should include the prostate gland.

Examine the mucosae of the bladder and urethra. If the bladder is contracted, its mucosa will be thrown into numerous folds, or **rugae**, as a result of its inelasticity.

Observe the entrance of the ureters into the bladder. These lie opposite each other near the neck of the organ. The **trigone of the bladder** is the dorsal triangular area located within the line drawn between the two ureteral openings and the lines connecting each ureteral opening with the urethral exit from the bladder.

The **rectum** (see Figs. 4-11, 4-41, 4-45, 4-46, 4-52, 4-53) continues the descending colon through the pelvis. It begins at the pelvic inlet. The **anal canal** (see Figs. 4-41, 4-46, 4-52) is a continuation of the rectum to the anus. It consists of three zones and begins with the columnar zone, where the mucosa of the rectum forms longitudinal folds. The longitudinal ridges are called *anal columns.* They terminate at the intermediate zone, or anocutaneous line, where small pockets, anal sinuses, are formed between the columns. Distal to this line is the larger **cutaneous zone** of the anal canal, which has fine hairs, microscopic circumanal glands, and, on each side, the prominent ventrolateral opening of the **paranal sinus** (anal sac). The anal canal is surrounded by both a smooth internal and a striated **external sphincter muscle** (see Figs. 4-45 through 4-47, 4-54). The external opening of the anal canal is the **anus**. Transect the external sphincter on the left and reflect it from the paranal sinus. This muscle receives its nerve supply from the caudal rectal nerve (pudendal) and its blood supply from the caudal rectal branch of the internal pudendal artery.

Observe the **paranal sinus** (see Figs. 4-41, 4-45, 4-46), expose its duct, and find the opening in the cutaneous zone of the anal canal. In the wall of this sinus are microscopic glands, the secretion of which accumulates in the lumen. The secretion is discharged through the duct of the paranal sinus. Open the sinus and examine its interior.

The **internal sphincter muscle** (see Fig. 4-45) of the anus is an enlargement of the smooth circular muscle coat of the anal canal. It is not as distinct as the external sphincter.

The **rectococcygeus muscle** (see Figs. 4-45, 4-47, 4-54) continues the longitudinal smooth muscle of the rectum to the ventral surface of the tail. Reflect the levator ani and coccygeus muscles from the left side of the rectum. Observe the rectococcygeus muscle arising from the dorsal surface of the rectum cranial to the sphincter muscles. Trace it caudally to its insertion on the caudal vertebrae.

Male

The **prostate gland** (see Figs. 4-39, 4-41, 4-42, 4-44) completely surrounds the neck of the bladder and the beginning of the urethra. Examine the surface, form, size, and location of the prostate on several specimens. The normal size and weight of the prostate vary greatly. The organ generally lies at the pelvic inlet. It is larger and extends farther into the abdomen in older dogs. The prostate is flattened dorsally and rounded ventrally and on the sides. It is heavily encapsulated. Muscle fibers from the bladder run caudally on its dorsal surface. A longitudinal septum leaves the ventral part of the capsule and extends dorsally to reach the prostatic part of the pelvic urethra, thus partially dividing the gland ventrally into right and left lobes. This is indicated on the ventral surface by a shallow but distinct longitudinal furrow. Notice that the urethra runs through the center of the gland. Open the urethra and examine its lumen from the ventral aspect.

The male **urethra** is composed of a **pelvic part** within the pelvis and a **penile part** within the penis. The pelvic part has preprostatic and prostatic components. The **urethral crest** (see Fig. 4-42) protrudes into the lumen from the dorsal wall of the

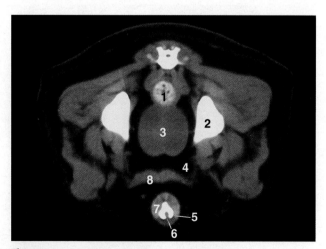

Fig. 4-44 CT image of male pelvic cavity.
1. Rectum
2. Ilium
3. Prostate
4. Peritoneal cavity
5. Os penis
6. Urethra and corpus spongiosum
7. Bulbus glandis
8. Caudal abdominal muscles

prostatic part of the pelvic urethra. Near its middle and protruding farthest into the lumen of the urethra is a hillock, the **colliculus seminalis**. On each side of this eminence the deferent ducts open. Many prostatic openings are found on both sides of the urethral crest and can usually be seen if the gland is compressed.

On the dorsal surface of the bladder, locate the two deferent ducts where they are joined by the **genital fold** (see Figs. 4-42, 4-43). Ventral to this fold is the **vesicogenital pouch** of the peritoneal cavity.

The **penis** is composed of a root, a body, and a glans (see Figs. 4-6, 4-39 through 4-42, 4-44, 4-47 through 4-51). The dorsal surface of the penis

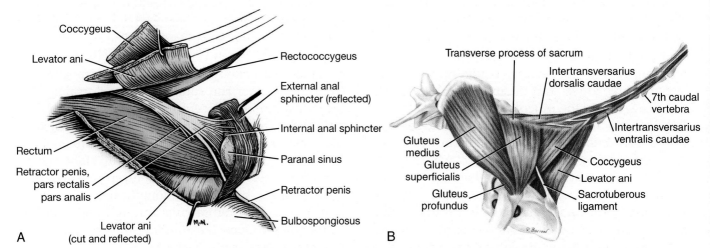

Fig. 4-45   A, Muscles of the anal region, left lateral aspect, in the male. **B,** Lateral aspect of the caudal and gluteal muscles. (Part **B** from Evans HE, de Lahunta A: *Miller's anatomy of the dog,* ed 4, St Louis, 2013, Saunders.)

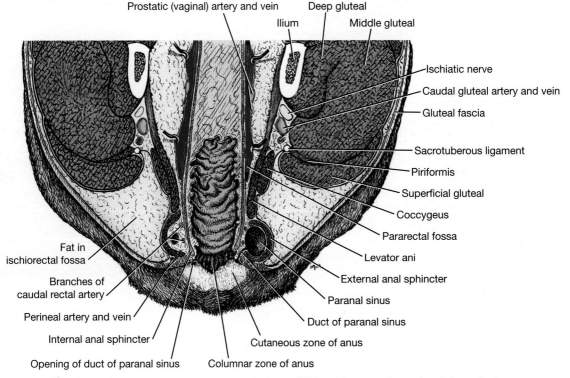

Fig. 4-46   Section through anus, dorsal plane. (Right side cut at lower level through duct of paranal sinus).

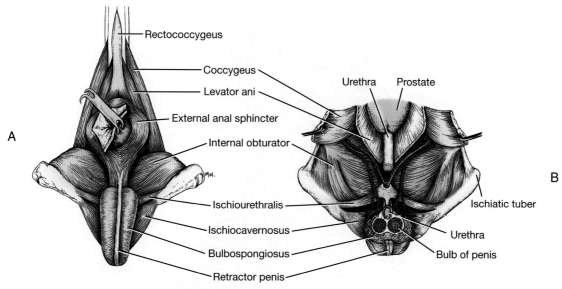

Fig. 4-47 Male perineum. **A,** Superficial muscles, caudal aspect. **B,** Dorsal section through pelvic cavity. The bilobed bulb of the penis is transected and the proximal portion is removed.

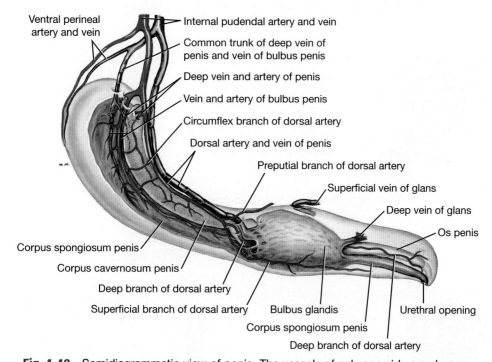

Fig. 4-48 Semidiagrammatic view of penis. The vessels of only one side are shown.

faces the pelvic symphysis and the abdominal wall. In the nonerect state the glans is entirely withdrawn into the prepuce.

The **prepuce** is a tubular sheath or fold of integument that is continuous with the skin of the ventral abdominal wall and is reflected over the glans (see Figs. 4-40, 4-41, 4-50). It has a smooth internal layer and a haired external layer, which meet at the preputial orifice. At its deepest

recess, the fornix of the prepuce, the internal layer is reflected onto the glans as the skin of the glans. In the erect state the fornix is eliminated, because the external layer of the prepuce is closely applied to the body of the penis. Open the prepuce by a midventral incision from the orifice to the fornix. Continue the midventral skin incision to the anus so as to expose the entire length of the penis (see Fig. 4-41, *B*).

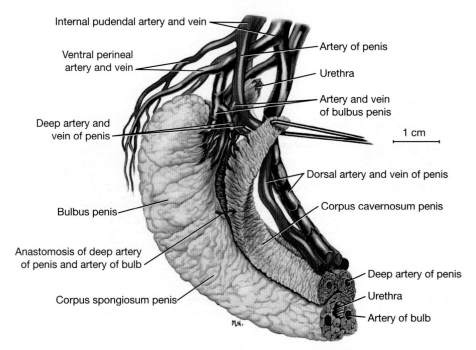

Internal pudendal artery and vein

Ventral perineal
artery and vein

Artery of penis

Urethra

Artery and vein
of bulbus penis

Deep artery and
vein of penis

1 cm

Dorsal artery and vein of penis

Corpus cavernosum penis

Bulbus penis

Anastomosis of deep artery
of penis and artery of bulb

Deep artery of penis

Urethra

Corpus spongiosum penis

Artery of bulb

Fig. 4-49   Corrosion preparation of proximal half of the penis.

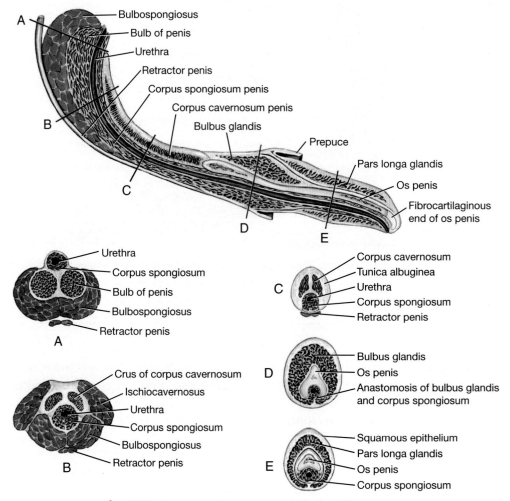

A

Bulbospongiosus

Bulb of penis

Urethra

Retractor penis

Corpus spongiosum penis

Corpus cavernosum penis

Bulbus glandis

Prepuce

Pars longa glandis

Os penis

Fibrocartilaginous
end of os penis

B

C

D

E

Urethra

Corpus spongiosum

Bulb of penis

Bulbospongiosus

Retractor penis

A

Corpus cavernosum

Tunica albuginea

Urethra

Corpus spongiosum

Retractor penis

C

Crus of corpus cavernosum

Ischiocavernosus

Urethra

Corpus spongiosum

Bulbospongiosus

Retractor penis

B

Bulbus glandis

Os penis

Anastomosis of bulbus glandis
and corpus spongiosum

D

Squamous epithelium

Pars longa glandis

Os penis

Corpus spongiosum

E

Fig. 4-50   Median and transverse sections of the penis.

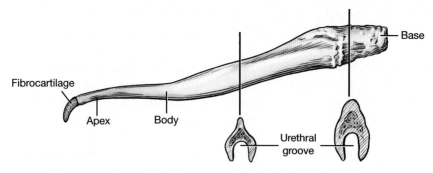

Fig. 4-51   Os penis with transverse sections, left lateral view.

The **root** of the penis is formed by right and left crura, which originate on the ischiatic tuberosity of each side. The root ends where the crura blend with each other on the midline to form the body. Each **crus** is composed of vascular cavernous tissue, **corpus cavernosum penis,** supplied by the deep artery of the penis and surrounded by a thick fibrous tunic, the **tunica albuginea.** Examine the root. The left crus was transected when the limb was reflected. The trabeculae and vascular spaces can be seen on the cut surface. Note the firm attachment of the right crus to the ischiatic tuberosity. The root of the penis includes the two crura and the bulb. The **ischiocavernosus muscle** (see Figs. 4-47, 4-50) arises from the ischiatic tuberosity, covers the origin of the crus, and inserts distally on the crus.

The **retractor penis muscle** (see Figs. 4-45, 4-47, 4-50) is an elongated slip of mixed smooth and striated muscle fibers. It originates from the ventral surface of the sacrum, or first two caudal vertebrae, blends with the external anal sphincter, and extends distally on the ventral surface of the penis to the level of the glans, where it inserts. In the region of the anal sphincter, there is muscle fiber exchange between the retractor penis muscle and the external anal sphincter. Observe the retractor muscle on the body of the penis.

The **bulbospongiosus muscle** (see Figs. 4-47, 4-50) bulges between the ischiocavernosus muscles ventral to the external anal sphincter. The fibers of the bulbospongiosus are transverse proximally, where they cover the **bulb** of the penis, and longitudinal distally, where they pass onto the body of the penis.

At the root of the penis between the crura is the **bulb of the penis** (see Figs. 4-47, 4-50) covered by the bulbospongiosus muscle. This bilobed dorsal expansion of the **corpus**

spongiosum penis surrounds the urethra and is located at the ischial arch. It is supplied by the artery of the bulb. Observe the penile bulb and its relationship to the urethra at the root of the penis. Make one or two transverse sections through the root of the penis to observe its components. A thin layer of corpus spongiosum penis surrounds the entire length of the urethra in the penis.

The **ischiourethralis muscle** (see Fig. 4-47) is a small transverse muscle that arises from the dorsal surface of the ischial tuberosity laterally and forms a fibrous ring with the opposing muscle at the pelvic symphysis that encircles the common trunk of the left and right dorsal veins of the penis. Contraction of the two muscles controls the venous return from the penis and helps maintain penile tumescence.

The **body** of the penis extends from the root, where the crura blend with each other, to the glans covering the os penis in the caudal portion of the prepuce (see Figs. 4-40, 4-48 through 4-50). Note that the region at the beginning of the body of the penis is compressed from side to side and wrapped by a thick tunic. It is capable of being bent without twisting when the male dismounts during coitus and remains "locked" for a variable period.

The **corpus cavernosum penis** (see Figs. 4-48 through 4-50) of each crus converges toward the midline and the two corpora extend side by side throughout the body to the os penis. A median septum completely separates the two corpora, and each is covered by a thick white capsule (tunica albuginea) throughout its length. The two corpora cavernosa form a groove ventrally that contains the urethra and the thin **corpus spongiosum** that surrounds the urethra. Make several incomplete transections through the body of the penis to study these structures.

The **glans** of the penis is composed of two parts—the proximal **bulbus glandis** and the distal, more elongate **pars longa glandis** (see Figs. 4-40, 4-44, 4-48 through 4-50). The bulbus glandis, surrounding the proximal end of the os penis, is a dorsal extension of the corpus spongiosum. It is an expansile vascular structure that is largely responsible for retaining the penis within the vagina during copulation. The pars longa glandis is a cavernous tissue structure that overlaps the distal half of the bulbus glandis and continues to the distal end of the penis, partially encircling the os penis and the urethra. The pars longa glandis has no direct arterial communication with the corpus spongiosum penis and is separated from the bulbus glandis by a layer of connective tissue. Venous channels drain the pars longa glandis into the bulbus glandis through this layer. Make a longitudinal incision on the dorsum of the penis through the glans to observe its structure.

The **os penis** (see Figs. 4-50, 4-51) is a long, ventrally grooved bone that lies almost entirely within the glans penis. It forms about a month after birth as an ossification of the fused distal ends of the corpora cavernosa penis. The expanded, rough, truncate base of the bone originates in the tunica albuginea of the corpora cavernosa penia. The body of the os penis extends through the glans penis. The base and body are grooved ventrally by the **urethral groove**, which surrounds the urethra and the corpus spongiosum on three sides. The bone ends as a long, pointed fibrocartilage in the tip of the glans, dorsal to the urethral opening.

At the level of the collar-like bulbus glandis of the glans of the penis, there is a communication between the corpus spongiosum penis and the bulbus glandis. The dorsal artery of the penis courses to the glans, where it supplies the prepuce, corpus spongiosum penis, and pars longa glandis.

Female

The **cervix** (see Figs. 4-24, 4-38, 4-52, 4-53) is the constricted caudal portion of the uterus. It forms a small palpable enlargement just caudal to the short body of the uterus. The **cervical canal** is in a nearly vertical position, with the uterine opening (internal uterine ostium) dorsal and the vaginal opening (external uterine ostium) ventral in position.

The **vagina** (see Figs. 4-24, 4-37, 4-38, 4-52, 4-54) is located between the uterine cervix and the vestibule. The most cranial part of the vagina is the fornix, which extends cranial to the cervix along its ventral margin. The mucosal lining of the remaining part of the vagina is thrown into longitudinal

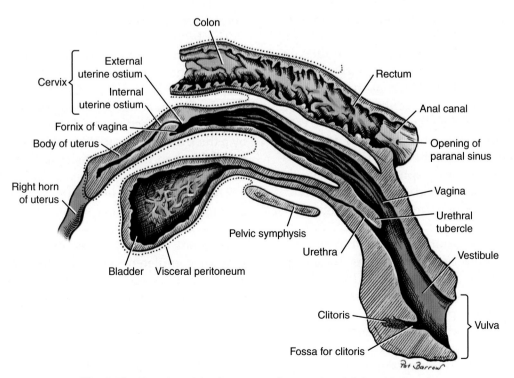

Fig. 4-52　Female pelvic viscera, median section, left lateral view.

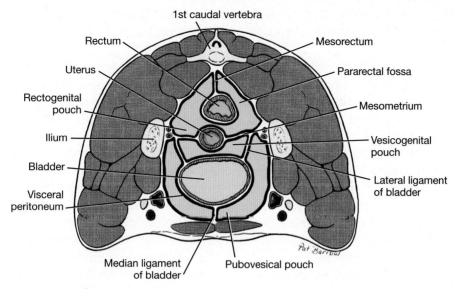

Fig. 4-53 Schematic transection of female pelvic cavity.

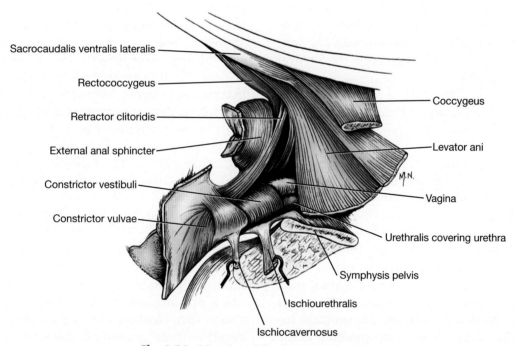

Fig. 4-54 Muscles of the female perineum.

folds that have small transverse folds. These are evidence of its ability to enlarge in both diameter and length. The longitudinal folds end dorsally at the level of the urethral orifice, where the vagina joins the vestibule. A prominent dorsal longitudinal fold in the cranial vagina nearly obscures the external uterine os and makes catheterization difficult. Note the caudoventral inclination of the vagina and the vestibule.

The **vestibule** (see Figs. 4-24, 4-52) is the cavity that extends from the vagina to the vulva. Open

the vestibule and vagina by a dorsal, midline longitudinal incision. The **urethral tubercle** projects from the floor of the cranial part of the vestibule. The urethra opens on this tubercle. This tubercle is at the level of the ischial arch. Note its relationship to the more ventrally placed vulva.

In the floor and ventrolateral wall of the vestibule, deep to the mucosa, are two elongated masses of erectile tissue, the **vestibular bulbs.** They are homologous to the bulbs of the penis of the male and lie in close proximity to the body of the clitoris. They are difficult to distinguish unless your incision passed through them.

The **clitoris** (see Figs. 4-24, 4-52) is the female homologue of the penis. It is a small structure located in the floor of the vestibule near the vulva. It is composed of paired crura, a short body, and a **glans clitoridis,** which are difficult to distinguish. The glans clitoridis is a very small erectile structure that lies in the **fossa clitoridis**. The fossa is a depression in the floor of the vestibule and should not be mistaken as the urethral opening. The dorsal wall of the fossa partly covers the glans clitoridis and is homologous to the male prepuce. Identify the fossa and glans clitoridis. Only rarely is an os clitoridis present in the glans.

The **retractor clitoridis muscle** (see Fig. 4-54), a homologue of the retractor penis in the male, originates on the first two caudal vertebrae, joins the external anal sphincter, blends with the constrictor vulvae, and continues onto the ventral surface of the clitoris.

The **vulva** (see Figs. 4-24, 4-52) includes the two labia and the external urogenital orifice that they bound, the rima pudendi. The labia fuse above and below the rima pudendi to form dorsal and ventral commissures. The dorsal commissure is ventral to a dorsal plane through the pelvic symphysis. The ventral commissure is directed caudoventrally.

Observe the course of the female urethra by passing a flexible probe through it. It extends from the bladder caudodorsally over the cranial edge of the pelvic symphysis to the genital tract caudal to the vaginovestibular junction. It ends at the external urethral orifice on the urethral tubercle, which is dorsal to the rima pudendi at the level of the ischial arch.

LIVE DOG

Abdominal palpation is an art that takes considerable experience to develop. It is dependent on your knowledge of the topographical anatomy of abdominal organs. Not all organs are palpable, and some cannot be felt in all dogs. In the standing dog, grasp the caudal abdomen gently with one hand and palpate the bladder ventrally and the descending colon above it. In the female the nonpregnant uterus can sometimes be felt between them. As the uterus enlarges with advanced gestation, it will be felt in the ventral abdomen. Dorsal to the colon, lumbar and iliac lymph nodes that are enlarged from disease can be felt.

Stand over or beside the standing dog and palpate the two sides simultaneously, starting cranially at the costal arch and progressing caudally. The liver is not usually felt. On the left side the empty stomach is not palpable, but the full stomach will be felt. The spleen should be felt on the left behind the costal arch. The left kidney is deeper but usually palpable. Cranially on the right, no specific organ is palpable. If pain is elicited, the organs to be considered as a source of irritation include the liver, pancreas, pylorus, and right kidney. Sometimes the descending duodenum can be felt on the right. The right kidney is not usually felt. Remember its close relationship with the caudate process of the caudate lobe of the liver. The descending colon can be felt on the left. In the ventral midabdominal region, you should be able to feel the coils of small intestine slip through your fingers. The ileum and cecum are not usually palpable. Deep in the midabdominal region, you may feel mesenteric lymph nodes, but only if they are enlarged from disease.

In the male palpate the root of the penis. Feel the ischiocavernosus muscles covering the crura on either side of the bulbospongiosus muscle that covers the penile bulb. Feel the slightly compressed, firm body of the penis formed by the paired corpora cavernosa penis and the groove ventrally that contains the urethra and corpus spongiosum penis. Bend the body of the penis and note its flexibility. In normal canine mating, the male will step over the female with one hindlimb and face in the opposite direction while still "locked" in copulation. The penis bends without twisting at the level of the penile body. Palpate the junction of the corpora cavernosa of the penis with the os penis. This is sometimes the site of blockage of the urethra with calculi. Palpate the length of the os penis and the two parts of the glans penis that cover it. Palpate the superficial inguinal lymph nodes in the skin fold that suspends the penis at the level of the bulbus glandis. These are normally flat and difficult to feel. Palpate the spermatic cord from the superficial inguinal ring to the testes. Palpate the testes and epididymis in the scrotum.

In the female open the vulva and observe the clitoral fossa. The urethral opening on its tubercle is dorsal to this at the level of the ischial arch and is not visible.

Gently extend the tail and observe the cutaneous zone of the anal canal. Find the openings of the paranal sinuses on either side of the cranial part of this zone. Feel the tense coccygeus and levator ani muscles. Press your finger into the ischiorectal fossa.

VESSELS AND NERVES OF THE PELVIC LIMB (Table 4-1)

Internal iliac artery
  Umbilical a.
  Internal pudendal a.
  Caudal gluteal a.
    Iliolumbar a.
    Cranial gluteal a.
    Lateral caudal a.
    Dorsal perineal a.

The **caudal gluteal artery** (see Figs. 4-38, 4-39, 4-40, 4-55, 4-58, 4-59) is the larger of the two terminal branches of the internal iliac artery. It arises opposite the sacroiliac joint and passes caudally across the greater ischiatic notch and over the ischiatic spine lateral to the coccygeus muscle, parallel to the internal pudendal artery. The branches of the caudal gluteal are the iliolumbar, cranial gluteal, lateral caudal, and dorsal perineal arteries (see Fig. 4-55). The veins (Fig. 4-56) will not be dissected. Observe the origin of the caudal gluteal artery on the medial aspect of the right ilium at the pelvic inlet. Pull the caudal gluteal artery away from the ilium and observe the iliolumbar branch coursing cranial to the wing of the ilium and the cranial gluteal branch coursing caudal to the wing of the ilium across the greater ischiatic notch (see Fig. 4-55).

Make a skin incision on the medial surface of the right thigh to the stifle. Encircle the stifle and reflect the skin from the lateral pelvis, rump, and thigh.

Expose the insertion of the superficial gluteal deep to the proximal edge of the biceps femoris. Transect the insertion at this level. Reflect the proximal portion of the superficial gluteal to its origin. Transect the middle gluteal muscle 1 cm from the crest of the ilium. Start at the cranial border of the bone and detach the muscle from the gluteal surface.

The **cranial gluteal artery** and **nerve** (see Figs. 4-55, 4-58, 4-59, 4-65, 4-66, 4-68 through 4-70)

Table **4-1**	Vessels and Nerves of the Pelvic Limb		
		Vessels	**Nerve**
Cranial Thigh Muscle			
Extension of stifle:		Lateral circumflex femoral	Femoral
Quadriceps femoris			
Medial Thigh Muscles			
Adductors of pelvic limb:		Deep femoral	Obturator
Gracilis		Caudal femorals	
Adductor			
Pectineus			
Caudal Thigh Muscles			
Flexors and extensors of stifle, extensors of hip:		Deep femoral	Sciatic
Biceps femoris		Caudal gluteal	
Semimembranosus		Caudal femorals	
Semitendinosus			
Cranial Muscles of Crus			
Flexors of tarsus:		Cranial tibial	Fibular
Cranial tibial			
Fibularis longus			
Extensor of digits:			
Long digital extensor			
Caudal Muscles of Crus			
Rotator of stifle:		Popliteal	Tibial
Popliteus		Distal caudal femoral	
Extensor of tarsus:			
Gastrocnemius			
Flexors of digits:			
Superficial digital flexor			
Deep digital flexors			

pass across the cranial part of the greater ischiatic notch of the ilium and between the middle and deep gluteal muscles, which they supply. The cranial gluteal nerve also continues into and innervates the tensor fasciae latae.

The **iliolumbar artery** (see Figs. 4-38, 4-39, 4-55, 4-58, 4-59, 4-68) arises close to the origin of the caudal gluteal artery or directly from the internal iliac. It passes across the cranioventral border of the ilium and supplies the psoas minor,

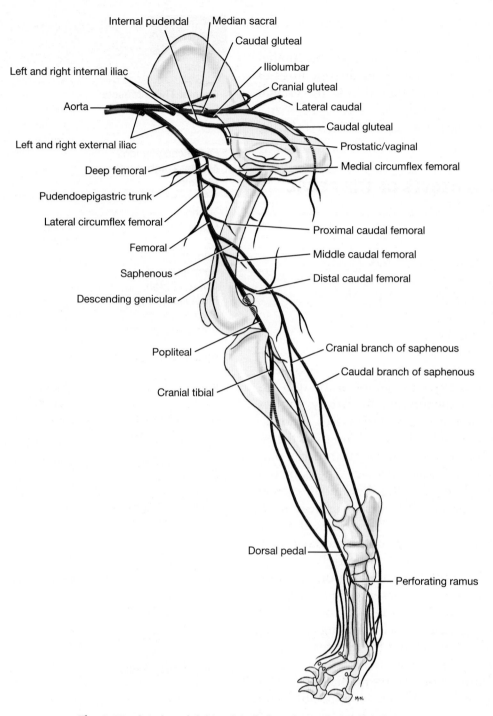

Fig. 4-55 Arteries of right pelvic limb, schematic medial view.

iliopsoas, sartorius, tensor fasciae latae, and middle gluteal muscles. On the lateral side, observe its terminal distribution to the deep surface of the cranial end of the middle gluteal.

Transect the biceps femoris midway between its origin and the stifle. Transect the semitendinosus 1 cm distal to the transection through the biceps.

Turn both muscles toward their origins. The caudal gluteal artery lies on the ventrocranial side of the sacrotuberous ligament and in this location gives off several small branches to adjacent muscles: the lateral caudal artery to the tail and the dorsal perineal artery to the perineum. These need not be dissected.

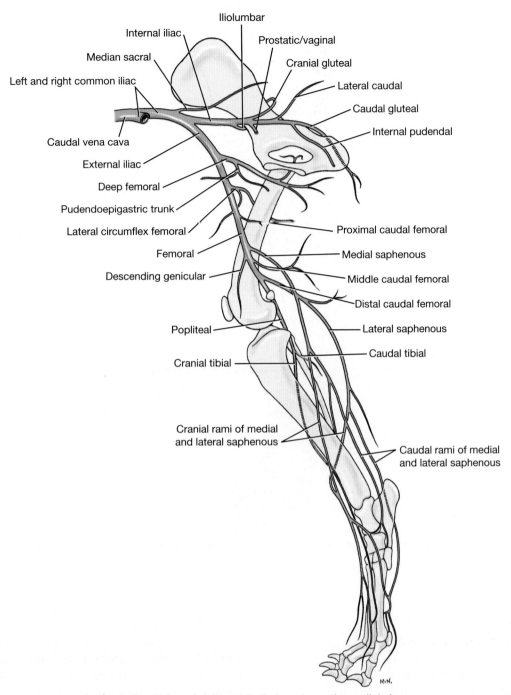

Fig. 4-56 Veins of right pelvic limb, schematic medial view.

Follow the caudal gluteal artery as it passes over the ischiatic spine with the sciatic nerve ventral to the sacrotuberous ligament (see Fig. 4-59). Here the artery supplies the superficial and middle gluteals, the rotators of the hip, and the adductor muscle. It divides into several branches, which supply the biceps femoris and the semitendinosus and semimembranosus muscles.

Turn the biceps femoris caudally to expose the caudal gluteal artery lying deep to it, close to the sacrotuberous ligament and ischiatic tuberosity.

External Iliac Artery and Primary Branches

External iliac a.

    Deep femoral a.

        Pudendoepigastric trunk

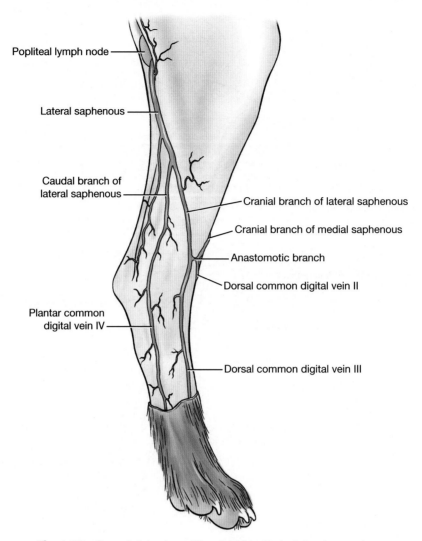

Popliteal lymph node

Lateral saphenous

Caudal branch of
lateral saphenous

Cranial branch of lateral saphenous

Cranial branch of medial saphenous

Anastomotic branch

Dorsal common digital vein II

Plantar common
digital vein IV

Dorsal common digital vein III

Fig. 4-57   Superficial veins of the right hindlimb, lateral aspect.

Caudal epigastric a.
External pudendal a.
Medial circumflex femoral a.
Femoral a.
  Superficial circumflex iliac a.
  Lateral circumflex femoral a.
  Proximal caudal femoral a.
  Saphenous a.
  Descending genicular a.
  Middle caudal femoral a.
  Distal caudal femoral a.
Popliteal a.
Cranial tibial a.
Dorsal pedal a.
  Arcuate a.
    Dorsal metatarsal aa.
      Perforating br.
Caudal tibial a.

The right **external iliac artery** (see Figs. 4-28, 4-33, 4-37 through 4-39, 4-55, 4-58, 4-60) arises from the aorta on a level with the sixth and seventh lumbar vertebrae. It runs caudoventrally and is related laterally near its origin to the common iliac vein and the psoas minor muscle. Farther distally it lies on the iliopsoas muscle. After passing through the abdominal wall, the external iliac becomes the femoral artery. The opening through which the external iliac artery passes is the **vascular lacuna**, located between the caudal border of the aponeurosis of the external abdominal oblique (inguinal ligament) and the pelvis (see Figs. 2-79, 2-80).

The **deep femoral artery** is the only branch of the external iliac artery and arises inside the abdomen near the vascular lacuna and courses caudally.

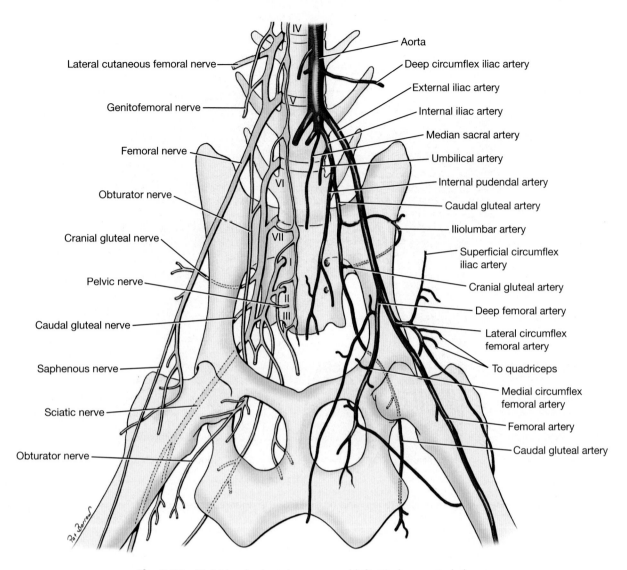

Fig. 4-58 Right lumbosacral nerves and left arteries, ventral view.

Two vessels leave the ventral surface of the deep femoral artery within the abdomen by a short pudendoepigastric trunk. These are the external pudendal and caudal epigastric arteries. The external pudendal artery passes through the inguinal canal and has already been dissected.

The **caudal epigastric artery** (see Figs. 4-33, 4-60) arises from the pudendoepigastric trunk and passes cranially on the dorsal surface of the rectus abdominis. It supplies the caudal half of the rectus abdominis and the ventral parts of the oblique and transverse muscles.

Expose the femoral artery and vein and the saphenous nerve in the **femoral triangle**. This triangle is bounded cranially by the sartorius, laterally by the vastus medialis and rectus femoris, and caudally by the pectineus and adductor.

After giving off the pudendoepigastric trunk, the deep femoral artery continues as the **medial circumflex femoral artery** (see Figs. 4-55, 4-58, 4-60, 4-63, 4-64), which leaves the abdomen through the vascular lacuna. It continues caudally between the quadriceps femoris and pectineus muscles and enters the adductor. Transect the pectineus at its origin and reflect it. Transect the origin of the gracilis and reflect the muscle caudally. Transect the origin of the adductor. Spare the branches of the medial circumflex femoral artery and obturator nerve that enter its cranial aspect. Remove portions of the adductor muscle to follow the distribution of the medial circumflex femoral artery.

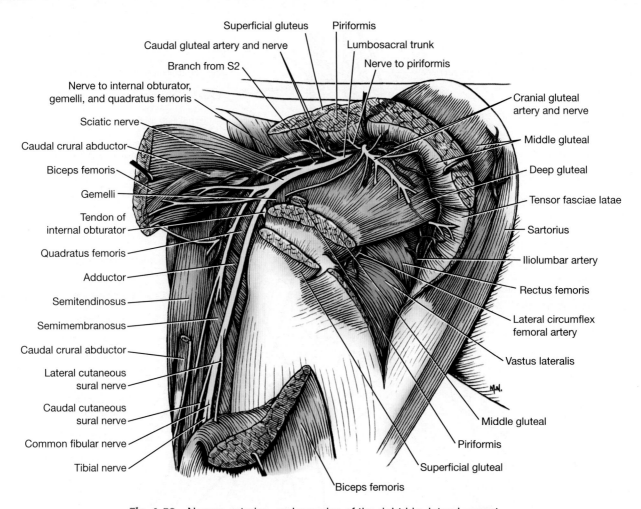

Fig. 4-59 Nerves, arteries, and muscles of the right hip, lateral aspect.

As the medial circumflex femoral artery approaches the large adductor muscle, it gives off a **deep branch** that descends distally between the adductor and vastus medialis muscles, both of which it supplies. Small branches of the medial circumflex femoral supply the obturator muscles and the hip joint capsule. The **transverse branch** passes caudally through the adductor muscle, which it supplies, and terminates in the semimembranosus muscle.

The **femoral artery** (see Figs. 4-55, 4-58, 4-60 through 4-64) is the continuation of the external iliac artery beyond the level of the vascular lacuna. The branches of the femoral artery in the order that they arise are superficial circumflex iliac, lateral circumflex femoral, proximal caudal femoral, saphenous, descending genicular, and middle and distal caudal femoral.

The **superficial circumflex iliac artery** (see Figs. 4-58, 4-63, 4-64) is a small branch that arises

from the lateral side of the femoral artery near or with the lateral circumflex femoral artery. The superficial circumflex iliac artery courses cranially and supplies both parts of the sartorius, the tensor fasciae latae, and the rectus femoris. It becomes superficial at the cranial ventral iliac spine of the tuber coxae. Transect both parts of the sartorius over the vessel and observe its branches.

The **lateral circumflex femoral artery** (see Figs. 4-55, 4-58, 4-59, 4-64) is a large branch that passes between the rectus femoris and the vastus medialis. Although most of the vessel arborizes in the quadriceps, it also supplies the tensor fasciae latae, the superficial and middle gluteals, and the hip joint capsule.

The **proximal caudal femoral artery** (see Figs. 4-55, 4-63, 4-64) leaves the caudal surface of the femoral artery distal to the origin of the lateral circumflex femoral in the midthigh region.

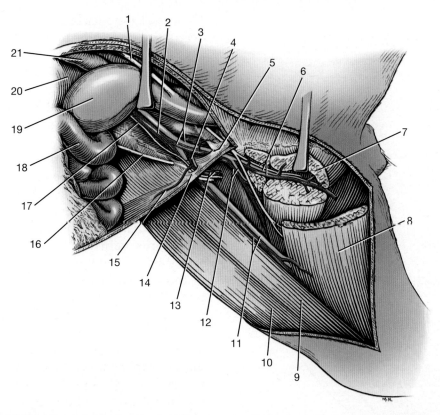

Fig. 4-60 Deep femoral artery, medial view, pectineus muscle removed, and adductor transected.

1. Left ureter
2. External iliac artery
3. Deep femoral a. and v.
4. Pudendoepigastric trunk
5. Prepubic tendon
6. Transverse branch of medial circumflex femoral a. and v. and obturator n.
7. Adductor
8. Gracilis
9. Caudal part sartorius
10. Cranial part sartorius
11. Femoral a. and v.
12. Deep branch of medial circumflex femoral a. and v.
13. External pudendal a. and v.
14. Deep inguinal ring
15. Caudal epigastric artery
16. Round ligament of uterus
17. Genitofemoral nerve
18. Small intestine
19. Bladder
20. Descending colon
21. Uterine horn

It extends distocaudally over the pectineus and adductor muscles, which it supplies, and enters the deep surface of the gracilis.

Make a skin incision from the stifle to the claw of the second digit. Remove the skin as far distally as the metatarsal pad. Try to leave the subcutaneous vessels on the limb.

The **saphenous artery** (see Figs. 4-55, 4-62 through 4-64), **nerve**, and **medial saphenous vein** continue distally between the converging borders of the caudal part of the sartorius and gracilis. Observe that the saphenous artery arises from the femoral artery, proximal to the stifle. The saphenous artery supplies the skin on the medial side of the stifle and terminates in a cranial and a caudal branch.

The **cranial branch** (see Figs. 4-55, 4-63, 4-71) of the saphenous artery arises opposite the proximal end of the tibia, obliquely crosses the medial surface of the tibia, and passes distally on the cranial tibial muscle. It crosses the flexor surface of the tarsus with this muscle. At the proximal part of the metatarsus, it terminates as the dorsal common digital arteries.

The **caudal branch** (see Figs. 4-55, 4-63, 4-73) of the saphenous artery arises at the proximal end of the tibia. It lies between the medial head of the gastrocnemius and the tibia. Distally, it is related to the flexors of the digits, and, with the tibial nerve, it crosses the medial plantar surface of the tarsus through the tarsal tunnel to enter the metatarsus.

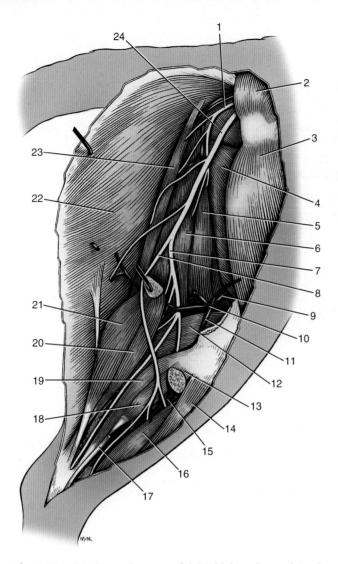

Fig. 4-61   Arteries and nerves of right thigh and crus, lateral view.
1. Sciatic nerve
2. Superficial gluteal m.
3. Vastus lateralis
4. Adductor
5. Semimembranosus
6. Semitendinosus
7. Tibial n.
8. Common fibular n.
9. Femoral a.
10. Distal caudal femoral a.
11. Popliteal a.
12. Gastrocnemius, medial head
13. Fibularis longus (muscle transected)
14. Cranial tibial muscle
15. Cranial tibial a.
16. Long digital extensor
17. Fibularis longus (tendon transected)
18. Lateral digital extensor
19. Lateral digital flexor
20. Superficial digital flexor
21. Gastrocnemius, lateral head
22. Biceps femoris (reflected)
23. Caudal crural abductor
24. Sciatic nerve

The vessel supplies branches to the tarsus and the deep structures of the proximal end of the metatarsus. In the metatarsus it supplies the paw by branches that give rise to the plantar common digital arteries. It also gives off deep branches that contribute to a deep plantar arch that is the source of plantar metatarsal arteries. These branches need not be dissected.

In some specimens the saphenous veins (see Figs. 4-56, 4-57) may be congested enough to be identified. The **medial saphenous vein** is similar to the saphenous artery in its origin in the paw and termination in the femoral vein. The **lateral saphenous vein** has no comparable saphenous artery. It is formed by cranial and caudal branches in the leg that arise from venous arcades in the paw. It terminates in the distal caudal femoral vein. The **cranial branch** of the lateral saphenous vein is often used for venipuncture. It arises from an anastomosis with the cranial branch of the medial saphenous vein on the dorsal aspect of the tarsus and courses proximocaudally across the lateral surface of the leg.

After the saphenous artery arises from the femoral, the latter disappears lateral to the semimembranosus. Transect and turn the distal end of the semimembranosus craniomedially and trace the femoral artery to the gastrocnemius muscle.

The **descending genicular artery** (see Figs. 4-55, 4-62 through 4-64) arises from the femoral distal to the origin of the saphenous and supplies the medial surface of the stifle.

The **middle caudal femoral artery** (see Figs. 4-55, 4-62, 4-64) arises distal to the descending genicular and saphenous arteries after the femoral artery passes lateral to the semimembranosus. It ramifies in the distal parts of the adductor and semimembranosus muscles.

The **distal caudal femoral artery** (see Figs. 4-55, 4-61, 4-62) is a large vessel that arises from the caudal surface of the last centimeter of the femoral. The femoral is continued by the popliteal artery on entering the gastrocnemius. Reflect the insertions of the gracilis, semimembranosus, and semitendinosus to uncover the medial head of the gastrocnemius muscle. Transect the medial head of the gastrocnemius and reflect it. This will expose the distal caudal femoral artery and its branches, which supply the biceps femoris, the semimembranosus, the semitendinosus, the gastrocnemius, and the digital flexors.

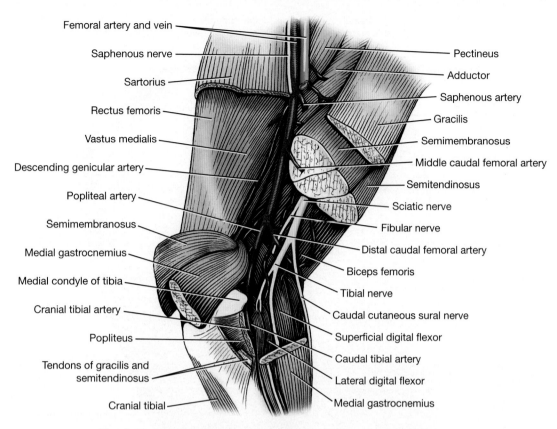

Fig. 4-62 Arteries and nerves of right popliteal region, medial view.

The **popliteal artery** (see Figs. 4-55, 4-61, 4-62), a continuation of the femoral artery, passes between the two heads of the gastrocnemius muscle, crosses the medial surface of the superficial digital flexor muscle, and courses over the flexor surface of the stifle and through the popliteal notch of the tibia. It inclines laterally under the popliteus muscle and perforates the lateral digital flexor to reach the interosseous space. The popliteal artery supplies the stifle, gastrocnemius, and popliteus muscles and terminates as cranial and caudal tibial arteries. The caudal tibial artery is a small vessel that leaves the caudal surface of the popliteal in the interosseous space. It need not be dissected.

Transect the popliteus where it covers the popliteal artery and follow the artery to the interosseous space.

The **cranial tibial artery** (see Figs. 4-55, 4-61, 4-62, 4-71, 4-72) passes between the tibia and the fibula. Reflect the fascia on the cranial aspect of the stifle and leg where it serves for the insertion of the biceps femoris. Separate the cranial tibial

and long digital extensor muscles throughout their length. Observe the cranial tibial artery between these two muscles. Transect the fibularis longus muscle at its origin and reflect it to expose the cranial tibial artery emerging from the interosseous space between the tibia and fibula. It supplies the fibularis longus, long digital extensor, and cranial tibial muscles. The termination of the artery will be dissected with the fibular nerve.

The **lumbosacral plexus** (see Figs. 4-58, 4-65, 4-66, 4-69) is diffuse and consists of the ventral branches of the lumbar and sacral spinal nerves. Of the nerves that arise from this plexus, the cranial and caudal iliohypogastric, the ilioinguinal, the lateral cutaneous femoral, and the genitofemoral have been dissected. The remainder will be dissected in the order of their accessibility.

1. The **obturator nerve** (see Figs. 4-58, 4-65 through 4-67, 4-69) arises from the fourth, fifth, and sixth lumbar spinal nerves. It is formed within the caudomedial portion of the iliopsoas muscle. It leaves the muscle dorsomedially, runs

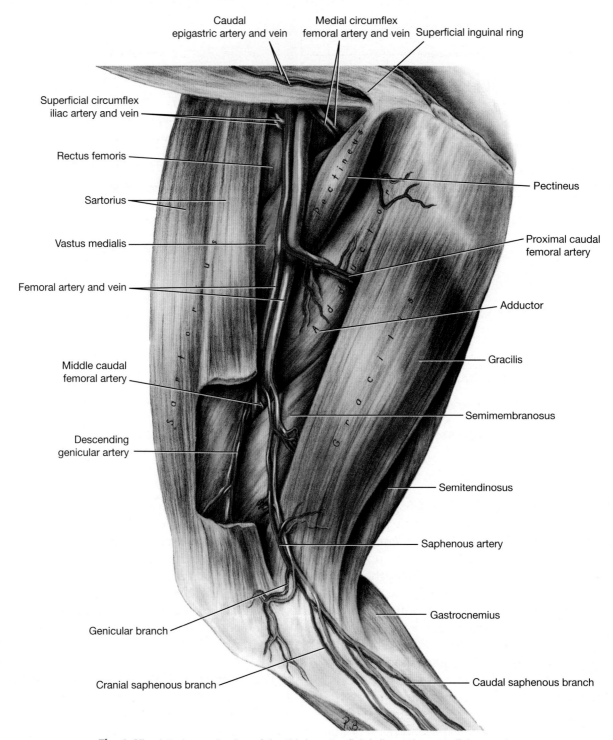

Fig. 4-63   Arteries and veins of the thigh, superficial dissection, medial aspect.

caudoventrally along the body of the ilium, penetrates the medial side of the levator ani muscle, and leaves the pelvis by passing through the cranial part of the obturator foramen. It supplies the adductor muscles of the

limb: the external obturator, the pectineus, the gracilis, and the adductor. Locate this nerve on the medial side of the right ilium. Find it as it emerges ventrally from the obturator foramen and arborizes in the adductor muscles

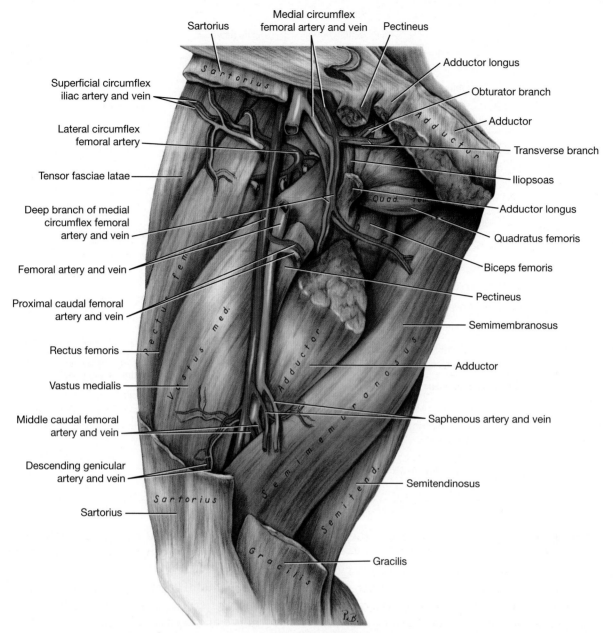

Fig. 4-64 Deep structures of the right thigh, medial view.

with the branches of the medial circumflex femoral artery.

2. The **femoral nerve** (see Figs. 4-58, 4-65 through 4-67, 4-69) arises primarily from the fourth, fifth, and occasionally the sixth lumbar spinal nerves. Find the femoral nerve with the lateral circumflex femoral artery. Observe its emergence from the iliopsoas muscle. Within the iliopsoas the saphenous nerve (see Figs. 4-65, 4-66) arises from the cranial side of the femoral nerve. The saphenous or femoral innervates the

sartorius muscle. The cutaneous portion of the saphenous nerve supplies the skin on the medial side of the thigh, the stifle, leg, tarsus, and remainder of the paw. Follow this nerve as far distally as the tarsus.

The femoral nerve supplies branches to the iliopsoas muscle. It enters the quadriceps muscle between the rectus femoris and vastus medialis and supplies all four heads of the quadriceps. It is responsible for stifle extension to support weight in the pelvic limb.

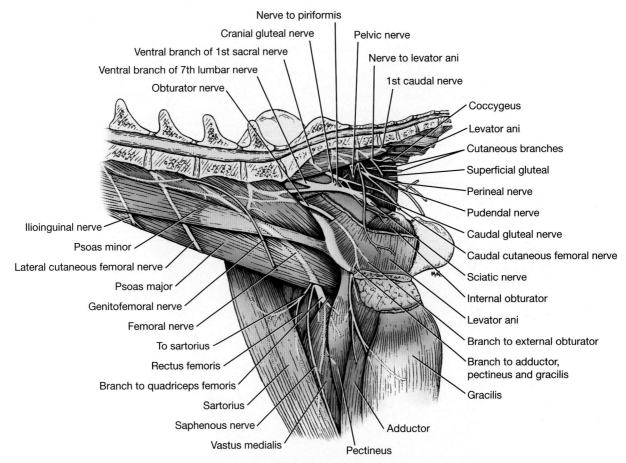

Nerve to piriformis
Cranial gluteal nerve
Ventral branch of 1st sacral nerve
Ventral branch of 7th lumbar nerve
Obturator nerve
Pelvic nerve
Nerve to levator ani
1st caudal nerve
Coccygeus
Levator ani
Cutaneous branches
Superficial gluteal
Perineal nerve
Pudendal nerve
Caudal gluteal nerve
Caudal cutaneous femoral nerve
Sciatic nerve
Internal obturator
Levator ani
Branch to external obturator
Branch to adductor, pectineus and gracilis
Gracilis
Ilioinguinal nerve
Psoas minor
Lateral cutaneous femoral nerve
Psoas major
Genitofemoral nerve
Femoral nerve
To sartorius
Rectus femoris
Branch to quadriceps femoris
Sartorius
Saphenous nerve
Vastus medialis
Adductor
Pectineus

Fig. 4-65 Lumbosacral plexus, right pelvic limb.

In the right ischiorectal fossa, identify the coccygeus muscle. Reflect the already transected superficial and middle gluteals to uncover the greater ischiatic notch. Transect and reflect the sacral attachment of the sacrotuberous ligament. This exposes the caudal gluteal artery and the sciatic nerve. Deep to these are the internal pudendal artery and pudendal nerve and the ventral branches of the sacral nerves. These ventral branches emerge from the two pelvic sacral foramina and the sacrocaudal intervertebral foramen to form the sacral plexus.

3. The **pudendal nerve** (see Figs. 4-65, 4-66, 4-68, 4-69) arises from all three sacral nerves. It passes caudolaterally, where it lies lateral to the levator ani and coccygeus muscles, medial to the superficial gluteal muscle, and dorsal to the internal pudendal vessels. It appears superficially in the ischiorectal fossa after emerging from the medial side of the superficial gluteal muscle and courses caudomedially toward the

pelvic symphysis at the ischial arch. The following branches arise from the pudendal nerve:

a. The **caudal rectal nerve** may arise from sacral nerves or may leave the pudendal nerve at the caudal border of the levator ani muscle. It innervates the external anal sphincter.

b. The **perineal nerves** arise from the dorsal surface of the pudendal nerve. They supply the skin of the anus and the perineum and continue to the scrotum or labium. Short nerves from the pudendal or perineal nerves supply the muscles of the penis or the vestibule and vulva.

c. The **dorsal nerve of the penis** in the male (or of the clitoris in the female) curves around the ischial arch and reaches the dorsal surface of the penis, where it courses cranially. It continues through the glans penis and ends in the skin covering the apex of the

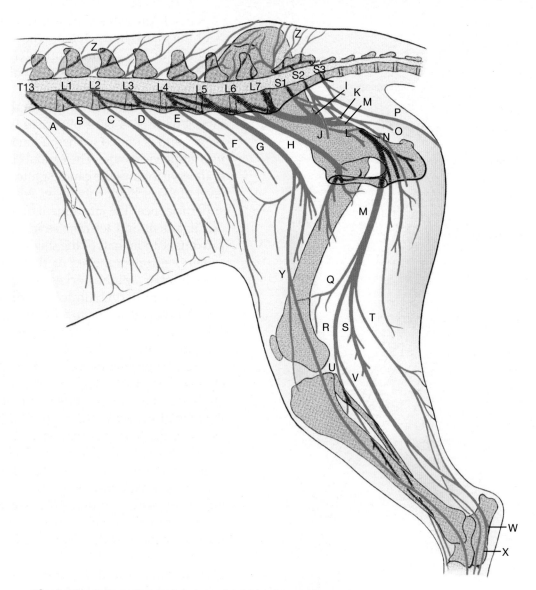

Fig. 4-66 Schematic medial view of right lumbar and sacral nerves.

A. 13th thoracic n., ventral br.
B. Cranial iliohypogastric n.
C. Caudal iliohypogastric n.
D. Ilioinguinal n.
E. Lat. cutaneous femoral n.
F. Genitofemoral n.
G. Femoral n.
H. Obturator n.
I. Cranial gluteal n.
J. Pelvic n.
K. Caudal gluteal n.
L. To obturator internus, gemelli, and
  quadratus femoris mm.
M. Sciatic n.

N. Pudendal n.
O. Perineal n.
P. Caudal cutaneous femoral n.
Q. Lat. cutaneous sural n.
R. Common fibular n.
S. Tibial n.
T. Caudal cutaneous sural n.
U. Deep fibular n.
V. Superficial fibular n.
W. Lateral plantar n.
X. Medial plantar n.
Y. Saphenous n.
Z. Dorsal branches of lumbar and sacral nn.

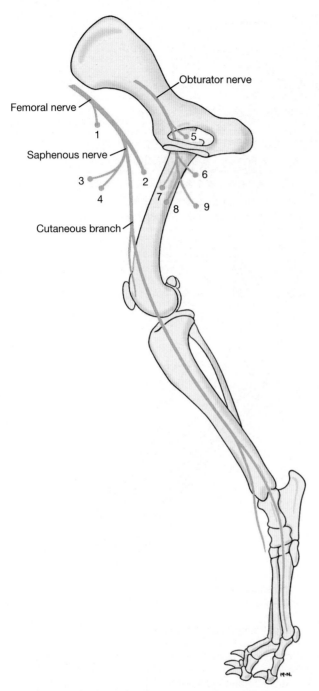

Fig. 4-67 Distribution of saphenous, femoral, and obturator nerves of right pelvic limb, schematic medial aspect. Muscles innervated by numbered nerves.
Femoral nerve
1. Iliopsoas
2. Quadriceps femoris
Saphenous nerve
3. Sartorius, cranial part
4. Sartorius, caudal part
Obturator nerve
5. External obturator
6. Adductor longus
7. Pectineus
8. Adductor magnus and brevis
9. Gracilis

penis. It provides sensory nerves to the skin of the glans. In the female the smaller dorsal nerve of the clitoris runs ventrally to the ventral commissure of the vulva, where it terminates in the clitoris.

4. The **caudal cutaneous femoral nerve** (see Figs. 4-65, 4-66, 4-68, 4-69) arises from the sacral plexus and is united to the pudendal for most of its intrapelvic course. The caudal cutaneous femoral nerve follows the caudal gluteal artery to the level of the ischiatic tuberosity, where it becomes superficial near the attachment of the sacrotuberous ligament and terminates in the skin on the proximal caudal half of the thigh.

The ventral branches of the sixth and seventh lumbar spinal nerves and the first two sacral spinal nerves unite to form a **lumbosacral trunk** adjacent to the greater ischiatic notch. The nerves that arise from this trunk are the caudal gluteal, cranial gluteal, and sciatic.

5. The **caudal gluteal nerve** (see Figs. 4-58, 4-59, 4-65, 4-66, 4-69, 4-70) passes over the ischiatic notch medial to the middle gluteal muscle and enters the medial surface of the superficial gluteal muscle. It is the sole innervation to the superficial gluteal. It has a variable origin from the seventh lumbar and first two sacral spinal nerves.

6. The **cranial gluteal nerve** (see Figs. 4-58, 4-59, 4-65, 4-66, 4-68 through 4-70) passes over the greater ischiatic notch, crosses the lateral surface of the ilium at the origin of the deep gluteal muscle, and innervates the middle and deep gluteal muscles and the tensor fasciae latae. It arises from the ventral branches of the sixth and seventh lumbar and first sacral spinal nerves. It was dissected with the cranial gluteal artery.

7. The **sciatic nerve** (see Figs. 4-58, 4-59, 4-61, 4-62, 4-65, 4-66, 4-68 through 4-70) arises from the last two lumbar and first two sacral spinal nerves. Isolate the nerve as it emerges from the lumbosacral trunk that passes over the greater ischiatic notch. Small branches leave within the pelvis to supply the internal obturator, gemelli, and quadratus femoris muscles. Do not dissect these branches. The sciatic nerve passes caudally over the hip medial to the greater trochanter, craniomedial to the tuber ischium, and then distally, caudal to the femur on the lateral side of the adductor muscle. A branch leaves the nerve at the level of the hip and innervates the biceps femoris, semitendinosus, and semimembranosus muscles.

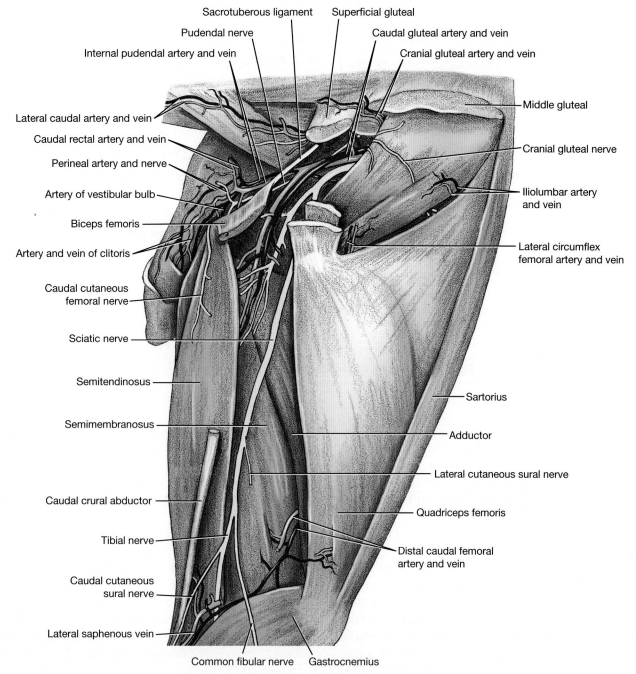

Sacrotuberous ligament

Superficial gluteal

Pudendal nerve

Caudal gluteal artery and vein

Internal pudendal artery and vein

Cranial gluteal artery and vein

Middle gluteal

Lateral caudal artery and vein

Caudal rectal artery and vein

Cranial gluteal nerve

Perineal artery and nerve

Artery of vestibular bulb

Iliolumbar artery and vein

Biceps femoris

Artery and vein of clitoris

Lateral circumflex femoral artery and vein

Caudal cutaneous femoral nerve

Sciatic nerve

Semitendinosus

Sartorius

Semimembranosus

Adductor

Lateral cutaneous sural nerve

Caudal crural abductor

Quadriceps femoris

Tibial nerve

Distal caudal femoral artery and vein

Caudal cutaneous sural nerve

Lateral saphenous vein

Common fibular nerve   Gastrocnemius

Fig. 4-68 Vessels and nerves of right thigh and perineum, lateral view.

There are **lateral** and **caudal cutaneous sural nerves** (see Figs. 4-59, 4-62, 4-66, 4-68, 4-70) that arise from the fibular and tibial components, respectively, of the sciatic nerve in the thigh and supply the skin on the lateral and caudal surfaces of the crus. The sciatic nerve terminates in the thigh as the common fibular and tibial nerves.

The **common fibular nerve** arises primarily from L6 and L7 spinal nerve ventral branches (see

Figs. 4-61, 4-62, 4-66, 4-68, 4-70). It is smaller than the tibial nerve and passes laterally, deep to the thin terminal part of the biceps femoris muscle. It crosses the lateral head of the gastrocnemius muscle and the proximal fibula and passes between the lateral digital flexor muscle caudally and the fibularis longus muscle cranially to enter the muscles on the cranial side of the crus. Here the common fibular nerve divides into superficial

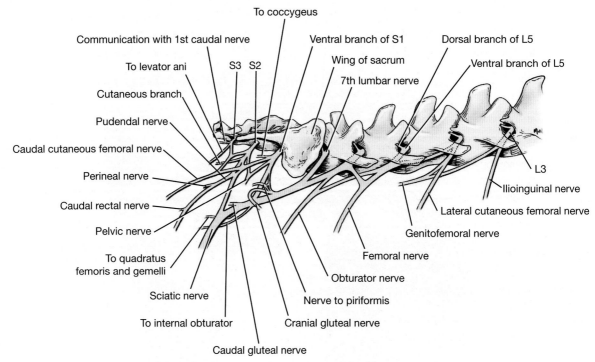

Fig. 4-69   Diagram of lumbosacral plexus, lateral aspect.

and deep fibular nerves. These nerves innervate the flexor muscles of the tarsus and extensor muscles of the digits. These include the cranial tibial, fibularis longus, and long digital extensor muscles.

The **superficial fibular nerve** (see Figs. 4-70, 4-71) leaves the lateral portion of the parent nerve below the stifle, where it lies between the lateral digital flexor caudally and the fibularis longus cranially. Expose the nerve and trace it as it curves distally, deep to the distal part of the fibularis longus. At the beginning of the distal third of the crus, it becomes subcutaneous and accompanies the cranial branch of the saphenous artery. Distal to the tarsus the superficial fibular nerve forms dorsal common digital nerves that innervate the paw (see Fig. 4-71).

The **deep fibular nerve** (see Figs. 4-70, 4-71) arises from the cranial surface of the parent nerve. It enters the muscles on the cranial part of the crus and courses distally in association with the cranial tibial artery. In the proximal half of the tarsus, they both lie in a groove formed by the tendons of the long digital extensor muscle laterally and by the cranial tibial muscle medially. Expose them by cutting the extensor retinaculum. At the tarsus the nerve divides into

dorsal metatarsal nerves that continue distally to innervate the dorsal aspect of the paw (see Fig. 4-71) along with the dorsal common digital nerves from the superficial fibular nerve. Follow the deep fibular nerve as the termination of the cranial tibial artery is now dissected.

The cranial tibial artery is continued opposite the talocrural joint as the **dorsal pedal artery** (see Figs. 4-55, 4-71, 4-72). Branches supply the tarsus, and the dorsal pedal artery terminates in the **arcuate artery** (see Figs. 4-71, 4-72) at the level of the tarsometatarsal joint. The arcuate artery runs transversely laterally through the ligamentous tissue at the proximal end of the metatarsus. It gives off **dorsal metatarsal arteries** that run distally to supply the paw dorsally. These need not be dissected. The **cranial branch of the saphenous artery** crosses the dorsal surface of the tarsus and in the metatarsus divides into three **dorsal common digital arteries.** In the distal metatarsus, the union of the dorsal common digital and dorsal metatarsal arteries results in the formation of the **dorsal proper digital arteries.**

A **perforating branch** (see Figs. 4-71 through 4-73) leaves dorsal metatarsal artery II, a branch of the arcuate artery, and courses distally in the space between the second and third metatarsal

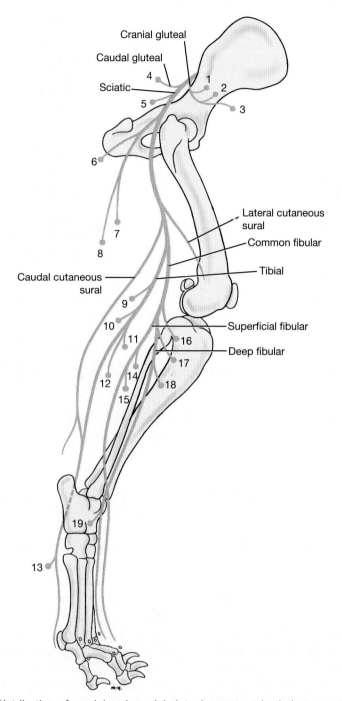

Fig. 4-70 Distribution of cranial and caudal gluteal nerves and sciatic nerve of right pelvic limb, schematic lateral view. Muscles innervated by numbered nerves.

Cranial gluteal nerve
1. Middle gluteal
2. Deep gluteal
3. Tensor fasciae latae
Caudal gluteal nerve
4. Superficial gluteal
Sciatic nerve
5. Gemelli, int. obturator, and quadratus femoris
6. Biceps femoris
7. Semimembranosus
8. Semitendinosus
Tibial nerve
9. Gastrocnemius

10. Superficial digital flexor
11. Popliteus
12. Deep digital flexors
13. Plantar muscles
Superficial fibular nerve
14. Lateral digital extensor
15. Fibularis brevis
Common fibular nerve
16. Fibularis longus
Deep fibular nerve
17. Cranial tibial and long digital extensor
18. Ext. digiti longus
19. Ext. digitorum brevis

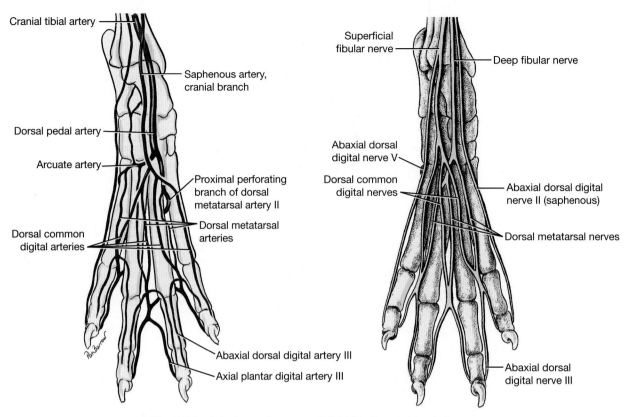

Fig. 4-71 Arteries and nerves of right hindpaw, dorsal view.

bones. This perforating branch passes from the dorsal to the plantar surface of the metatarsus in the proximal end of this space. It anastomoses with the branches of the caudal branch of the saphenous artery to contribute to the **plantar metatarsal arteries** that supply the paw. This is the largest source of blood to the digits of the paw. Expose the arcuate artery and the perforating branch. Remove the proximal half of the interosseous muscle covering the plantar side of the second metatarsal bone to observe the perforating metatarsal branch that emerges between the second and third metatarsal bones (see Fig. 4-73).

The **caudal branch of the saphenous artery,** previously observed in the crus, continues across the tarsus as the medial plantar artery. In the midmetatarsus this medial plantar artery divides into three **plantar common digital arteries.** The union of the plantar common digital arteries with the plantar metatarsal arteries provides for the origin of the **plantar proper digital arteries.**

The **tibial nerve** arises primarily from L7 and S1 spinal nerve ventral branches and is the

caudal portion of the sciatic nerve (Figs. 4-61, 4-62, 4-66, 4-68, 4-70, 4-73). It separates from the common peroneal nerve in the thigh. At the stifle it passes between the two heads of the gastrocnemius muscle. The tibial nerve supplies the muscles caudal to the tibia and fibula, which include the extensors of the tarsus and flexors of the digits, and sends branches to the stifle. It innervates both heads of the gastrocnemius muscle and the superficial digital flexor, the popliteus, and both deep digital flexor muscles. The tibial nerve is continued beyond these branches on the lateral digital flexor muscle. It emerges from the deep surface of the medial head of the gastrocnemius and continues distally along the medial side of the caudal surface of the tibia. Proximal to the tarsocrural joint, the tibial nerve divides into the medial and lateral plantar nerves. These cross the tarsus medial to the tuber calcanei through the tarsal tunnel and terminate as the plantar common digital and plantar metatarsal nerves, respectively, which are sensory to the plantar surface

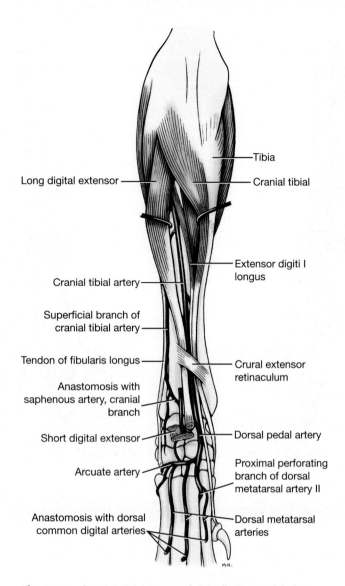

Fig. 4-72   Cranial tibial artery of right limb, cranial view.

of the paw. The **tarsal tunnel** is formed by the sustentaculum tali dorsally, the calcanean tuber laterally, and the flexor retinaculum on the plantar side. It contains the tendon of the lateral digital flexor with its synovial sheath, the medial and lateral plantar nerves, and the caudal branch of the saphenous artery.

Blood supply and innervation of the digits of the pelvic limb are summarized in Table 4-2.

LIVE DOG
Place the palm of your hand over the cranial thigh with your fingers on the medial side and palpate the borders of the femoral triangle. Feel

the pulse in the femoral artery. This is the most common site to determine the pulse rate and quality in a physical examination. The pulse can also be felt at two other sites in the pelvic limb. One is where the cranial branch of the saphenous artery crosses the medial side of the middle third of the tibia. Both the bone and the artery are subcutaneous here. The other is from the dorsal pedal artery, where it crosses the dorsal surface of the tarsus.

Trace the course of the sciatic nerve and appreciate where the nerve is close to bones that can fracture and injure it or close to the sites of intramuscular injections. The common fibular

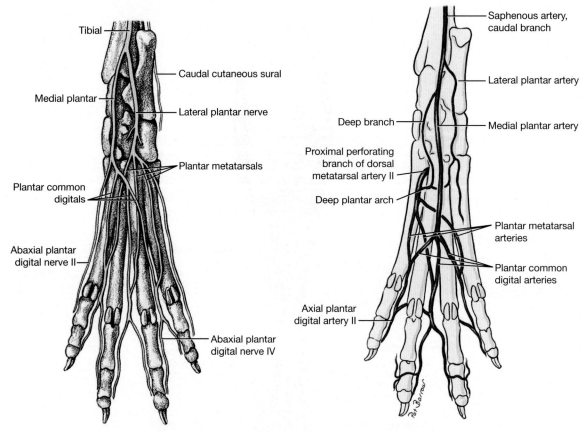

Fig. 4-73 Arteries and nerves of right hindpaw, plantar view.

Table 4-2	Blood Supply and Innervation of the Digits of the Pelvic Limb			
Dorsal Surface				
Vessels				
Superficial	Cranial br. saphenous		Dorsal common digitals	Axial or abaxial dorsal digital a., v.
Deep	Cranial tibial		Dorsal metatarsals	
	Dorsal pedal—arcuate			
Nerves				
Superficial	Superficial fibular		Dorsal common digitals	Axial or abaxial dorsal digital a., v.
Deep	Deep fibular		Dorsal metatarsals	
Plantar Surface				
Vessels				
Superficial	Caudal br. saphenous		Plantar common digitals	Axial or abaxial plantar digital a., v.
	Medial plantar			
Deep	Deep plantar arch		Plantar metatarsals	
	Perforating ramus from dorsal pedal; lateral plantar from caudal br. saphenous			
Nerves				
Superficial	Tibial—medial plantar		Plantar common digitals	Axial or abaxial plantar digital n.
Deep	Tibial—lateral plantar		Plantar metatarsals	

nerve is palpable where it crosses the proximal end of the fibula. Feel the head of the fibula and stroke the skin from proximal to distal to roll the nerve on the bone here. The tibial nerve can be felt proximal to the tarsus between the skin layers cranial to the common calcanean tendon. It is accompanied by saphenous vessels here.

Study Fig. 4-74 and identify the autonomous zones of the nerves in the pelvic limb on the live dog.

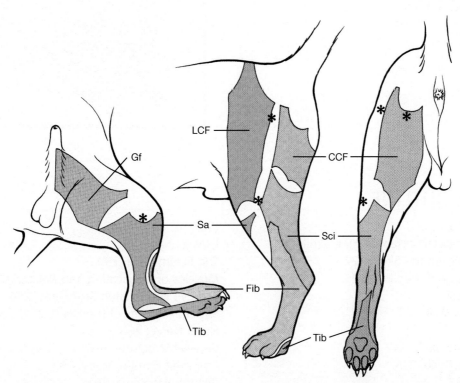

Fig. 4-74 Autonomous zones of cutaneous innervation of the pelvic limb. Medial, lateral, and caudal aspects. *CCF*, Caudal cutaneous femoral; *Gf*, genitofemoral; *LCF*, lateral cutaneous femoral; *Fib*, fibular; *Sa*, saphenous; *Sci*, sciatic; *Tib*, tibial. *Asterisks* indicate palpable bony landmarks—medial and lateral tibial condyles, greater trochanter, and lateral end of tuber ischiadicum. The sciatic nerve autonomous zone is for lesions proximal to the greater trochanter and includes the zones for the fibular and tibial nerves. For sciatic nerve lesions caudal to the femur, the autonomous zone varies, depending on how many of its cutaneous branches are affected. (After Kitchell RL et al: Electrophysiologic studies of cutaneous nerves of the thoracic limb of the dog, *Am J Vet Res* 41:61–76, 1980.)

The Head

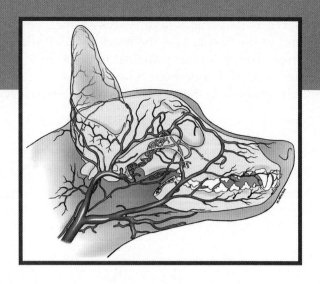

CHAPTER OUTLINE

THE SKULL

The **skull** is a complex of bones formed in both membrane and cartilage. Those that surround the brain make up the **cranium.** These include the dermal bone roof, the **calvaria,** fused with the cartilage-bone walls and floor. The skull bones that surround the entrances into the digestive and respiratory systems make up the bones of the **face.** Articulated with the cranial bones are the mandibles of the jaw, the ear ossicles, and the hyoid apparatus.

Various skull elements fuse with one another during development or have been lost phylogenetically, with the result that each species of mammal has distinctive features that may not be present in others. The dog's skull varies more in shape among the different breeds than does the skull of other species of domestic animals.

Dorsal and Lateral Surfaces of the Skull
(Figs. 5-1 through 5-4)

Cranium

The paired frontal and parietal bones form the dorsum of the cranium or calvaria. The **parietal bone** joins the frontal bone rostrally and its fellow medially. Caudally, the parietal bone meets the occipital bone, which forms the caudal surface of the skull. The unpaired interparietal bone fuses with the occipital bone prenatally and appears as a process extending rostrally. The ventral border of the parietal bone joins the squamous temporal and basisphenoid bones. Rostral to the parietal bone is the **frontal bone,** which forms the dorsomedial part of the orbit.

The **external sagittal crest** is a median ridge formed by the parietal and interparietal bones. It varies in height and may be absent. In most

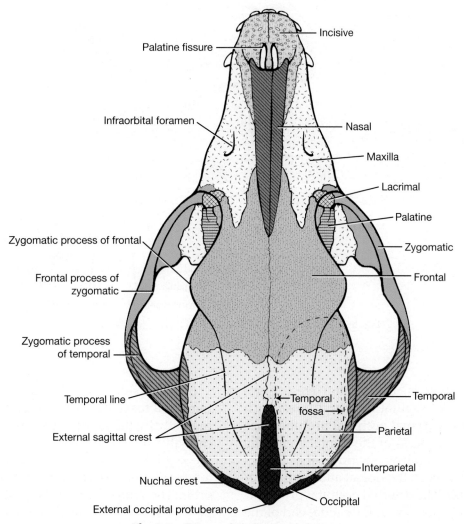

Fig. 5-1 Bones of skull, dorsal view.

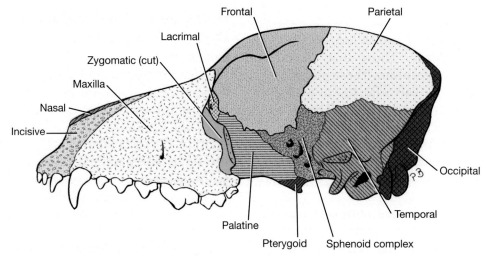

Fig. 5-2   Bones of skull, lateral view, zygomatic arch removed.

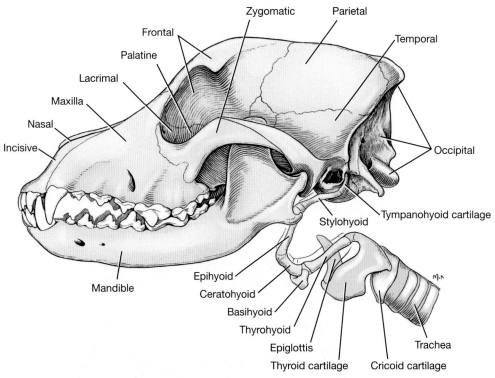

Fig. 5-3   Skull, hyoid apparatus, and larynx, lateral view.

brachycephalic breeds, the sagittal crest is replaced by a pair of sagittal **temporal lines.** Each extends from the **external occipital protuberance** to the zygomatic process of the frontal bone. The **nuchal crest** is a transverse ridge that marks the transition between the dorsal and caudal surfaces of the skull. The external occipital protuberance is median in position at the caudal end of the sagittal crest.

On each side of the dorsum of the skull is the **temporal fossa.** The fossa is convex. It is bounded medially by the sagittal crest or the temporal line, caudally by the nuchal crest, and ventrally by the zygomatic process of the temporal bone. The temporal fossa is continuous rostrally with the orbit. The temporal muscle arises from this temporal fossa on the frontal, parietal, and squamous temporal bones.

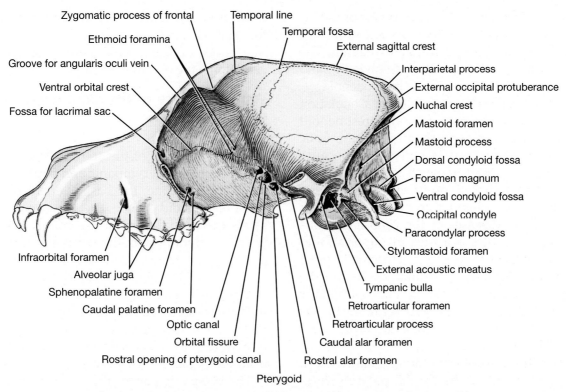

Zygomatic process of frontal
Ethmoid foramina
Groove for angularis oculi vein
Ventral orbital crest
Fossa for lacrimal sac
Temporal line
Temporal fossa
External sagittal crest
Interparietal process
External occipital protuberance
Nuchal crest
Mastoid foramen
Mastoid process
Dorsal condyloid fossa
Foramen magnum
Ventral condyloid fossa
Occipital condyle
Paracondylar process
Stylomastoid foramen
External acoustic meatus
Tympanic bulla
Retroarticular foramen
Retroarticular process
Caudal alar foramen
Rostral alar foramen
Infraorbital foramen
Alveolar juga
Sphenopalatine foramen
Caudal palatine foramen
Optic canal
Orbital fissure
Rostral opening of pterygoid canal
Pterygoid

Fig. 5-4 Skull with foramina, lateral aspect. (Zygomatic arch removed.)

Lateral portions of the frontal and parietal bones form the lateral surface (see Fig. 5-3) of the cranium. The caudoventral part of the lateral surface of the skull is composed largely of the **temporal bone.** This compound bone comprises **squamous, tympanic,** and **petrous** parts.

The **squamous part** forms the ventral portion of the temporal fossa and bears a **zygomatic process,** which forms the caudal part of the zygomatic arch. It articulates dorsally with the parietal bone, rostrally with the basisphenoid wing, and caudally with the occipital bone.

Rostral to the squamous temporal bone, the ventrolateral surface of the cranium is formed by the wings of the **basisphenoid** and **presphenoid.** The wing of the basisphenoid articulates caudally with the squamous part of the temporal bone, dorsally with the parietal and frontal bones, and rostrally with the wing of the presphenoid.

Facial Bones

The facial part of the dorsal surface of the skull is formed by parts of the frontal, nasal, maxillary, and incisive bones. All are paired. The **nasal bone** meets its fellow on the midline, the frontal bone caudally, and the **maxilla** and incisive bone laterally. The maxilla contains the upper cheek teeth and upper canine. The **incisive bone** bears the three upper incisor teeth and has a long nasal process that articulates with the maxilla and nasal bone. The **nasal aperture** is bounded by the incisive and nasal bones. It is nearly circular in brachycephalic breeds and is oval in the dolichocephalic breeds.

The **orbit** is the cavity in which the eye is situated. A portion of it is bony. The **orbital margin** is formed by the frontal, lacrimal, and zygomatic bones. The lateral margin of the orbit is formed by the **orbital ligament,** which extends from the frontal process of the zygomatic bone to the zygomatic process of the frontal bone. The medial wall of the orbit is formed by the orbital surfaces of the frontal, lacrimal, presphenoid, and palatine bones.

The **zygomatic arch** is formed by the zygomatic process of the maxilla, the zygomatic bone, and the zygomatic process of the temporal bone. The arch serves as an origin for the masseter muscle, which closes the mouth.

The **pterygopalatine fossa** is located ventral to the orbit. The maxilla, palatine bone, and zygomatic bone bound the rostral part. The caudal part is bounded by the palatine and pterygoid bones and the wings of the sphenoid bones. The pterygoid muscles arise from this fossa.

The three openings in the caudal part of the orbit are, from rostral to caudal, the **optic canal,** the **orbital fissure,** and the **rostral alar foramen.** The optic canal passes through the presphenoid, and the alar canal passes through the basisphenoid.

The orbital fissure is formed in the articulation between the basisphenoid and presphenoid bones. The optic nerve passes through the optic canal. The term *optic nerve* is a misnomer, because the axons in this structure never leave the central nervous system. Based on their development, myelination by oligodendrocytes and their susceptibility to diseases of the central nervous system, this structure is a tract of the brain and should be referred to as the prechiasmatic optic tract. Passing through the orbital fissure are the oculomotor, trochlear, abducent, and ophthalmic nerves and some vessels. Emerging from the rostral alar foramen are the maxillary artery and the maxillary nerve.

In the rostral part of the pterygopalatine fossa are several foramina. The **caudal palatine foramen** and **sphenopalatine foramen** are closely related openings of about equal size located on the rostromedial wall of the fossa. The sphenopalatine foramen is dorsal to the caudal palatine. The major palatine artery, vein, and nerve enter the palatine canal through the caudal palatine foramen and together course to the hard palate. The sphenopalatine artery and vein and the caudal nasal nerve enter the nasal cavity via the sphenopalatine foramen. Rostrolateral to these is the **maxillary foramen,** the caudal opening of the infraorbital canal. The infraorbital artery, vein, and nerve course rostrally through this canal. A small part of the rostromedial wall of the pterygopalatine fossa, just caudal to the maxillary foramen, often presents an open defect that is normally occupied by a thin plate of bone, which serves as the origin of the ventral oblique eye muscle. Caudal to the maxillary foramen are a number of small openings, most of them for the small nerves and vessels that pass through their respective **alveolar canals** to the roots of the two molar teeth and the caudal root of the last premolar. Dorsal to the maxillary foramen in the lacrimal bone is the shallow **fossa for the lacrimal sac.** The fossa is continued rostrally by the nasolacrimal canal for the nasolacrimal duct.

The facial part of the lateral surface of the skull rostral to the orbit includes the lateral surface of the maxilla and the incisive bone. Dorsal to the

third premolar tooth is the **infraorbital foramen,** the rostral opening of the infraorbital canal. The roots of the cheek teeth produce lateral elevations, the **alveolar juga.**

Ventral Surface of the Skull (Figs. 5-4 through 5-8, 5-14)

Cranium

The ventral aspect of the cranium consists of the basioccipital bone, tympanic and petrosal parts of the temporal bone, the basisphenoid bone, and the presphenoid bone. The basioccipital bone forms the caudal third of the cranial base. It articulates laterally with the tympanic and petrous parts of the temporal bone and rostrally with the body of the basisphenoid. Caudally, the occipital condyle articulates with the atlas. The **paracondylar process,** a ventral projection of the **occipital bone,** articulates with the caudolateral part of the tympanic bulla. The digastricus muscle arises from the paracondylar process.

The **tympanic part** of the temporal bone has a bulbous enlargement, the **tympanic bulla,** which encloses the middle ear cavity and its **ossicles.** On the lateral side of the bulla is the **external acoustic meatus** (see Fig. 5-3). In life, the tympanic membrane closes this opening and the annular cartilage of the external ear attaches around its periphery.

The **petrosal part** of the temporal bone contains the membranous and bony labyrinths of the **inner ear.** The major portion of this bone is visible inside the cranial cavity. The tympanic bulla has been removed on one side. This exposes a barrel-shaped eminence, the **promontory,** on the ventral surface of the petrosal part of the temporal bone. The promontory contains the **cochlear window,** which is closed in life by a membrane. The **vestibular window** lies dorsal to the promontory and contains the footplate of the **stapes.** The stapes articulates with the **incus,** which in turn articulates with the **malleus.** The malleus is attached to the medial side of the tympanic membrane. The **mastoid process** is the only part of the petrosal portion of the temporal bone to reach the exterior. It is small and lies caudal to the external acoustic meatus lateral and dorsal to the root of the prominent paracondylar process. The mastoid parts of the cleidocephalicus, sternocephalicus, and splenius muscles terminate on the mastoid process.

The **basisphenoid** articulates caudally with the basioccipital and rostrally with the presphenoid and pterygoid bones. The oval foramen,

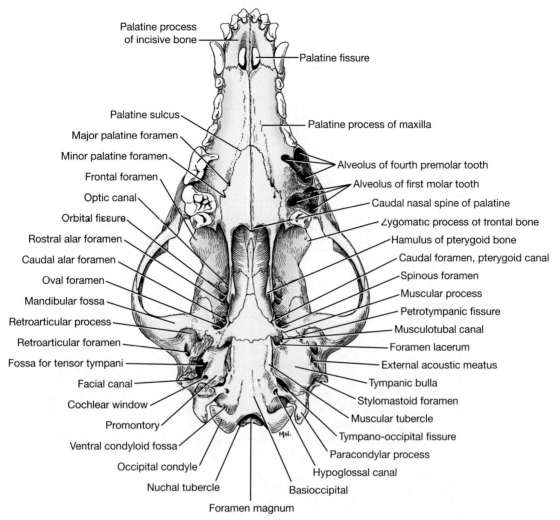

Palatine process of incisive bone
Palatine fissure
Palatine sulcus
Major palatine foramen
Minor palatine foramen
Frontal foramen
Optic canal
Orbital fissure
Rostral alar foramen
Caudal alar foramen
Oval foramen
Mandibular fossa
Retroarticular process
Retroarticular foramen
Fossa for tensor tympani
Facial canal
Cochlear window
Promontory
Ventral condyloid fossa
Occipital condyle
Nuchal tubercle
Foramen magnum
Palatine process of maxilla
Alveolus of fourth premolar tooth
Alveolus of first molar tooth
Caudal nasal spine of palatine
Zygomatic process of frontal bone
Hamulus of pterygoid bone
Caudal foramen, pterygoid canal
Spinous foramen
Muscular process
Petrotympanic fissure
Musculotubal canal
Foramen lacerum
External acoustic meatus
Tympanic bulla
Stylomastoid foramen
Muscular tubercle
Tympano-occipital fissure
Paracondylar process
Hypoglossal canal
Basioccipital

Fig. 5-5   Skull, ventral view, with right tympanic bulla removed.

round foramen, and alar canal pass through the basisphenoid bone. The **presphenoid** articulates caudally with the basisphenoid and pterygoid, laterally with the perpendicular part of the palatine, and rostrally with the vomer. Only a small median portion of the presphenoid is exposed on the ventral surface of the cranium. The optic canals pass through the orbital wing of the presphenoid.

The **rostral alar foramen,** caudoventral to the orbital fissure, is the rostral opening of the **alar canal.** The caudal opening of this short canal is the **caudal alar foramen.** The **round foramen** opens from the cranial cavity into the alar canal. The maxillary nerve from the trigeminal nerve enters the alar canal from the cranial cavity through this round foramen. The nerve courses rostrally and leaves the alar canal by the rostral alar foramen. In addition, the maxillary artery traverses the full length of the alar canal.

The **oval foramen,** a direct opening into the cranial cavity, is caudolateral to the caudal alar foramen. The mandibular nerve from the trigeminal nerve leaves the cranial cavity through this opening.

The **foramen lacerum** lies at the rostromedial edge of the tympanic bulla. A loop of the internal carotid artery protrudes through this opening. This loop is between the part of the internal carotid that is coursing rostrally in the carotid canal and the part that returns through the foramen lacerum and enters the cavernous sinus on the floor of the cranial cavity.

The **musculotubal canal** lies lateral to the foramen lacerum and caudal to the oval foramen. It is the bony enclosure of a cartilaginous tubular connection, the auditory tube, which runs from the middle ear to the nasopharynx.

The **tympano-occipital fissure** is an oblong opening between the basilar part of the occipital bone and the tympanic part of the temporal bone.

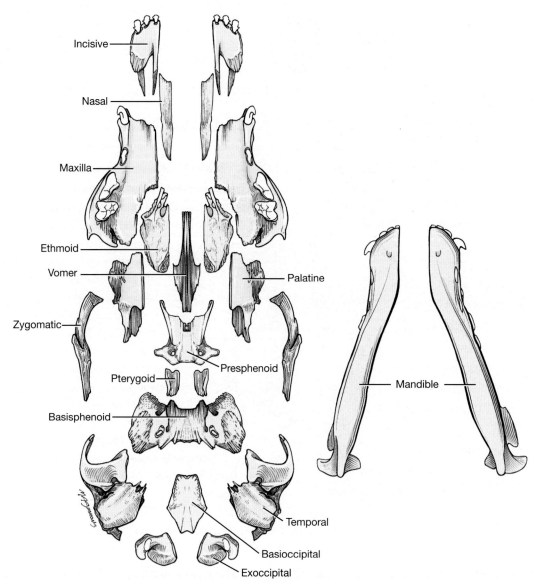

Incisive

Nasal

Maxilla

Ethmoid

Vomer

Palatine

Zygomatic

Presphenoid

Pterygoid

Mandible

Basisphenoid

Temporal

Basioccipital

Exoccipital

Fig. 5-6 Disarticulated puppy skull, ventral view.

The petro-occipital canal and the carotid canal leave the depths of the fissure at about the same place. The carotid canal transmits the internal carotid artery. The petro-occipital canal transmits the ventral petrosal venous sinus. Neither canal can be adequately demonstrated on an articulated skull. The glossopharyngeal, vagus, and accessory nerves course peripherally from the jugular foramen through the tympano-occipital fissure. Also passing through this fissure are the internal carotid artery, venous radicles of the vertebral and internal jugular veins, and sympathetic postganglionic axons from the cranial cervical ganglion.

The **hypoglossal canal,** for the passage of the hypoglossal nerve, lies caudomedial to the tympano-occipital fissure in the occipital bone.

The **mandibular fossa** of the zygomatic process of the temporal bone articulates with the condyle of the mandible to form the temporomandibular joint. The **retroarticular process** forms the caudal wall of the medial aspect of the mandibular fossa. The **retroarticular foramen** caudal to this process conducts the emissary vein from the temporal venous sinus.

Between the tympanic bulla and the mastoid process of the temporal bone is the **stylomastoid foramen.** This is the opening of the facial canal

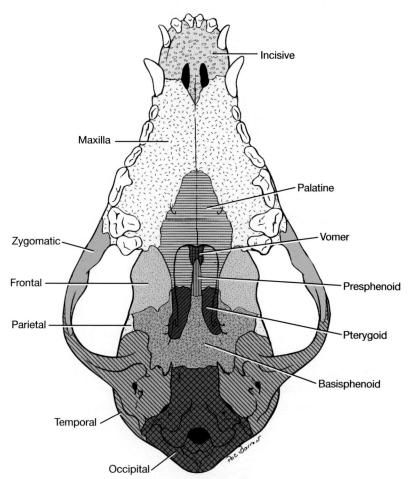

Fig. 5-7 Bones of skull, ventral view.

that conducts the facial nerve peripherally through the petrosal part of the temporal bone.

Facial Bones

The ventral surface of the facial part of the skull is characterized by the teeth and hard palate. There is a superior (maxillary) and an inferior (mandibular) dental arch. Each tooth lies in an alveolus or socket. **Interalveolar septae** separate the alveoli of adjacent teeth. An alveolus is subdivided by **interradicular septae** for those teeth with more than one root. In the superior dental arch single alveoli are present in the incisive bones for the incisor teeth and in the maxilla for the canine and first premolar teeth. There are two alveoli in the maxilla for the second premolar and two for the third. The fourth premolar and the two molars each have three alveoli in the maxilla. The **hard palate** is composed of the horizontal parts of the palatine, maxillary, and the incisive bones. An opening, the **palatine fissure,** is located

on each side of the midline between the canine teeth.

The palatine bones form the caudal third of the hard palate. The **major palatine foramen** is medial to the fourth cheek tooth. Caudal to this is the **minor palatine foramen.** The major palatine artery, vein, and nerve and their branches emerge through these foramina. The **choanae** are the openings of the right and left nasal cavities into the nasopharynx. They are located at the caudal end of the hard palate, where the vomer articulates with the palatine bones.

Caudal Surface of the Skull (Figs. 5-3, 5-4, 5-8, 5-9)

During development the occipital bone is formed by paired exoccipitals (which bear the condyles), a supraoccipital, and a basioccipital. The lateral borders form a **nuchal crest** where the occipital meets the parietal and squamous temporal bones. Mid-dorsally, an **external occipital protuberance**

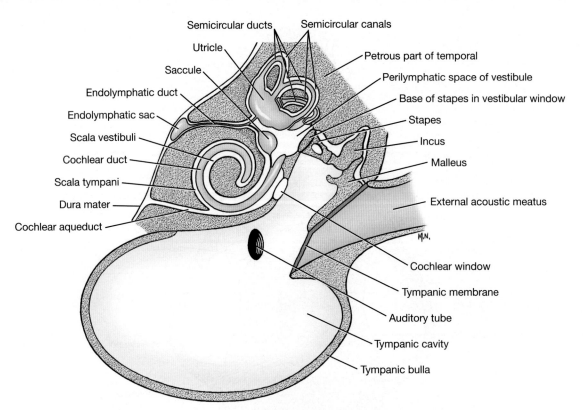

Fig. 5-8 Diagrammatic transverse section of middle and inner ear.

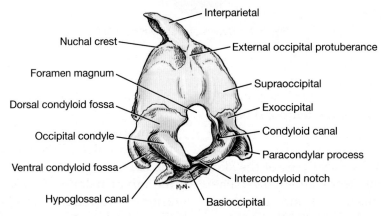

Fig. 5-9 Occipital bones, caudolateral aspect.

is formed where the interparietal bone is fused to the occipital at the caudal end of the sagittal crest. The **foramen magnum** is the large opening from the cranial cavity through which the medulla of the brain stem is continued as the spinal cord. The **mastoid foramen** is located in the occipitotemporal suture, dorsolateral to the occipital condyle. It transmits the caudal meningeal artery and vein. The rest of the caudal surface of the skull is roughened for muscular attachment.

If a disarticulated skull is available for study, try to locate each of the bones in the whole skull (see Figs. 5-1 to 5-6). Being able to visualize one bone in relation to another aids in radiographic interpretation of normal features. Several of the skull bones overlap each other to a considerable degree, so that it is not always possible to see the boundaries of an individual bone in situ. The **presphenoid bone,** through whose orbital wings the prechiasmatic optic tracts (optic nerve) pass, is a good example. Identify the **optic canal** of an intact skull and note the outline of the presphenoid sutures with adjacent bones. Orient an individual presphenoid bone in a similar position. Do the same for the more caudally located basisphenoid bone with its temporal wings and for the basioccipital bone, which is part of the occipital ring. These three bones form the basicranial axis of the skull upon which the brain rests (Figs. 5-5, 5-7, 5-14). Study the components of the disarticulated ethmoid bone, which would be located at the rostral end of the basicranial axis. The bone is described under Nasal Cavity, which is part of the section Cavities of the Skull.

With the aid of diagrams of the disarticulated skull (see Figs. 5-6, 5-10), try to locate the other bones on the intact skull.

Mandible

The two **mandibles** (Figs. 5-11, *A*, 5-12) compose the lower jaw. Each mandible bears the inferior teeth and articulates with the mandibular fossa of the zygomatic process of the temporal bone. The two mandibles join rostrally at the intermandibular articulation. Each mandible can be divided into a body, or horizontal part, and a **ramus,** or perpendicular part. The **alveolar border** of the mandible contains alveoli for the roots of the teeth. The incisors, canine, first premolar, and third molar have one root each. The last three premolars and first two molars have two roots each.

On the lateral surface of the ramus of the mandible is the triangular **masseteric fossa** for the insertion of the masseter muscle. The dorsal half of the ramus is the **coronoid process**. Its medial surface has a shallow depression for insertion of the temporal muscle. Ventral to this is the **mandibular foramen.** This foramen is the caudal opening of the **mandibular canal,** which is located in the ramus and body of the mandible. It transmits the inferior alveolar artery and vein and the inferior alveolar nerve. It opens rostrally at the three **mental foramina,** where mental nerves supply sensory innervation to the adjacent lower lip and chin. The pterygoid muscles insert on the medial surface of the mandible and on the angular process, ventral to the insertion of the temporal muscle.

The **condylar process** helps form the **temporomandibular joint.** Between the condylar process and the coronoid process is a U-shaped depression,

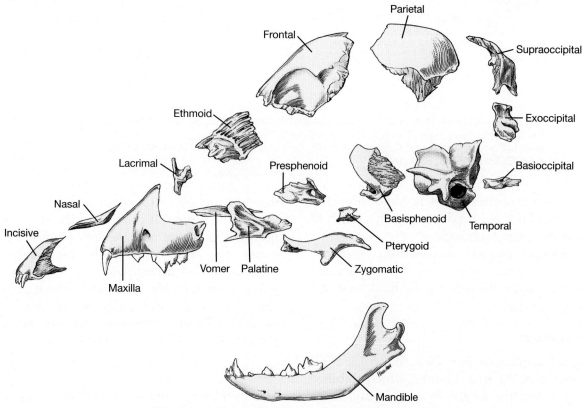

Fig. 5-10 Disarticulated puppy skull, left lateral view.

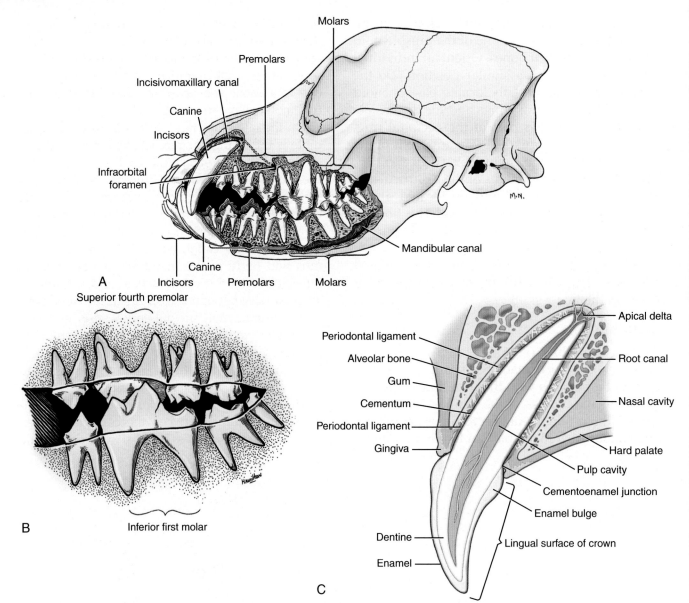

Molars

Premolars

Incisivomaxillary canal

Canine

Incisors

Infraorbital
foramen

Mandibular canal

Canine

A   Incisors   Premolars   Molars

Superior fourth premolar

B   Inferior first molar

Apical delta

Periodontal ligament

Alveolar bone

Gum

Cementum

Periodontal ligament

Gingiva

Root canal

Nasal cavity

Hard palate

Pulp cavity

Cementoenamel junction

Enamel bulge

Dentine

Lingual surface of crown

Enamel

C

Fig. 5-11 A, Teeth of an adult dog. Sculptured to show roots. **B,** Bite of the shearing teeth. Medial view, right direction. **C,** Diagrammatic section through a superior canine of an adult dog. (Parts **B** and **C** from Evans HE, de Lahunta A: *Miller's anatomy of the dog,* ed 4, St Louis, 2013, Saunders.)

known as the **mandibular notch.** Motor branches of the mandibular nerve pass across this notch to innervate the masseter muscle.

The **angular process** is a hooked eminence ventral to the condylar process. It serves for the attachment of the pterygoids medially and the masseter laterally.

Hyoid Bones

The **hyoid apparatus** (see Figs. 5-3, 5-13, 5-27) is composed of the hyoid bones, which stabilize the tongue and the larynx by suspending them from the skull. This apparatus extends from the mastoid process of the skull to the thyroid cartilage of the larynx. It consists of the short **tympanohyoid cartilage** and the following articulated bones: the **stylohyoid, epihyoid, ceratohyoid, basihyoid,** and **thyrohyoid.** All of the bones are paired except for the basihyoid, which unites the elements of the two sides in the root of the tongue. Examine these on the wet specimens provided, as well as on your own specimen.

Teeth

The teeth are arranged in superior (upper) and inferior (lower) arches that face each other. The

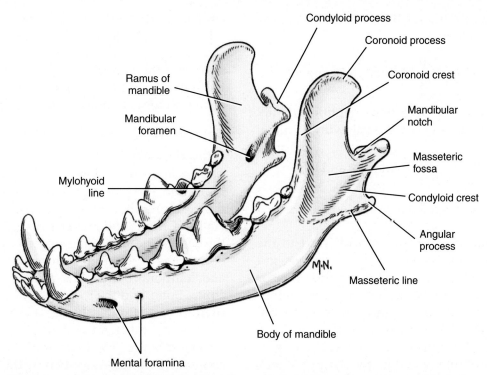

Fig. 5-12 Left and right mandibles, dorsal lateral aspect. (From Evans HE, de Lahunta A: *Miller's anatomy of the dog,* ed 4, St Louis, 2013, Saunders.)

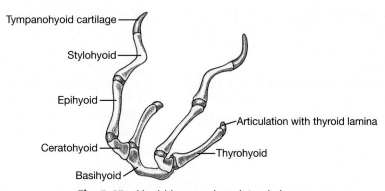

Fig. 5-13 Hyoid bones, dorsolateral view.

inferior arch is narrower than the superior (see Figs. 5-3, 5-5, 5-11, *A-C).*

The upper teeth are contained in the incisive and maxillary bones. Those whose roots are embedded in the incisive bone are known as the **incisor teeth.** Caudal to these and separated from them by a space is the **canine tooth.** Behind this are the **cheek teeth,** which are divided into **premolars** and **molars.** The inferior incisors, canine tooth, and inferior cheek teeth are all in the mandible. They are generally similar to the superior teeth. There is one more molar tooth in each mandible than in the corresponding maxilla. Some of the teeth—the incisors, the fourth premolar, and the molars—usually meet those of the opposite arch when the mouth is closed. The superior fourth premolar and first molar shear along the first inferior molar. The first three premolars fail to meet during normal closure, and the opening between the teeth is called the *premolar carrying space.* In dogs with long muzzles, there may be a considerable interval between teeth, supernumerary teeth may be present, and some premolars do not occlude. In short-muzzle breeds the teeth are usually crowded, have shallow roots, and are all in wear. In addition, most of the teeth are set obliquely and some may be missing.

The dental formula for the permanent teeth of the dog is as follows:

$$I\frac{3}{3}C\frac{1}{1}P\frac{4}{4}M\frac{2}{3} = \frac{10}{11}42 \quad \text{total right and left.}$$

The temporary or deciduous dentition ("milk teeth") can be expressed by the following formula:

$$I\frac{3}{3}C\frac{1}{1}P\frac{3}{3} = \frac{7}{7}28 \quad \text{total right and left.}$$

The deciduous teeth are erupted between 4 and 8 weeks.

The first incisor tooth (central) is next to the median plane and is followed by the second incisor (intermediate) and the third incisor (corner). In the permanent dentition the premolar and molar teeth are numbered from rostral to caudal; thus the tooth nearest the canine is number one. The fourth premolar is the largest cheek tooth of the maxilla; the largest cheek tooth of the mandible is the first molar. These are known as the *sectorial* or *shearing teeth.*

The first premolar and all of the molar teeth in the dog have no deciduous predecessor. The teeth of the permanent set are much larger than those of the deciduous set. The last permanent tooth erupts at 6 or 7 months.

Each tooth possesses a **crown** and a **root** (or roots), which is embedded in an alveolus of the jaw. The junction of root and crown is the **neck** of the tooth.

The roots of the teeth are fairly constant. The incisors and canines of both jaws have one each. In the maxilla the first premolar has one root; the second and third have two each; the fourth premolar and the first and second molars have three each. The mandibular cheek teeth have two roots each, except the first premolar and third molar, which have one. The **superior shearing tooth,** which is the fourth premolar, has two rostral roots in a transverse plane and a large caudal root. Notice that the lateral roots of the fourth premolar lie ventrolateral to the infraorbital canal and that the medial root of the rostral pair lies ventromedial to the infraorbital foramen.

The outer surface of the teeth is the **vestibular surface,** and the inner surface is the **lingual surface** for mandibular teeth or the **palatine surface** for maxillary teeth. The sides of a tooth that lie in contact with or face an adjacent tooth are the **contact surfaces.** On the first incisor, the **mesial**

contact surface is next to the median plane, whereas on all other teeth the mesial contact surface is directed toward the first incisor; the **distal surface** is the opposite surface. The surface of the tooth that faces the opposite dental arch is known as the **occlusal** or **masticating surface.**

Cavities of the Skull

Cranial Cavity

The cranial cavity (Figs. 5-14, 5-15) contains the brain and its coverings and vessels. The roof of the cranium, the calvaria, is formed by the parietal and frontal bones. The rostral two thirds of the base of the cranium is formed by the sphenoid bones. The caudal third is formed by the occipital and temporal bones. The caudal wall is the occipital bone, and the rostral wall is the **cribriform plate** of the ethmoid bone. The lateral walls are formed by the temporal, parietal, frontal, and sphenoid bones. The interior of the cranial cavity contains impressions formed by the gyri and sulci of the brain. Arteries leave grooves on the cerebral surface of the bones, whereas many of the veins lie in the diploë between the outer and inner tables of the bones. The base of the cranial cavity is divided into rostral, middle, and caudal cranial fossae.

The **rostral cranial fossa** is located rostral to the optic canals. The floor of this fossa is formed by the presphenoid bone and the cribriform plate of the ethmoid. It is bounded laterally by the frontal bone. The olfactory bulbs and the rostral parts of the frontal lobes of the brain lie in this fossa. The numerous foramina in the cribriform plate transmit blood vessels and olfactory nerves from the olfactory epithelium of the caudal nasal cavity to the olfactory bulbs of the brain. The much perforated cribriform plate of the ethmoid bone separates the cranium from the nasal cavity. (It can be the route of invasive organisms via the nasal cavity.) It is concave on its caudal surface and can be seen in a skull through the foramen magnum. On its rostral side it has many ethmoturbinate scrolls that project into and fill the caudal part of the nasal cavity and floor of the frontal sinus. In life, these thin ossified scrolls are covered by olfactory mucosa. The **optic canal** is a short passage in each orbital wing of the presphenoid bone through which the prechiasmatic optic tract (optic nerve) courses.

The **middle cranial fossa** extends caudally from the optic canals to the petrosal crests and the

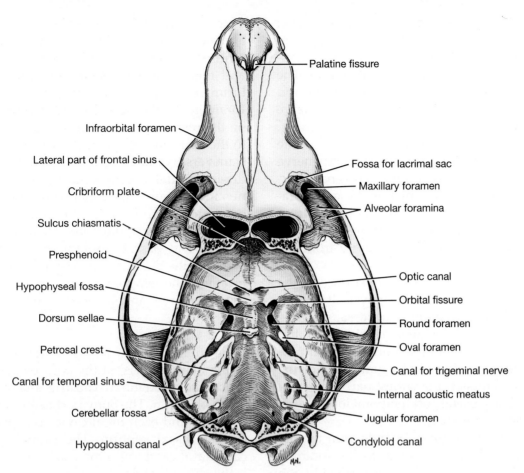

Fig. 5-14 Skull with calvaria removed, dorsal view.

Palatine fissure

Infraorbital foramen

Lateral part of frontal sinus

Cribriform plate

Sulcus chiasmatis

Presphenoid

Hypophyseal fossa

Dorsum sellae

Petrosal crest

Canal for temporal sinus

Cerebellar fossa

Hypoglossal canal

Fossa for lacrimal sac

Maxillary foramen

Alveolar foramina

Optic canal

Orbital fissure

Round foramen

Oval foramen

Canal for trigeminal nerve

Internal acoustic meatus

Jugular foramen

Condyloid canal

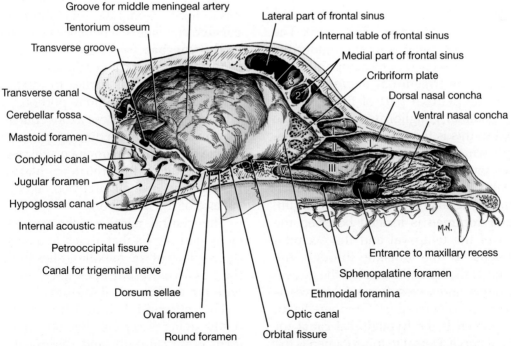

Groove for middle meningeal artery

Tentorium osseum

Transverse groove

Transverse canal

Cerebellar fossa

Mastoid foramen

Condyloid canal

Jugular foramen

Hypoglossal canal

Internal acoustic meatus

Petrooccipital fissure

Canal for trigeminal nerve

Dorsum sellae

Oval foramen

Round foramen

Orbital fissure

Optic canal

Ethmoidal foramina

Sphenopalatine foramen

Entrance to maxillary recess

Lateral part of frontal sinus

Internal table of frontal sinus

Medial part of frontal sinus

Cribriform plate

Dorsal nasal concha

Ventral nasal concha

Fig. 5-15 Sagittal section of skull, medial view. Roman numerals *I, II, III, IV* indicate endoturbinates in the nasal cavity; Arabic numerals *1, 2, 3* are ectoturbinates located in the frontal sinus.

dorsum sellae. It is situated on a more ventral level than the rostral cranial fossa. Several paired foramina are found on the floor of this fossa. Caudal to the optic canal is the **orbital fissure.** The oculomotor, trochlear, and abducent nerves and the ophthalmic nerve from the trigeminal nerve leave the cranial cavity through this opening. Caudal and lateral to the orbital fissure is the **round foramen** that transmits the maxillary nerve from the trigeminal nerve to the alar canal. Caudolateral to the round foramen is the **oval foramen** that transmits the mandibular nerve from the trigeminal nerve and the middle meningeal artery, which enters the cranial cavity from the maxillary artery.

The **sella turcica,** on the dorsal surface of the basisphenoid, contains the hypophysis. It is composed of a shallow **hypophyseal fossa,** which is limited rostrally by the presphenoid bone and bounded caudally by a raised quadrilateral process, the **dorsum sellae.** The caudal part of the middle cranial fossa is the widest part of the cranial cavity. The parietal and temporal lobes of the cerebrum are located here.

The **caudal cranial fossa** extends from the petrosal crests and dorsum sellae to the foramen magnum. The floor of this fossa is formed by the basioccipital bone and petrosal parts of the temporal bones. It contains the cerebellum, the pons, and the medulla.

Study the foramina and canals on the floor and sides of the braincase (see Figs. 5-14, 5-15). The opening of the carotid canal is located under the rostral tip of the petrosal part of the temporal bone.

The **canal for the trigeminal nerve** is in the rostral end of the petrosal part of the temporal bone. The trigeminal ganglion is located in the canal. Caudal to this is the **internal acoustic meatus,** through which the facial and vestibulocochlear nerves pass. Dorsocaudal to the internal acoustic meatus is the **cerebellar fossa,** which contains a small lateral portion of the cerebellum.

The **jugular foramen** is located between the petrosal part of the temporal and the occipital bones. It opens to the outside through the tympano-occipital fissure and transmits the glossopharyngeal, vagus, and accessory cranial nerves as well as the sigmoid venous sinus. Caudomedial to the jugular foramen is the **hypoglossal canal** for the hypoglossal nerve. Dorsal to this foramen is the **condyloid canal,** which transmits a venous sinus.

Projecting rostroventrally from the caudal wall of the cranial cavity is the **tentorium osseum.** This is composed of processes from the parietal and occipital bones. The dural membrane, the **tentorium cerebelli,** attaches to the petrosal crests and the tentorium osseum, separating the cerebrum from the cerebellum. A relatively median **foramen for the dorsal sagittal sinus** is located on the rostral surface of the occipital bone dorsal to the tentorium osseum. It opens into the paired **transverse canals.** This foramen transmits the dorsal sagittal venous sinus to the transverse sinus in the transverse canal. The transverse sinus continues ventrolaterally through the **transverse groove** of the occipital bone. Then, as the temporal sinus, it passes through the temporal bone lateral to the petrous portion. At the retroarticular foramen, the temporal sinus communicates with the maxillary vein via the emissary vein.

Nasal Cavity

There are two nasal cavities. Each begins rostrally at the nostril (naris) at the apex of the nose. The groove between the two nostrils and superior lips is the philtrum. The bony part begins at the **nasal aperture** and each nasal cavity is separated by a median **nasal septum.** The caudal opening of each nasal cavity into the common nasopharynx is the **choana.** The two choanae, at the caudal end of the nasal septum, open into the single **nasopharynx.** On a skull split on the median plane, study the bony scrolls or **conchae,** which lie in the nasal fossa. Compare them with the mucosa-covered conchae of a hemisected embalmed head.

The **conchae** (see Figs. 5-15, 5-16, 5-17, *A, B,* 5-20, 5-25) project into each nasal cavity and, with their mucosa, act as baffles to warm and cleanse inspired air. Their caudal portions also contain olfactory neurons, whose axons course to the olfactory bulbs of the brain through the cribriform plate.

The **dorsal nasal concha** originates as the most dorsal scroll on the cribriform plate and extends rostrally as a shelf attached along the medial surface of the nasal bone.

The **ventral nasal concha** consists of several elongated scrolls that attach to a crest on the medial surface of the maxilla. It lies in the middle of the nasal cavity but does not come into contact with the median nasal septum.

The **ethmoidal labyrinth** is composed of many delicate scrolls that attach to the cribriform plate caudally and occupy the fundus of each nasal cavity. Dorsally, the scrolls extend as **ectoturbinates** into the rostral portion of the frontal sinus. Ventrally, as **endoturbinates,** the

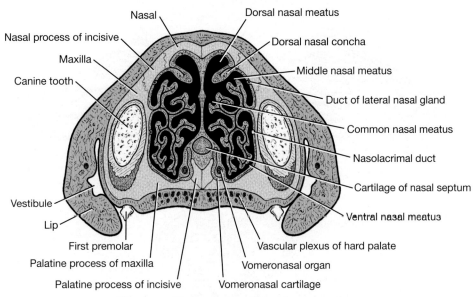

Fig. 5-16 Transverse section of nasal cavity.

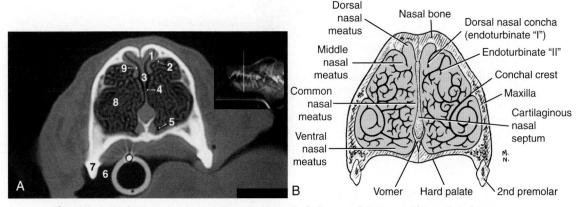

Fig. 5-17 A, CT image of midnasal cavities. **B,** Scheme of the ventral conchae in cross-section. (Part **B** from Evans HE, de Lahunta A: *Miller's anatomy of the dog,* ed 4, St Louis, 2013, Saunders.)
1. Dorsal nasal meatus
2. Middle nasal meatus
3. Nasal septum
4. Common nasal meatus
5. Ventral nasal meatus
6. Oral cavity
7. 2nd premolar
8. Ventral concha
9. Dorsal concha

scrolls attach to the vomer, which separates the entire ethmoidal labyrinth from the nasopharynx. The endoturbinates usually extend into the presphenoid bone.

The **ethmoid bone** complex is located between the cranium and the facial part of the skull (see Fig. 5-18). It consists of the ethmoidal labyrinth, the cribriform plate caudally, a median bony perpendicular plate of the nasal septum, and the orbital laminae laterally. The ethmoid bone complex is surrounded by the frontal bone dorsally, the maxilla laterally, and the vomer and the palatine ventrally. The ethmoidal labyrinth, consisting of ectoturbinates and endoturbinates attached to the cribriform plate, has an orbital lamina on each side that forms the medial wall of the maxillary recess (see Fig. 5-20).

The **nasal septum** separates the right and left nasal cavities. It is composed of cartilage and bone. The cartilaginous part, the **septal cartilage,** forms the rostral two thirds of this median partition. It

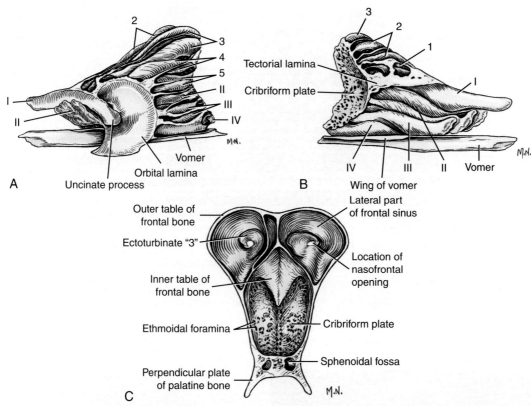

Fig. 5-18 A, Vomer and left ethmoid, lateral aspect. Roman numerals indicate endoturbinates. Arabic numbers indicate ectoturbinates. **B,** Vomer and medial aspect of left ethmoid. Perpendicular plate removed. Roman numerals indicate endoturbinates. Arabic numbers indicate ectoturbinates. **C,** Transverse section of the skull caudal to the cribriform plate. (From Evans HE, de Lahunta A: *Miller's anatomy of the dog,* ed 4, St Louis, 2013, Saunders.)

articulates with other cartilages at the nares, which prevent collapse of the nostrils. Ventrally, the septal cartilage fits into a groove formed by the vomer; dorsally, it articulates with the nasal bones where they meet at the midline. The osseous part of the nasal septum is formed by the perpendicular plate of the ethmoid bone, the septal processes of the frontal and nasal bones, and the sagittal portion of the vomer.

In each nasal cavity, the shelflike dorsal nasal concha and the scrolls of the ventral nasal concha divide the cavity into four primary passages known as *meatuses* (see Figs. 5-16, 5-17). The **dorsal nasal meatus** lies between the nasal bone and the dorsal nasal concha. The small **middle nasal meatus** lies between the dorsal nasal concha and the ventral nasal concha, whereas the **ventral nasal meatus** is dorsal to the hard palate. Because the conchae do not reach the nasal septum, a vertical space, the **common nasal meatus,** is formed on each side of the nasal septum. This space extends from the nasal aperture to the choanae in a longitudinal direction and from the nasal bone to the hard palate in a vertical direction.

Paranasal Sinuses
There are three frontal sinuses (see Figs. 5-14, 5-15) located between the outer and inner tables of the frontal bone. They are designated lateral, rostral, and medial. The **lateral frontal sinus** is much larger than the others and is the only one of clinical relevance. Its size and shape vary with the type of skull. It occupies the zygomatic process and extends caudally, bounded laterally by the temporal line and medially by the median septum. It may be partially divided by bony septa extending into it. Ethmoidal ectoturbinates project into the rostral floor of the sinus. The **rostral frontal sinus** is small and lies between the median plane and the orbit. The ethmoid labyrinth bulges into this sinus. The **medial frontal sinus** lies between the median septum and the walls of the other two sinuses. It is very small and may be absent. All three sinuses communicate with the nasal cavity.

The **maxillary recess** (see Figs. 5-15, 5-20) communicates with the nasal cavity. Its opening lies in a transverse plane through the rostral roots of the superior fourth premolar tooth.

The recess continues caudally to a plane through the last molar tooth. The walls of the maxillary recess are formed laterally and ventrally by the maxilla and medially by the orbital lamina of the ethmoid bone. The **lateral nasal gland** occupies the rostral portion of this recess. Its duct opens rostrally into the dorsal vestibule, and its secretion prevents desiccation caused by nasal panting.

Tympanic Cavity

The tympanic cavity is the cavity of the middle ear. It houses the auditory ossicles and communicates with the nasopharynx via the auditory tube. It is bounded ventrally by the tympanic bulla and dorsally by the petrosal part of the temporal bone. Laterally, the external acoustic meatus is closed by the tympanic membrane (see Figs. 5-5, 5-19).

Joints of the Head

The atlanto-occipital joint was described with the vertebrae. The **temporomandibular joint** is between the condylar process of the mandible and the mandibular fossa of the zygomatic process of the squamous part of the temporal bone. The articulation is elongated transversely. There is a thin cartilaginous **articular disc** that separates the articular surfaces of each bone and divides the joint capsule into two compartments. Lateral and caudal ligaments strengthen the joint capsule.

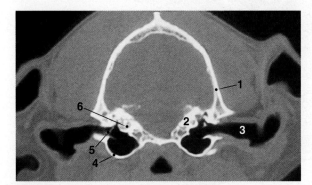

Fig. 5-19 CT image of caudal nasal cavities.
1. Squamous temporal bone
2. Petrous part of temporal bone
3. External acoustic meatus
4. Tympanic bulla
5. Malleus at tympanum
6. Cochlea

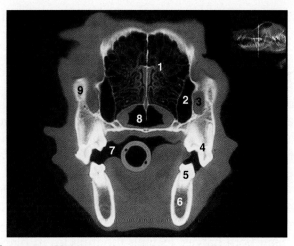

Fig. 5-20 CT image of caudal nasal cavities.
1. Ethmoidal labyrinth
2. Maxillary recess
3. Maxillary foramen
4. Superior molar 1
5. Inferior molar 1
6. Body—mandible
7. Oral cavity
8. Rostral nasopharynx just caudal to choanae
9. Zygomatic bone

The **intermandibular articulation** is a synchondrosis with an interdigitating surface that persists throughout life in most dogs.

LIVE DOG

Palpate the features of the skull of the dog's head. The widest part of the head is the palpable zygomatic arch. Palpate the zygomatic process of the frontal bone (its widest point) and the orbital ligament between it and the frontal process of the zygomatic bone. This ligament forms the lateral border of the rostral part of the orbit. Follow the frontal bone caudally to the temporal line and sagittal crest. Feel the external occipital protuberance and follow the nuchal crest ventrally on each side to the mastoid process of the temporal bone. Flex and extend the atlanto-occipital joint. Follow the frontal bones rostrally to the nose and maxillary bones. Feel the infraorbital foramen on the side of the maxilla at the level of the rostral roots of the fourth premolar. Reflect the lip and study the crowns and necks of the teeth of each dental arch. Find the shearing teeth and note how they come into contact with each other.

Palpate the coronoid process of the mandible medial to the zygomatic arch and the angular process ventrally. Feel the body of the mandible and move the temporomandibular joint by opening the mouth. Palpate the mental foramina, which lie rostrally on the lateral side of the body of the mandible. Palpate the hyoid bones.

STRUCTURES OF THE HEAD

To facilitate the dissection of the head, it should be removed and divided on the median plane. Using a hand saw, make a complete transection of the neck at the level of the fourth cervical vertebra.

Section the head and attached portion of the neck on the median plane using a band saw. Wash the cut surface to remove bone dust and hair.

Skin both halves, leaving the muscles in place. Leave a narrow rim of skin around the margin of the eyelids and at the edge of the lips. Preserve the nose and the **philtrum,** which is the median groove separating the right and left parts of the nose and superior lips. Skin only the base of the ear.

The right side of the head will be used for the dissection of vessels and nerves, whereas the left side will be used for muscles. At the end of each dissection period, wrap the head in cheescloth moistened with 1% phenol water or 2% phenoxyethanol before covering your specimen. A plastic bag is useful to prevent desiccation.

Muscles of the Face

The muscles of the face function to open, close, or move the lips, eyelids, nose, and ear. They are all innervated by the facial (seventh cranial) nerve, with the exception of an elevator of the upper eyelid.

Cheek, Lips, and Nose (Fig. 5-21)

The **superior** (upper) and **inferior** (lower) **lips** (labia oris) form the lateral wall of the **vestibule,** which is the space bounded medially by the teeth and gums. Caudal to the lips the **cheek** (buccae) forms the lateral wall of the vestibule. The **nose** is the region rostral to the orbits that bounds the rostral portion of the respiratory passageway.

The **platysma** (Fig. 5-21) is a cutaneous muscle that passes from the dorsal median raphe of the neck to the angle of the mouth, where it radiates into the orbicularis oris in the lips. It is the most superficial muscle, covering the ventrolateral surface of the face. Transect this muscle and reflect it.

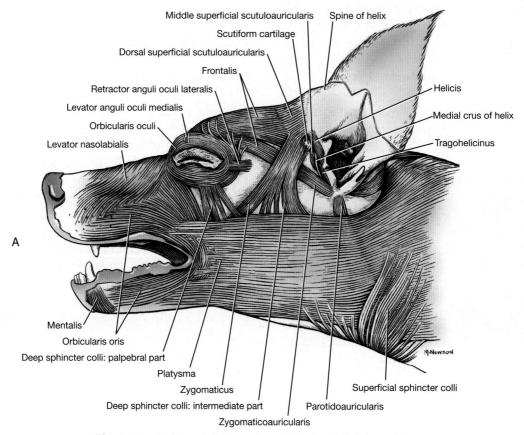

Fig. 5-21 **A,** Superficial muscles of the head, left lateral view.

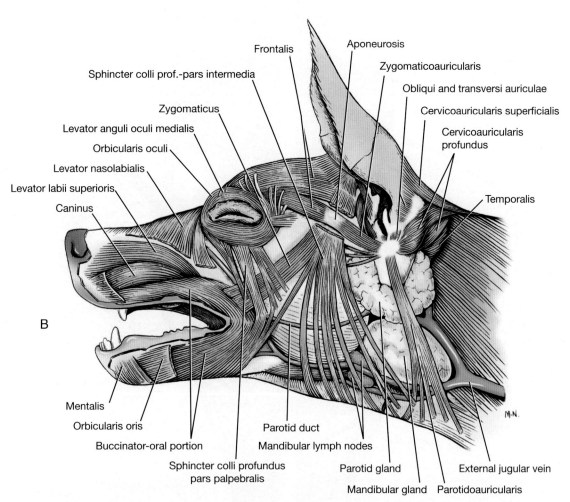

Frontalis

Aponeurosis

Zygomaticoauricularis

Sphincter colli prof.-pars intermedia

Obliqui and transversi auriculae

Cervicoauricularis superficialis

Zygomaticus

Cervicoauricularis profundus

Levator anguli oculi medialis

Orbicularis oculi

Levator nasolabialis

Levator labii superioris

Temporalis

Caninus

B

Mentalis

Orbicularis oris

Buccinator-oral portion

Parotid duct

Mandibular lymph nodes

Sphincter colli profundus pars palpebralis

Parotid gland

Mandibular gland

Parotidoauricularis

External jugular vein

Fig. 5-21, cont'd   B, Superficial muscles of the head, lateral aspect. (Platysma and sphincter colli superficialis removed.)

Continued

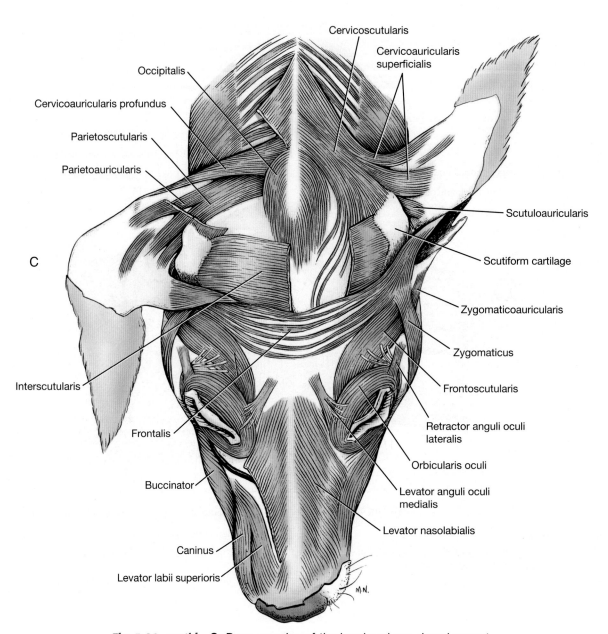

Cervicoscutularis

Cervicoauricularis
superficialis

Occipitalis

Cervicoauricularis profundus

Parietoscutularis

Parietoauricularis

Scutuloauricularis

Scutiform cartilage

C

Zygomaticoauricularis

Zygomaticus

Interscutularis

Frontoscutularis

Retractor anguli oculi
lateralis

Frontalis

Orbicularis oculi

Buccinator

Levator anguli oculi
medialis

Caninus

Levator nasolabialis

Levator labii superioris

M.N.

Fig. 5-21, cont'd   C, Deep muscles of the head and ear, dorsal aspect.

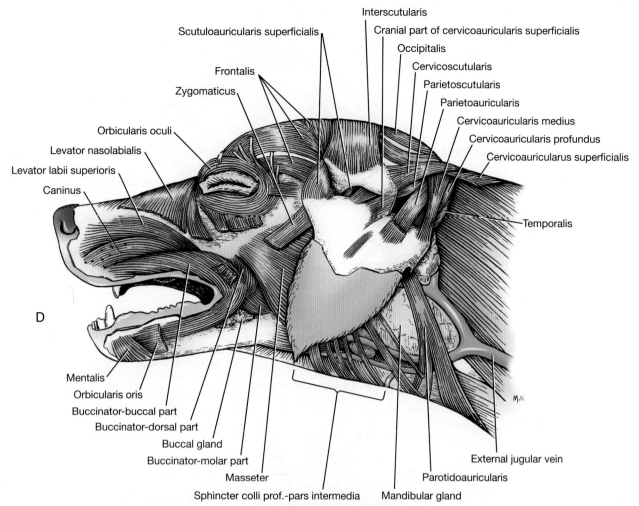

Interscutularis
Scutuloauricularis superficialis
Cranial part of cervicoauricularis superficialis
Frontalis
Occipitalis
Zygomaticus
Cervicoscutularis
Parietoscutularis
Orbicularis oculi
Parietoauricularis
Levator nasolabialis
Cervicoauricularis medius
Levator labii superioris
Cervicoauricularis profundus
Caninus
Cervicoauricularus superficialis
Temporalis
D
Mentalis
Orbicularis oris
Buccinator-buccal part
Buccinator-dorsal part
Buccal gland
Buccinator-molar part
External jugular vein
Masseter
Parotidoauricularis
Sphincter colli prof.-pars intermedia
Mandibular gland

Fig. 5-21, cont'd D, Deep muscles of the head and ear, lateral aspect. (**B-D** From Evans HE: *Miller's anatomy of the dog,* ed 4, St Louis, 2013, Saunders.)

The **orbicularis oris** lies near the free borders of the lips and extends from one lip to the other around the angle of the mouth. The fibers of each side end at the median plane of both the superior and inferior incisor regions.

The **buccinator muscle** is a thin, wide muscle that forms the foundation of the cheek. It attaches to the alveolar margins of the mandible and maxilla and the adjacent buccal mucosa. It may be found between the rostral border of the masseter muscle and the orbicularis oris. Place your finger within the cheek and press outward. This will help define the buccinator. A portion of the buccinator lies deep to the orbicularis oris muscle and is difficult to separate from it. It functions to return food from the vestibule to the occlusal surface of the teeth.

The **levator nasolabialis** is a flat muscle lying beneath the skin on the lateral surface of the maxillary bone. It arises from the maxillary bone, courses rostroventrally, and attaches to the edge of the superior lip and on the **naris,** the external opening of each half of the nasal cavity. It dilates the nostril and raises the superior lip.

Eyelids (Figs. 5-22 to 5-24)

Before dissecting the eyelids, **palpebrae,** observe their external features. The **superior and inferior palpebrae** (upper and lower eyelids) border the **palpebral fissure.** They join at either end of the fissure to form the **medial** and **lateral palpebral commissures.** Each commissure is attached by ligaments to adjacent bone. The **medial palpebral ligament** is well developed and attaches the medial commissure to the frontal bone near the nasomaxillary suture. The **lateral palpebral ligament** is poorly developed and attaches to the zygomatic bone at the orbital ligament.

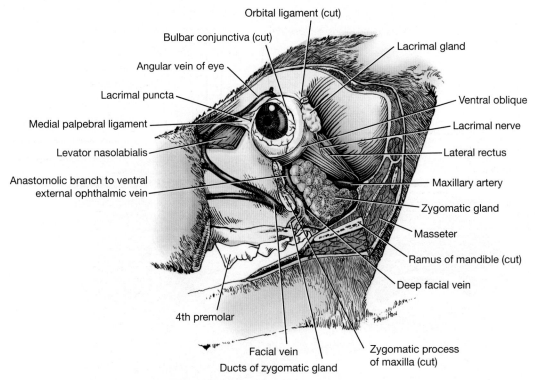

Orbital ligament (cut)

Bulbar conjunctiva (cut)

Angular vein of eye

Lacrimal puncta

Medial palpebral ligament

Levator nasolabialis

Anastomolic branch to ventral
external ophthalmic vein

Lacrimal gland

Ventral oblique

Lacrimal nerve

Lateral rectus

Maxillary artery

Zygomatic gland

Masseter

Ramus of mandible (cut)

Deep facial vein

4th premolar

Facial vein

Ducts of zygomatic gland

Zygomatic process
of maxilla (cut)

Fig. 5-22 Lateral aspect of orbit.

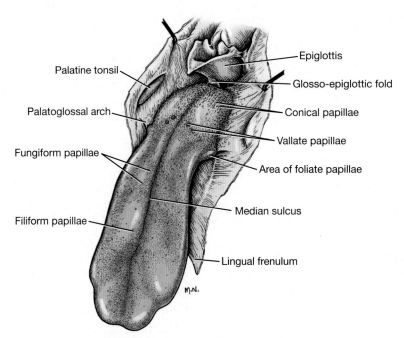

Palatine tonsil

Palatoglossal arch

Fungiform papillae

Filiform papillae

Epiglottis

Glosso-epiglottic fold

Conical papillae

Vallate papillae

Area of foliate papillae

Median sulcus

Lingual frenulum

Fig. 5-23 Tongue, dorsal aspect.

The upper eyelid bears cilia (eyelashes) on its free border. The lower eyelid lacks cilia. The cutaneous or external surface of the eyelid is covered by hair. The posterior or inner surface is covered by a mucous membrane, the **palpebral conjunctiva** (see Fig. 5-38). Follow the palpebral conjunctiva posteriorly to its reflection from the eyelids onto the globe of the eye, which is the **bulbar conjunctiva**. The angle formed by this reflection is called the **fornix**. The cavity thus formed, the **conjunctival sac,** is open rostrally at the palpebral fissure. It is bounded externally by the palpebral conjunctiva and internally by the bulbar conjunctiva adjacent to the sclera.

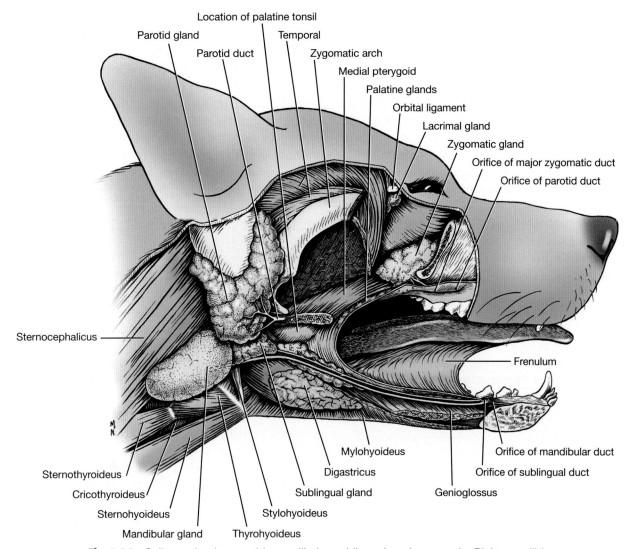

Fig. 5-24 Salivary glands: parotid, mandibular, sublingual, and zygomatic. Right mandible removed.

At the medial commissure, observe the triangular prominence of finely haired skin, the **lacrimal caruncle**. The **lacrimal punctum** (see Figs. 5-22, 5-37) of each lid is the beginning of the dorsal and ventral lacrimal ducts. Each is a small opening on the conjunctival margin of the lid a few millimeters from the medial commissure. The puncta may be difficult to see without the aid of magnification. They are easier to see in a live dog. The **lacrimal gland** (see Figs. 5-22, 5-24, 5-51, 5-55), located ventral to the zygomatic process of the frontal bone, secretes through many duct openings into the dorsolateral part of the conjunctival sac. After this serous fluid has passed across the cornea, it is collected by the puncta and passes in succession through the **lacrimal duct** of each lid, the **lacrimal sac,** and the **nasolacrimal duct** to the ventral nasal meatus of the rostral part of each nasal cavity. There, evaporation of the lacrimal secretion takes place. A significant contribution to tear secretion comes from the gland of the third eyelid, conjunctival goblet cells, and tarsal glands of the eyelids. The lacrimal gland and the rostral opening of the nasolacrimal duct will be seen later.

The **plica semilunaris,** or **third eyelid** (see Fig. 5-37), is a concave fold of palpebral conjunctiva and cartilage that protrudes from the medial angle of the eye. The cartilage is T-shaped, with an expanded portion in the medial canthus and a stem that extends ventrally into the orbit. It is surrounded by a body of fat and glandular tissue, the **superficial gland of the third eyelid**. This will be dissected shortly. Its serous secretion enters the conjunctival sac under the third eyelid at the medial commissure. Lift the third eyelid from the bulbar conjunctiva and examine its bulbar (lateral) surface. Note the slightly raised lymphoid tissue.

There are several muscles associated with the eyelids. The **orbicularis oculi** (see Fig. 5-21) lies partly in the eyelids and is attached medially to the medial palpebral ligament. Laterally, the fibers of the muscle blend with those of the **retractor anguli oculi lateralis,** which covers the lateral palpebral ligament. The action of the muscle is to close the palpebral fissure. The **levator palpebrae superioris** arises deep within the orbit and will be dissected with the muscles of the eyeball. It elevates the superior lid.

The External Ear

The **rostral auricular muscles** (see Fig. 5-21) include those muscles that lie on the forehead caudal to the orbit and converge toward the auricular cartilage. Transect the muscles at their origins and turn them toward the auricular cartilage. Notice that the mid-dorsal part arises from its fellow of the opposite side.

The **scutiform cartilage** is a small, boot-shaped, cartilaginous plate located in the muscles rostral and medial to the external ear. It is an isolated cartilage interposed in the auricular muscles.

The **caudal auricular muscles** are the largest group. Most of these muscles arise from the median raphe of the neck and attach directly to the auricular cartilage. Transect the caudal auricular muscles and turn the external ear ventrally to expose the temporal muscle. The other superficial muscles of the face, all innervated by the facial nerve, will not be dissected. They are collectively referred to as the *mimetic muscles* or *muscles of facial expression.*

Oral Cavity

The **oral cavity,** or mouth, is divided into the **vestibule** and the oral cavity proper. The vestibule is the cavity lying outside the teeth and gums and inside the lips and cheeks. The ducts of the parotid and zygomatic salivary glands open into the dorsocaudal part of the vestibule. The **parotid duct** opens through the cheek on a small papilla located opposite the caudal end of the upper fourth premolar or shearing tooth. The **ducts of the zygomatic gland** (see Figs. 5-22, 5-24) open into the vestibule lateral to the last upper molar tooth.

The **oral cavity proper** is bounded dorsally by the hard palate and a small part of the adjacent soft palate, laterally and rostrally by the dental arches, and ventrally by the tongue and adjacent mucosa. Its caudal boundary ventrally is the body of the tongue at the palatoglossal arch. Pull the tongue away from one mandible and note the fold of tissue that extends from the body of the tongue to the beginning of the soft palate; this is the **palatoglossal arch** (see Fig. 5-23). The oral cavity communicates freely with the vestibule by numerous interdental spaces and is continued caudally by the oropharynx.

Tongue

Examine the tongue (see Fig. 5-23). It is a muscular organ composed of the interwoven bundles of intrinsic and extrinsic muscles. These will be dissected later. It is divided into a **root,** which composes its caudal third; a **body,** which is the long, slender, rostral part of the tongue; and a free extremity, the **apex.** The mucosa covering the dorsum of the tongue is modified to form various types of papillae. A dissecting microscope facilitates examination of these structures. Five types of papillae are recognized by their shape. The **filiform papillae** are found predominantly on the body and apex of the tongue. They are arranged in rows like shingles, with their multiple pointed tips directed caudally. At the root of the tongue, the filiform papillae are replaced by **conical papillae,** which have only one pointed tip. The **fungiform papillae** have a smooth, rounded surface and are fewer in number. They are located among the filiform papillae. A few may be scattered caudally among the conical papillae. The **foliate papillae** are found on the lateral margins of the root of the tongue, rostral to the palatoglossal arch. They are leaf-like but appear as a row of parallel grooves in the fixed specimen. The **vallate papillae** are located at the junction of the body and root of the tongue. There are four to six in the dog, and they are arranged in the form of a V with the apex directed caudally. They are larger than the others, have a circular surface, and are surrounded by a sulcus. There are taste buds on vallate, foliate, and fungiform papillae.

The tongue is attached rostrally to the floor of the oral cavity by a ventral median fold of mucosa, the **lingual frenulum** (see Fig. 5-24). Examine the medial cut surface of the apex of the tongue. On the midline, just under the mucosa, is the **lyssa** (Fig. 5-25). This fusiform fibrous spicule extends from the apex to the level of the attachment of the frenulum. Expose the lyssa.

Salivary Glands

Turn the tongue medially and observe the slightly raised elevation of mucosa that is lateral to the rostral part of the frenulum and protrudes from the floor of the oral cavity. This is the **sublingual caruncle**. Extending caudally from the caruncle is the **sublingual fold**. (This is easier to see in the

live animal.) The **mandibular duct** and **major sublingual duct** (see Figs. 5-24, 5-48) are found in this fold. They course rostrally to open on or beside the sublingual caruncle, separately or through a common opening. Carefully incise the mucosa over these ducts from the caruncle to the root of the tongue at the palatoglossal arch. Bluntly reflect the mucosa to expose the ducts and associated salivary tissue. The major sublingual duct is connected caudally with the monostomatic sublingual gland. This is closely associated with the mandibular salivary gland. There

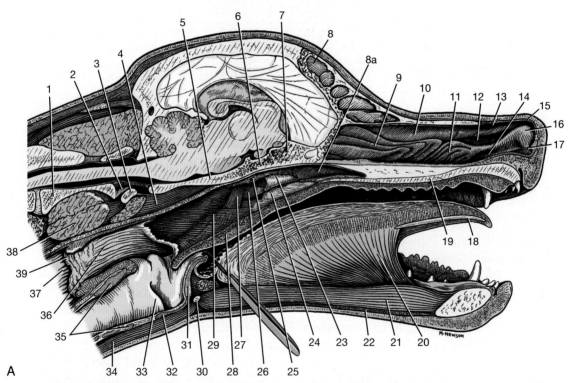

Fig. 5-25 A, Midsagittal section of head.

1. Axis
2. Dens
3. Atlas
4. Longus capitis
5. Basioccipital
6. Basisphenoid
7. Presphenoid
8. Frontal sinus
8a. Nasopharynx
9. Ethmoid labyrinth
10. Dorsal nasal concha
11. Ventral nasal concha
12. Middle nasal meatus
13. Dorsal nasal meatus
14. Ventral nasal meatus
15. Dorsal lateral nasal cartilage
16. Alar fold
17. Nasolacrimal duct orifice
18. Lyssa
19. Hard palate
20. Genioglossus
21. Geniohyoideus
22. Mylohyoideus
23. Pterygoid bone
24. Tensor veli palatini
25. Pharyngeal orifice of auditory tube
26. Pterygopharyngeus
27. Levator veli palatini
28. Soft palate
29. Palatopharyngeus
30. Basihyoid
31. Epiglottis
32. Thyroid cartilage
33. Vocal fold
34. Sternohyoideus
35. Cricoid cartilage
36. Laryngopharynx
37. Esophagus
38. Longus colli
39. Pharyngoesophageal limen

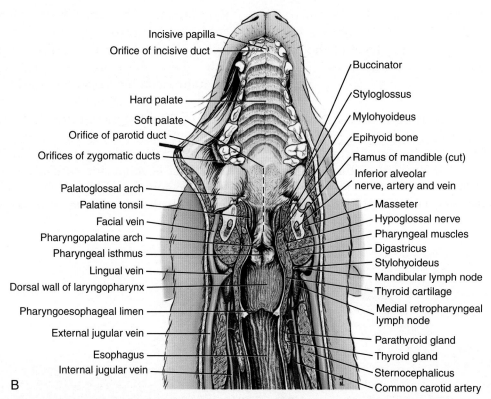

Incisive papilla
Orifice of incisive duct

Hard palate
Soft palate
Orifice of parotid duct
Orifices of zygomatic ducts

Palatoglossal arch
Palatine tonsil
Facial vein
Pharyngopalatine arch
Pharyngeal isthmus
Lingual vein
Dorsal wall of laryngopharynx
Pharyngoesophageal limen
External jugular vein
Esophagus
Internal jugular vein

Buccinator
Styloglossus
Mylohyoideus
Epihyoid bone
Ramus of mandible (cut)
Inferior alveolar
nerve, artery and vein
Masseter
Hypoglossal nerve
Pharyngeal muscles
Digastricus
Stylohyoideus
Mandibular lymph node
Thyroid cartilage
Medial retropharyngeal
lymph node
Parathyroid gland
Thyroid gland
Sternocephalicus
Common carotid artery

B

Fig. 5-25, cont'd   B, Dorsal plane section of head and neck through the digestive tube, ventral aspect. (From Evans HE, de Lahunta A: *Miller's anatomy of the dog*, ed 4, St Louis, 2013, Saunders.)

are also sublingual gland lobules (the polystomatic sublingual gland) deep to the mucosa of the sublingual fold. These have independent microscopic ducts opening into the oral cavity. Follow the mandibular and major sublingual ducts to the root of the tongue. Their origin will be seen when these glands are dissected from the lateral side of the head.

Expose the **mandibular salivary gland** (see Figs. 2-12, 5-24, 5-48) on the lateral side of the head just caudal to the angle of the mandible, where it lies between the maxillary and linguofacial veins. It is covered by a thick capsule that also includes the caudal part of the monostomatic **sublingual gland** (see Figs. 5-24, 5-48). Incise the capsule that surrounds these two glands and free the caudal portion by elevating it from the capsule.

Locate the division between the rostrally located sublingual gland, which is roughly triangular, and the larger ovoid mandibular gland. The ducts of both glands leave the rostromedial surface and enter the space between the masseter and the digastricus muscles. These ducts course rostrally beside the frenulum to open in the oral cavity at the sublingual caruncle. Lobules of the sublingual gland continue into the oral cavity

with these ducts, where they can be seen beneath the oral mucosa.

The **parotid salivary gland** (see Figs. 2-12, 5-24) lies between the mandibular gland and the ear. It is closely applied to the base of the auricular cartilage of the ear. A small **parotid lymph node** may be found along the rostral border of this gland. The **parotid duct** (see Figs. 5-24, 5-43) is formed by two or three converging radicles, which unite and leave the rostral border of the gland. It grooves the lateral surface of the masseter muscle as it passes to the cheek. It opens into the vestibule on a small papilla at the level of the caudal margin of the fourth upper premolar. Evert the upper lip near the commissure and find the small opening into the vestibule. The **zygomatic salivary gland** is medial to the zygomatic bone between the eyeball and the pterygoid muscle where it will be dissected with the eye. The **ducts of the zygomatic salivary gland** open into the vestibule near the last molar, caudal to the parotid duct.

Palate

The palate is a partly bony membranous partition between the rostral portions of the respiratory and digestive systems. The nasal cavities and nasopharynx are dorsal to the palate and the oral cavity and oropharynx are ventral to it. The hard palate is formed by the palatine, maxillary, and incisor bones on each side. Examine the roof of the oral cavity. The hard palate is crossed by approximately eight transverse ridges (see Figs. 5-25, 5-26, *B*). A small eminence, the **incisive papilla,** is located just caudal to the central incisor teeth. The fissure on either side of this papilla is the oral opening of the **incisive duct**. The incisive duct passes through the palatine fissure and opens into the ventral nasal meatus. Extending caudally from the incisive duct, close to its entrance into the nasal cavity, is the **vomeronasal organ** (see Fig. 5-16). This tubular structure about 2 cm long lies at the base of the nasal septum dorsal to the hard palate and is an olfactory receptor of sexual stimuli. It can sometimes be seen on the sagittal section of the head if the cut was made slightly to one side of the midline. The soft palate is caudal to the hard palate and consists of a relatively thick membrane that is primarily situated between the nasopharynx and the oropharynx.

Pharynx

The pharynx (see Figs. 5-25, 5-26, *A*) is a passage that is common, in part, to both the respiratory and digestive systems. It is located between the oral cavity and esophagus and is divided into

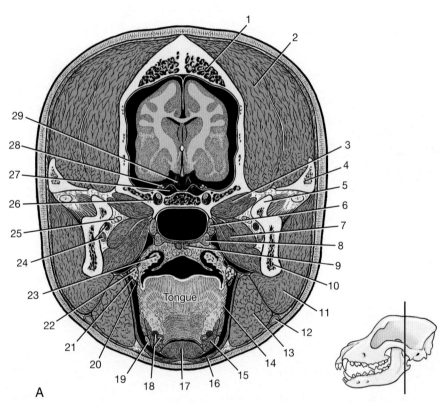

Fig. 5-26 **A,** Transection of head through palatine tonsil.

1. Diploë
2. Temporal m.
3. Lateral pterygoid m.
4. Zygomatic process of temporal bone
5. Condylar process
6. Tensor veli palatini
7. Medial pterygoid m.
8. Pterygopharyngeus m.
9. Palatinus m.
10. Mandible
11. Masseter m.
12. Facial vein
13. Digastricus m.
14. Styloglossus m.
15. Hyoglossus m.
16. Mylohyoideus m.
17. Geniohyoideus m.
18. Lingual a. and v.
19. Hypoglossal n.
20. Mandibular duct
21. Major sublingual duct
22. Sublingual salivary gland
23. Palatine tonsil in tonsillar fossa
24. Inferior alveolar a. and v.
25. Mylohyoid, inferior alveolar, and lingual nn.
26. Maxillary a., v., and n. in alar canal
27. Internal carotid a. in cavernous sinus
28. Cranial nerves III, IV, and VI and ophthalmic division of V
29. Cerebral arterial circle—caudal communicating a.

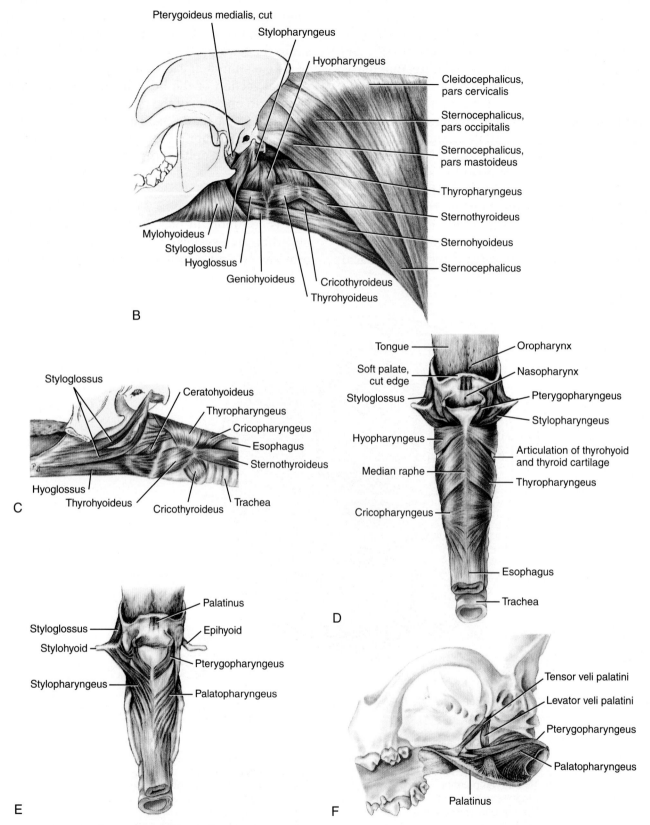

Fig. 5-26, cont'd   B, The hyoid muscles and muscles of the neck, lateral aspect. (Stylo-hyoideus and digastricus removed.) **C,** Muscles of the tongue and pharynx, deep dissection, lateral aspect. **D,** Muscles of the pharynx, dorsal aspect. **E,** Muscles of the pharynx, deep dissection, dorsal aspect. **F,** Muscles of the pharynx and palate, deep dissection, ventrolateral aspect. (Parts **B-F** from Evans HE, de Lahunta A: *Miller's anatomy of the dog,* ed 4, St Louis, 2013, Saunders.)

oral, nasal, and laryngeal parts. The **oropharynx** extends from the level of the palatoglossal arches to the caudal border of the soft palate and the base of the epiglottis at the caudal end of the root of the tongue. The dorsal and ventral boundaries of the oropharynx are the soft palate and the root of the tongue. The lateral wall of the oropharynx contains the palatine tonsil in the tonsillar fossa.

The **palatine tonsil** (see Figs. 5-23, 5-24, 5-26) is elongated and is located caudal to the palatoglossal arch. The medial wall of the fossa, which partially covers the tonsil, is the **semilunar fold**. The tonsil is attached laterally throughout its entire length. Reflect the tonsil from the fossa.

The two nasal cavities extend from the nares to the choanae. They are separated by the **nasal septum**. Each nasal cavity is divided into four meatuses. These were described with the bones of the nasal cavity and should be reviewed now. On the floor of the rostrolateral end of the ventral meatus, find the **opening of the nasolacrimal duct** on the ventral aspect of the alar fold (see Fig. 5-25). It may be necessary to remove the rostral end of the cartilaginous septum to see the opening. This duct comes from the lacrimal sac at the medial commissure of the eye.

The **nasopharynx** extends from the choanae to the junction of the palatopharyngeal arches at the caudal border of the soft palate. A **palatopharyngeal arch** extends caudally on each side from the caudal border of the soft palate to the dorsolateral wall of the nasopharynx. It is a fold of mucosa that covers the palatopharyngeus muscle. On the lateral wall of the nasopharynx, dorsal to the middle of the soft palate, is an oblique, slitlike opening, the pharyngeal opening of the **auditory tube**.

The **laryngopharynx** (see Fig. 5-25) is dorsal to the larynx. It extends from the palatopharyngeal arches to the beginning of the esophagus. The esophagus begins at an annular constriction at the level of the cricoid cartilage, the **pharyngoesophageal limen**.

Pharyngeal Muscles (Figs. 5-25, 5-26, 5-33)

The pharyngeal muscles aid directly in swallowing. The **cricopharyngeus** arises from the lateral surface of the cricoid cartilage. Its fibers are inserted on the median dorsal raphe of the laryngopharynx. Caudally, its fibers blend with the esophagus.

The **thyropharyngeus** arises from the lateral side of the thyroid lamina and is inserted on the median dorsal raphe of the pharynx. This muscle is rostral to the cricopharyngeus and caudal to the hyopharyngeus.

The **hyopharyngeus** is in two parts as it arises from the lateral surface of the thyrohyoid bone and the ceratohyoid bone. This origin was previously transected. The fibers of both parts form a muscle plate that passes dorsally over the larynx and pharynx to be inserted on the median dorsal raphe of the pharynx with its fellow from the opposite side. These pharyngeal muscles are all innervated by pharyngeal branches of the glossopharyngeal and vagus nerves. The remaining pharyngeal muscles and muscles of the palate listed here need not be dissected.

The **palatopharyngeus** passes from the soft palate into the lateral and dorsal wall of the pharynx. Its border is in the palatopharyngeal arch. The **pterygopharyngeus** arises from the pterygoid bone, passes caudally, and is inserted in the dorsal wall of the pharynx. These muscles constrict and shorten the pharynx.

The **stylopharyngeus** arises from the stylohyoid bone and passes caudolaterally deep to the hyopharyngeus and thyropharyngeus muscles to be inserted in the dorsolateral wall of the pharynx. It acts to dilate the pharynx.

The **levator veli palatini** arises from the tympanic part of the temporal bone and passes ventrally to enter the soft palate caudal to the pterygoid bone. It raises the caudal end of the soft palate.

The **tensor veli palatini** arises mainly from the cartilaginous wall of the auditory tube and is inserted on the pterygoid bone and medially on the soft palate.

Larynx

Cartilages of the Larynx (Figs. 5-27 to 5-30)

Study the cartilages of the larynx on the hemisected head and on specimens from which the muscles have been removed. Visualize their topography in your bisected specimen and palpate them through the laryngeal mucosa. The laryngeal cartilages that will be dissected include the paired arytenoid and the unpaired epiglottic, thyroid, and cricoid cartilages.

The **epiglottic cartilage** lies at the entrance to the larynx. Its lingual surface is attached to the

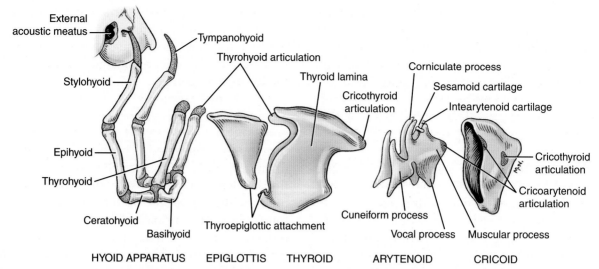

Fig. 5-27 Cartilages of disarticulated larynx with hyoid apparatus intact, left lateral view.

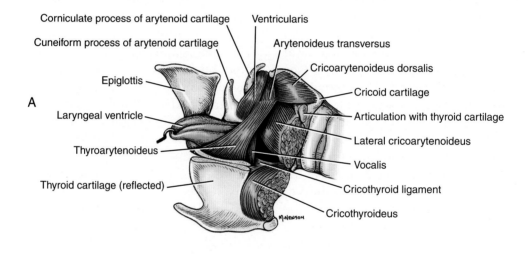

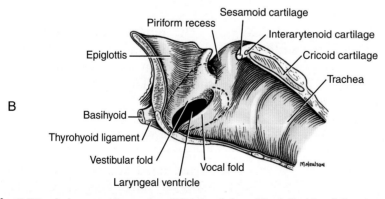

Fig. 5-28 **A,** Laryngeal muscles, left lateral view. The left side of the thyroid cartilage is reflected. The left laryngeal ventricle has been everted. **B,** Median section of the larynx. (The *dotted line* indicates the extent of the lateral ventricle and the laryngeal ventricle.) (From Evans HE: *Miller's anatomy of the dog,* ed 4, St Louis, 2013, Saunders.)

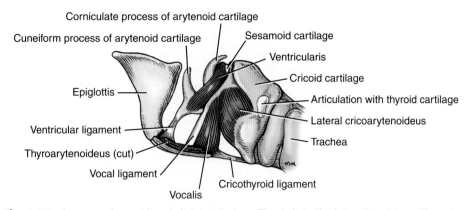

Fig. 5-29 Laryngeal muscles, left lateral view. The left half of the thyroid cartilage has been removed along with the thyroarytenoideus, arytenoideus transversus, and cricoarytenoideus dorsalis.

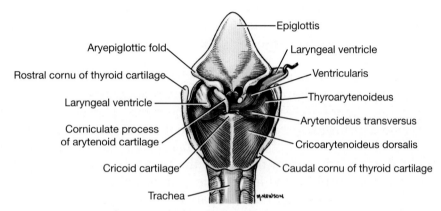

Fig. 5-30 Laryngeal muscles, dorsal view.

basihyoid bone and faces the oropharynx. The apex lies just dorsal to the edge of the soft palate. The lateral margin is attached by mucosa to the cuneiform process of the arytenoid to form the **aryepiglottic fold**. Caudally, the epiglottis attaches to the body of the thyroid cartilage.

The **thyroid cartilage** forms a deep trough, which is open dorsally. The **rostral cornu** articulates with the thyrohyoid bone; the **caudal cornu** articulates with the caudal aspect of the cricoid cartilage. Ventrally, the caudal border is notched by a median **caudal thyroid incisure**. The **cricothyroid ligament** attaches the caudal border to the ventral arch of the cricoid cartilage.

The **cricoid cartilage** forms a complete ring that lies partially within the trough of the thyroid cartilage. It has a wide dorsal plate, or lamina, and a narrow ventral arch. Near the caudal border at the junction of the lamina and the arch, there is a lateral facet for articulation with the caudal cornu of the thyroid cartilage. On the cranial border of the lamina, there is a prominent

pair of lateral facets for articulation with the arytenoid cartilages.

The **arytenoid cartilage** is paired, irregular in shape, and located in a sagittal plane. Each articulates medially with a facet on the rostral border of the cricoid lamina and has a lateral **muscular process** and a ventrally directed **vocal process**. The **vocal fold** is attached between the vocal process of the arytenoid and the midventral part of the thyroid cartilage. The arytenoid cartilage bears a **corniculate process** dorsally. Rostral to this process, the **cuneiform process** is attached to the arytenoid. The **vestibular fold** extends between the thyroid cartilage ventrally and the ventral portion of the cuneiform process dorsally and forms the rostral boundary of the laryngeal ventricle. The **laryngeal ventricle** is a diverticulum of the laryngeal mucosa bounded laterally by the thyroid cartilage and medially by the arytenoid cartilage. It opens into the larynx between the vestibular fold rostrally and vocal fold caudally. Observe these folds and the laryngeal ventricle on the medial side of your specimen.

The **glottis** consists of the vocal folds, the vocal processes of the arytenoid cartilages, and the **rima glottidis,** which is the narrow passageway through the glottis. At this level the size and shape of the air passageway can be altered by muscular activity.

Muscles of the Larynx (Figs. 5-28 through 5-30)

The **cricothyroid muscle** (see Fig. 5-28) lies ventral to the insertion of the sternothyroideus muscle and passes from the cricoid cartilage to the thyroid lamina. It tenses the vocal fold indirectly by drawing the ventral parts of the cricoid and thyroid cartilages together. It is innervated by the cranial laryngeal nerve, a branch of the vagus. Observe this on the lateral side.

On the medial side of the specimen reflect the mucosa of the laryngopharynx from the dorsal aspect of the larynx. Separate the thyroid lamina from the cricoid and arytenoid cartilages to expose the muscles.

The **cricoarytenoideus dorsalis** arises from the dorsolateral surface of the cricoid cartilage and inserts on the muscular process on the lateral surface of the arytenoid cartilage. It rotates the arytenoid so that the vocal process moves laterally, opening the glottis. It is the only laryngeal muscle that functions primarily to open the glottis. Transect the muscle and examine the articular surface of the cricoarytenoid joint. On the intact specimen of laryngeal cartilages, grasp the muscular process of the arytenoid with forceps and pull it caudomedially as it would be pulled by the functioning cricoarytenoideus dorsalis muscle. Observe the abduction of the vocal process and fold that widens the glottal opening.

The **cricoarytenoideus lateralis** arises from the lateral surface of the cricoid cartilage and inserts on the arytenoid cartilage between the cricoarytenoideus dorsalis and the vocalis. It acts to close the glottis by pulling the muscular process ventrally and thus moving the vocal process medially. Expose this muscle by reflecting the cricoid medially away from the thyroid lamina.

The **thyroarytenoideus** is the parent muscle that gives rise to the vocalis muscle medially and ventricularis muscle rostrally. It arises along the internal midline of the thyroid cartilage and inserts on the arytenoid cartilage. Its function is to relax the vocal fold and to constrict the glottis.

The **vocalis** is a medial division of the thyroarytenoid muscle. It arises on the internal midline of the thyroid cartilage and inserts on the vocal process of the arytenoid cartilage. Cut the laryngeal mucosa of the vocal fold and observe the medial side of this muscle. Attached along its rostral border is the **vocal ligament**.

The cricoarytenoideus dorsalis and lateralis and the thyroarytenoideus muscles are innervated by the caudal laryngeal nerve from the recurrent laryngeal nerve. The ventricularis and arytenoideus transversus will not be dissected. Notice the relationship of the laryngeal ventricles to the laryngeal muscles. From its laryngeal opening, the ventricle runs rostrally between the thyroid lamina and thyroarytenoideus laterally and the vestibular fold, the cuneiform process, and the ventricularis medially.

The External Ear (Fig. 5-31)

The external ear (Fig. 5-31) consists of the auricle and the external acoustic meatus (ear canal). The external acoustic meatus is mostly cartilaginous but has a short osseous part on the lateral aspect of the tympanic bulla. The cartilaginous part of the meatus makes a right-angle turn in the deeper part of its course and extends to the tympanic membrane.

Except for one small annular cartilage adjacent to the skull, the external ear consists of a single auricular cartilage that is rolled into a tube ventromedially. The tubular part becomes the external acoustic meatus. Remove the skin from the base of the auricular cartilage. The **auricular cartilage** is funnel-shaped. Its external, convex surface faces caudally; its internal, concave surface faces rostrally. It has a slightly folded medial and lateral margin called the **helix**. The auricular cartilage is thin and pliable except proximally, where it thickens and rolls into a tube. On its internal, concave wall at the level of the beginning of the external acoustic meatus, there is a transverse ridge, the **anthelix**. Opposite the anthelix the rostral boundary of the initial part of the ear canal is formed by a thick, quadrangular plate of the auricular cartilage, the **tragus**. Projecting caudally from the tragus and completing the lateral boundary of the external ear canal is a thin, elongate piece of cartilage, the **antitragus**. The **intertragic incisure** separates these two parts of the auricular cartilage.

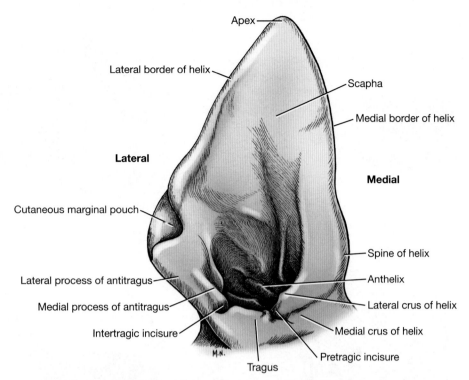

Fig. 5-31   Right external ear, rostral surface.

The lateral portion of the helix is indented proximally by an incisure. At this point the skin forms a pouch, the **marginal cutaneous sac**.

The medial helix is nearly straight. An abrupt angle in this border at its proximal end forms the **spine of the helix**. Between the spine of the helix and the tragus the medial border of the ear canal is formed by two curved portions of the cartilage, the **medial** and **lateral crura** of the helix. They both end laterally in a free border separated from the tragus by the **pretragic incisure**.

Incise the lateral wall of the ear canal by two parallel incisions starting at the intertragic and pretragic incisures. Reflect the isolated piece of the lateral wall to observe the course of the external acoustic meatus to the **tympanic membrane**.

Interposed between the auricular cartilage and the bony external acoustic meatus of the temporal bone is the **annular cartilage**. This is a band of cartilage that overlaps the bony projection of the meatus.

Muscles of Mastication and Related Muscles

On the left half of the head, cut all of the attachments of the temporal and masseter muscles to the zygomatic arch. Cut through the arch rostrally and caudally and remove all of the arch rostral to the temporomandibular joint.

The **temporalis muscle** (see Figs. 5-24, 5-26, 5-32) arises from the temporal fossa and inserts on the coronoid process of the mandible. Remove the muscle from its wide origin by scraping it off the bone with a blunt instrument, such as a scalpel handle, and reflect it. Be vigorous; there is a large amount of muscle to remove. The temporal and masseter muscles fuse between the zygomatic arch and the coronoid process.

The **masseter muscle** (see Figs. 2-12, 5-21, *D*, 5-26, 5-32) arises from the zygomatic arch, where its deep portion is intermingled with the fibers of the temporal muscle. It inserts in the masseteric fossa, the ventrolateral surface of the ramus of the mandible, and the angular process. The muscle is covered by a strong, glistening aponeurosis and contains many tendinous intermuscular strands.

Transect the temporal muscle as close to its insertion as possible. With bone cutters, remove the coronoid process and the remaining attached muscles. Observe the dorsal surface of the pterygoid muscles, which are now exposed in the ventral orbit.

Between the eyeball and the pterygoid muscles is the **zygomatic salivary gland** (see Figs. 5-22, 5-24, 5-48). It is hidden laterally by the zygomatic bone. The gland opens into the vestibule by one

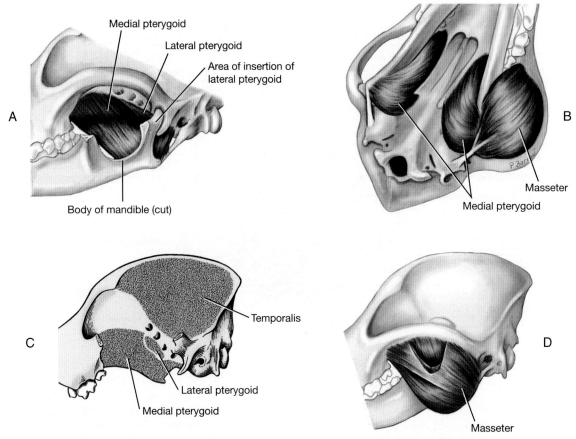

Fig. 5-32   Muscles of mastication. **A,** Pterygoideus medialis and lateralis. **B,** Masseter and pterygoideus medialis. **C,** Areas of origin of temporalis, pterygoideus medialis, and lateralis. **D,** Masseter cut to show the deep portion.

main and several minor ducts lateral to the last superior molar tooth.

The **medial** and **lateral pterygoid muscles** (see Figs. 5-24, 5-26, 5-32, 5-48, 5-55) arise from the pterygopalatine fossa and insert on the medial surface and caudal margin of the ramus of the mandible and angular process, ventral to the insertion of the temporal muscle. The muscles need not be distinguished from each other. The bulk of the muscle mass is the medial pterygoid. On the medial side of your specimen, cut the mucosa of the oropharynx from the rostral end of the palatine tonsil to the midline at the junction of the soft and hard palates. Reflect the cut edges to expose the ventral surface of the medial pterygoid muscle. On a dog skull, remove the mandible and place your thumb in the pterygopalatine fossa to appreciate the position of this muscle. The eyeball and its periorbital sheath would rest on your thumb.

The temporal, masseter, and pterygoid muscles (see Fig. 5-32) function to close the mouth. They are innervated by the mandibular nerve, a branch of the trigeminal nerve (cranial nerve V).

Reflect the mandibular and parotid salivary glands to expose the digastricus muscle.

The **digastricus** (see Figs. 2-12, 5-24, 5-26) arises from the paracondylar process of the occipital bone and is inserted on the body of the mandible. A tendinous intersection crosses its belly and divides it into rostral and caudal parts. Transect it and expose its attachments. It acts to open the mouth. The rostral portion is innervated by the mandibular nerve (a branch of the trigeminal, cranial nerve V), whereas the caudal belly is innervated by the facial nerve (cranial nerve VII).

Lingual Muscles (Figs. 5-25, 5-26, 5-33)
The muscles of the tongue may be divided into extrinsic and intrinsic groups. Three paired extrinsic muscles enter the tongue. The styloglossus and hyoglossus muscles are best exposed on the lateral side, the genioglossus on the medial side.

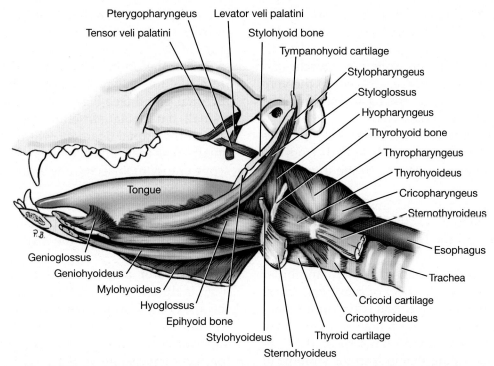

Fig. 5-33 Muscles of pharynx and tongue, left lateral view, left mandible removed.

The **styloglossus** arises from the stylohyoid bone, passes rostroventrally lateral to the palatine tonsil, and inserts in the middle of the tongue. It retracts and elevates the tongue.

The **hyoglossus** arises from the thyrohyoid and the basihyoid and passes into the root of the tongue. It lies medial to the styloglossus and retracts and depresses the tongue.

The **genioglossus** arises from the intermandibular articulation and adjacent surface of the body of the mandible. It joins its fellow at the median plane and is bounded medially by the geniohyoideus and laterally by the hyoglossus. Its caudal fibers protrude the tongue, and its rostral ones retract the apex. It lies partly in the frenulum. These muscles are all innervated by the hypoglossal nerve (cranial nerve XII).

Hyoid Muscles (Figs. 5-33, 5-34)

The hyoid muscles are associated with the hyoid apparatus, which suspends the larynx and anchors the tongue. They function in swallowing, lolling, lapping, and retching. All muscles of this group have names with the suffix *hyoideus*. The prefixes of the hyoid muscles designate the bone or part from which they arise. Dissect the following hyoid muscles from the lateral side.

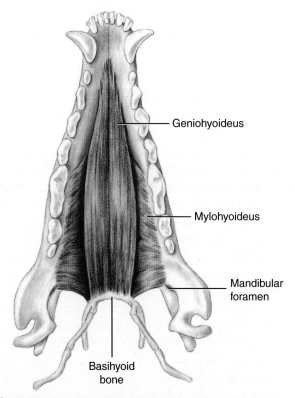

Fig. 5-34 Muscles of mandible and basihyoid bone, dorsal aspect. (From Evans HE, de Lahunta A: *Miller's anatomy of the dog,* ed 4, St Louis, 2013, Saunders.)

The **sternohyoideus,** from its origin on the sternum and first costal cartilage, is fused to the deeper sternothyroideus for the first third of its length. It then separates from this muscle and runs an independent course, adjacent to the ventral midline, to insert on the basihyoid bone. Its origin was previously dissected.

The **thyrohyoideus** is a short muscle that lies dorsal to the sternohyoideus. It extends from the thyroid cartilage of the larynx to the thyrohyoid bone.

The sternohyoideus and thyrohyoideus muscles are innervated by ventral branches of cervical spinal nerves and the hypoglossal nerve (cranial nerve XII).

The **mylohyoideus** spans the intermandibular space. It arises as a thin sheet of transverse fibers from the medial surface of the body of the mandible. It is inserted on its fellow muscle at the midventral raphe. Caudally, it inserts on the basihyoid. It forms a sling that aids in the support of the tongue. It is innervated by the mandibular nerve of the trigeminal.

The **geniohyoideus** lies deep to the mylohyoideus. It is a muscular strap that arises on and adjacent to the intermandibular articulation. It parallels its fellow along the median plane and attaches to the basihyoid. Contraction of the geniohyoideus draws the hyoid apparatus and larynx rostrally. It is innervated by the hypoglossal nerve.

The Eye and Related Structures

The **orbit** is a conical cavity containing the eyeball and ocular adnexa. These were exposed when the muscles of mastication were dissected. The orbital margin is formed by the frontal, lacrimal, maxillary, and zygomatic bones and the orbital ligament laterally. The medial wall of the orbit is formed by parts of the frontal, presphenoid, and lacrimal bones. The ventral wall includes the zygomatic salivary gland and the pterygoid muscles. The dorsal and lateral walls are formed primarily by temporal muscle.

The **periorbita** (see Fig. 5-55) is a cone-shaped sheath of connective tissue and smooth muscle that encloses the eyeball and its muscles, vessels, and nerves. Where the periorbita contacts the bone medially, it is the periosteum of the orbit. Its apex is caudal where it attaches to the bony margin of the optic canal and the orbital fissure. Here it is continuous with the dura intracranially.

Rostrally, it widens to blend with the periosteum of the face. Orbital fat may be observed on both sides of the periorbita.

Reflect the orbital ligament and the periorbita from the dorsolateral surface of the eyeball. The **lacrimal gland** (see Figs. 5-22, 5-24, 5-51, 5-55) is a small, flat lobular structure lying on the medial side of the orbital ligament within the periorbita. Small ducts that cannot be seen without a microscope empty their secretions into the conjunctival sac at the dorsal fornix.

Incise the periorbita longitudinally on its lateral side and reflect it to expose the eyeball muscles and the levator of the superior eyelid (see Figs. 5-35, 5-56).

The **levator palpebrae superioris** (Figs. 5-35, 5-56) is thin, narrow, and superficial. It begins at the apex of the orbit, extends over the dorsal rectus, and widens to insert as a flat tendon in the superior eyelid. It is innervated by the oculomotor nerve (cranial nerve III).

There are seven extrinsic muscles of the eyeball (see Figs. 5-35, 5-36, 5-51, 5-56): two **obliquus muscles,** four **rectus muscles,** and the **retractor bulbi.** All of these extrinsic muscles insert on the fibrous coat of the eyeball, the sclera, near the equator of the eyeball. The rectus muscles insert closer to the corneoscleral junction than the retractor muscles.

The four rectus muscles are the **dorsal rectus, medial rectus, ventral rectus,** and **lateral rectus.** As they course rostrally from their small area of origin around the optic canal and orbital fissure, they diverge and attach to the sclera on an imaginary line encircling the eyeball at its equator. In the spaces between the rectus muscles, parts of the **retractor bulbi** can be seen. The retractor bulbi muscle consists of four fascicles that surround the prechiasmatic optic tract (optic nerve), a dorsal pair and a ventral pair. The retractor bulbi and lateral rectus are innervated by the abducent nerve (cranial nerve VI). The other three recti are innervated by the oculomotor nerve.

The **dorsal oblique** ascends on the dorsomedial side of the extraocular muscles dorsal to the medial rectus. Roll the dorsal aspect of the eyeball laterally to expose these muscles. The dorsal oblique is a narrow muscle that forms a long tendon rostrally that passes through a groove in the trochlea. The **trochlea** is a cartilaginous plaque attached at the level of the medial angle of the eye to the wall of the orbit. This must be

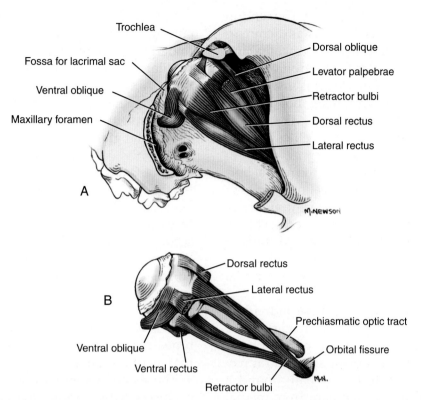

Fig. 5-35 **A,** Extrinsic muscles of left eyeball, dorsolateral view. **B,** Retractor bulbi muscle exposed, lateral view.

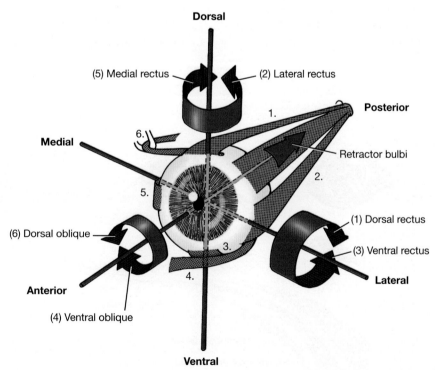

Fig. 5-36 Schema of extrinsic ocular muscles and their action on the left eyeball.

detached to roll the eyeball laterally. The tendon of the dorsal oblique muscle turns and courses laterally after passing around the trochlea and attaches to the sclera under the tendon of insertion of the dorsal rectus muscle. This insertion is difficult to distinguish and need not be dissected (see Figs. 5-35, 5-36, 5-56). The dorsal oblique is innervated by the trochlear nerve (cranial nerve IV).

The **ventral oblique** arises from the rostral border of the palatine bone at the level of the maxillary foramen, passes ventral to the ventral rectus, and is inserted on the sclera at the insertion of the lateral rectus. This is the only extraocular muscle that does not arise from the apex of the orbit. It is innervated by the oculomotor nerve (cranial nerve III).

To understand the action of these individual muscles, consider the eyeball as having three imaginary axes that cross in the center of the globe (see Fig. 5-36). The dorsal and ventral rectus muscles would rotate the eyeball around a horizontal axis through the equator from medial to lateral. The medial and lateral rectus muscles would rotate it around a vertical axis through the equator from dorsal to ventral. The oblique muscles would rotate the eyeball around a longitudinal axis passing from anterior to posterior through the center of the eyeball.

Enlarge the opening of the palpebral fissure by cutting through the lateral commissure and the underlying conjunctiva to the eyeball. This will facilitate exposure of the third eyelid in the medial angle.

Elevate the third eyelid and observe the lymph nodules on its bulbar conjunctival surface and the **superficial gland of the third eyelid** (Fig. 5-37).

Bulbus Oculi

In the following dissection, leave the bulbus oculi, or eyeball, in the orbit. Many of these structures are best observed in a fresh eye under a dissecting microscope. Freeze-dried preparations of the opened eyeball are instructive for seeing the zonular fibers that suspend the lens. Directional terms used with reference to the eyeball are anterior and posterior and superior and inferior. The wall is composed of three layers: an external fibrous coat, a vascular coat, and an internal coat that includes the retina (Figs. 5-38 through 5-40).

1. The **external fibrous coat** is composed of the **cornea,** which forms the anterior one fourth, and the **sclera,** which forms the posterior three fourths. The cornea is transparent and circular. It meets the dense, opaque sclera peripherally at the corneoscleral junction, or **limbus,** of the cornea. The sclera is dull gray-white. Anteriorly, it is covered by bulbar conjunctiva. Posterior

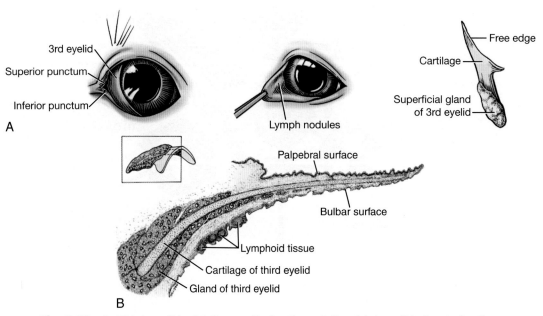

Fig. 5-37 A, Third eyelid of left eye. **B,** Section of the third eyelid. *Inset:* Cartilage and superficial gland of third eyelid showing plane of section. (Part **B** from Evans HE, de Lahunta A: *Miller's anatomy of the dog,* ed 4, St Louis, 2013, Saunders.)

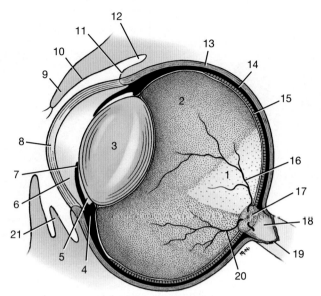

Fig. 5-38 Sagittal section of eyeball.

1. Tapetum lucidum
2. Nontapetal nigrum
3. Lens
4. Ciliary body
5. Posterior chamber
6. Anterior chamber
7. Iris
8. Cornea
9. Superior eyelid
10. Palpebral conjunctiva
11. Bulbar conjunctiva

12. Fornix
13. Sclera
14. Choroid
15. Retina
16. Superior retinal vein
17. Optic disk
18. Prechiasmatic optic tract
19. Dura—arachnoid
20. Inferior medial retinal vein
21. Third eyelid

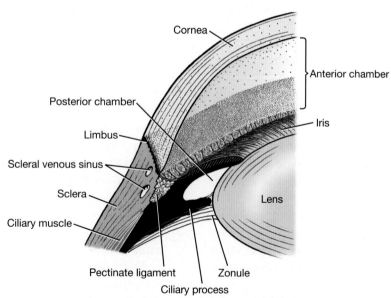

Fig. 5-39 Section of eyeball at iridocorneal angle.

to this, the extrinsic ocular muscles insert in its wall, and it is penetrated by blood vessels and nerves, including the large prechiasmatic optic tract posteriorly. Transect and reflect the attachments of the lateral rectus and retractor bulbi

muscles on the eyeball and observe the prechiasmatic optic tract on the posterior surface of the globe.

2. The **middle vascular coat** (the **uvea**) is deep to the sclera and consists of three continuous

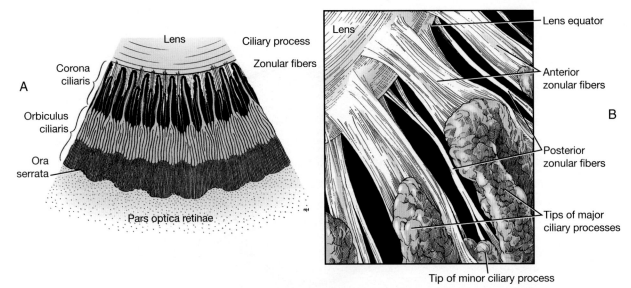

Fig. 5-40   A, Inner surface of a ciliary body segment. **B,** Zonular fibers passing along ciliary processes before attaching to lens, anterior view.

parts from posterior to anterior: the choroid, ciliary body, and iris. The **iris,** which has circular and radial smooth muscles, can be seen through the cornea as a pigmented diaphragm with a central opening, the **pupil.** While the eyeball is in the orbit, use a sharp scalpel or razor blade to make a sagittal cut through the eyeball from anterior to posterior pole and remove the lateral half of the eyeball.

The **choroid** is the posterior portion of the vascular coat and is firmly attached to the sclera. It is pigmented and lines the internal surface of the sclera as far anterior as the ciliary body posterior to the lens. The junction of the choroid and the ciliary body, called the **ora serrata** (see Fig. 5-40, *A*), is seen as an undulating line in the overlying retina. The **fundus** is the posterior or deep portion of the eyeball that is seen with the ophthalmoscope. The light-colored, reflective area in the dorsal part of the fundus is the **tapetum lucidum** (see Fig. 5-38) of the choroid. This is a specialized layer of cells in the choroid behind the retina that reflects light rays.

The vascular coat forms a thick circular mound at the level of the limbus. This is the **ciliary body** (see Fig. 5-38). The ciliary body, located between the iris and choroid, contains numerous muscle bundles that function in the regulation of the shape of the lens. The internal surface of the ciliary body is marked by longitudinal folds, the **ciliary processes** (see

Figs. 5-39, 5-40, *A* and *B*). Observe these on the lateral portion of the eyeball that was removed. These processes surround but do not attach to the lens at its equator. They consist of several hundred pigmented folds alternating in length, which are small at their posterior border near the ora serrata but enlarge anteriorly as they approach the lens.

The **zonule** is the suspensory apparatus of the lens (see Figs. 5-39, 5-40). It is composed of numerous fine strands, **zonular fibers,** which pass from the region of the ora serrata along the ciliary processes to the equator of the lens. The lens is suspended from the ciliary processes by the zonular fibers. Contraction of the ciliary muscles pulls the ciliary body and processes toward the lens and therefore relaxes the tension on the zonular fibers attached to the lens. This allows the elastic lens to become more spherical and accommodate for near vision. (In other words, contraction of the ciliary muscle is required for near vision.)

The **lens** in an embalmed specimen is firm and opaque. In life, it is transparent and elastic. It is bounded posteriorly by the transparent jelly-like **vitreous body,** which fills the **vitreous chamber** posterior to the lens. Anteriorly, the lens is bounded by the iris and the **aqueous humor.** The aqueous humor fills the space between the cornea and the lens. This space is divided by the iris into two chambers. The **anterior chamber** is the space between the cornea and the iris. The **posterior chamber** is a narrow cavity between the iris and the lens. Aqueous humor is continually produced by the ciliary epithelium covering the ciliary processes. It circulates through the zonular fibers into the posterior chamber before passing through the pupil into the anterior chamber. From the anterior chamber the aqueous humor is drained through a trabecular meshwork at the **iridocorneal angle** (see Fig. 5-39), where it passes into the venous system via the venous **scleral sinus**. The iridocorneal angle is traversed by a meshwork of fibers with intervening spaces. This meshwork of the angle is referred to as the **pectinate ligament** (see Fig. 5-39). The integrity of this angle is critical in the drainage of aqueous humor from the eyeball. Failure in the drainage results in increased intraocular pressure, which is known as *glaucoma.* Remove the lens. Note the zonular fibers as they stretch and break.

3. The **internal coat** of the eye, the "nervous coat," consists of the **retina** and its associated blood vessels and the neuronal processes surrounding the vitreous body. That portion of the retina containing the light-sensitive rods and cones, the bipolar cells, and the ganglion cells is the **pars optica retinae**. It covers the internal surface of the choroid from the point where the prechiasmatic optic tract enters to the level of the ciliary body. From this boundary, called the *ora serrata* (see Fig. 5-40), there is a thin non–light-receptive portion of the retina that passes anteriorly over the posterior surface of the ciliary body as the **pars ciliaris retinae** and continues on the posterior surface of the iris as the **pars iridica retinae**. The ciliary portion of the retina is two layers thick and forms the blood-aqueous barrier, through which aqueous fluid is secreted into the posterior chamber. The iridial portion of the retina is also a double cell layer consisting of pigment cells, which give the iris its color, and myoepithelial cells, which form the **dilator pupillae**.

In the embalmed specimen the nervous layer of the pars optica retinae has a gray-white appearance, and it readily peels away from the single layer of pigmented epithelial cells on its posterior surface, which remains attached to the choroid. This pigmented layer of the retina and the pigment of the choroid give the interior of the eyeball a brown to black appearance except where the specialized layer of the choroid, the **tapetum lucidum,** is located. This tapetal area exhibits a variety of brilliant colors from silver to blue to green or orange. In this area there is no pigment in the pigment epithelial cells of the retina covering the tapetum lucidum. The brown-black portion of the interior of the eyeball is sometimes referred to as the *nontapetal area* or *nontapetal nigrum.*

Notice the emergence of the prechiasmatic optic tract from the posterior aspect of the eyeball. This is the **optic disk**. With careful observation of the disk, you may see the retinal vessels that enter with it to supply the internal surface of the retina. The posterior portion of the eyeball that includes the area of the optic disk, tapetum lucidum, and adjacent nontapetal nigrum is referred to as the **fundus** of the eyeball. The optic disk may be found in the interior region of the tapetum lucidum or at or below its inferior border. This varies with the breed of dog.

Superficial Veins of the Head

The **external jugular vein** (Figs. 5-41 through 5-43) is formed by the confluence of the linguofacial and maxillary veins caudal to the mandibular salivary gland, which lies between these two veins.

The **lingual vein** (see Fig. 5-42) is the first large tributary that enters the **linguofacial vein** ventrally. Its radicles drain blood from the tongue, the larynx, and part of the pharynx. These radicles will not be dissected.

The **facial vein** is the other tributary of the linguofacial. The radicles that form the facial vein lie on the dorsal surface of the muzzle. One of these, the **dorsal nasal,** runs caudally from the nares, whereas another, the **angularis oculi,** passes rostrally from the medial aspect of the orbit, where it is continuous with the ophthalmic plexus within the periorbita (see Fig. 5-42). Blood may drain from the face in either direction through the angularis oculi. There is also a large communication between the ophthalmic plexus and the facial vein, via the **deep facial vein,** which is ventral to the zygomatic bone. Identify these veins. The remaining branches will not be dissected, for to do so would sacrifice nerves and arteries. These branches drain the lateral muzzle and the upper and lower lips. The facial vein generally follows the rostral and ventral borders of the masseter muscle before it meets the lingual vein. Note the two or three small mandibular lymph nodes

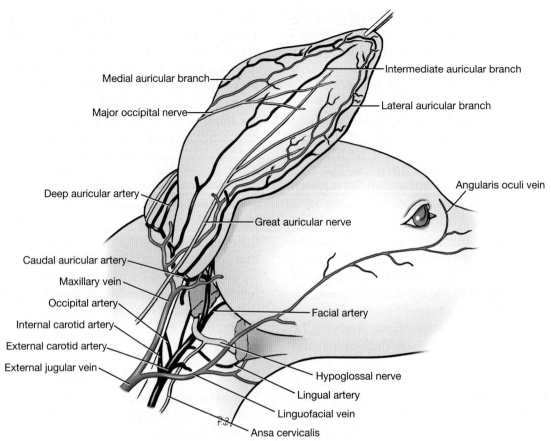

Medial auricular branch
Major occipital nerve
Intermediate auricular branch
Lateral auricular branch
Deep auricular artery
Angularis oculi vein
Great auricular nerve
Caudal auricular artery
Maxillary vein
Occipital artery
Internal carotid artery
External carotid artery
External jugular vein
Facial artery
Hypoglossal nerve
Lingual artery
Linguofacial vein
Ansa cervicalis

Fig. 5-41   Vessels and nerves of external ear, with a portion of digastricus removed.

along the linguofacial vein just rostroventral to the mandibular salivary gland.

The **maxillary vein** drains the ear, orbit, palate, nasal cavity, cheek, and mandible as well as the cranial cavity.

Facial Nerve

The **facial, or seventh cranial, nerve** (see Figs. 5-43, 5-49, 5-50) innervates all of the superficial muscles of the head as well as the caudal belly of the digastricus and the platysma of the neck. The nerve enters the petrosal part of the temporal bone through the internal acoustic meatus, courses through the facial canal of that bone, and leaves the skull at the stylomastoid foramen just caudal to the external acoustic meatus, where it divides into several branches.

Reflect the parotid gland. Dissect deep between the parotid and sublingual glands to expose the facial nerve arising from the stylomastoid foramen caudal to the horizontal portion of the ear canal. The maxillary vein may be transected as it crosses the lateral surface of the nerve at this site. Dissect the following branches of the facial nerve.

The **auriculopalpebral nerve** arises as the facial nerve curves rostrally ventral to the external acoustic meatus. Dissect deep to the rostral edge of the parotid gland to locate the nerve. **Rostral auricular branches** course through the parotid gland and are distributed to the rostral auricular muscles. The auriculopalpebral nerve crosses the zygomatic arch, supplies branches to the rostral auricular plexus, and continues to the orbit to supply **palpebral branches** to the orbicularis oculi. Beyond this, a branch passes medial to the orbit and continues rostrally on the nose to supply the muscles of the nose and upper lip.

Two **buccal branches** of the facial nerve course across the masseter muscle to innervate the muscles of the cheek, the superior and inferior lips, and the lateral surface of the nose. The dorsal buccal branch is dorsal to the parotid duct. The ventral buccal branch is ventral to the parotid duct, near the ventral border of the masseter. Identify these two branches and the parotid duct.

A branch of the mandibular nerve from the **trigeminal or fifth cranial nerve,** known as the **auriculotemporal nerve,** is apparent in the dissection

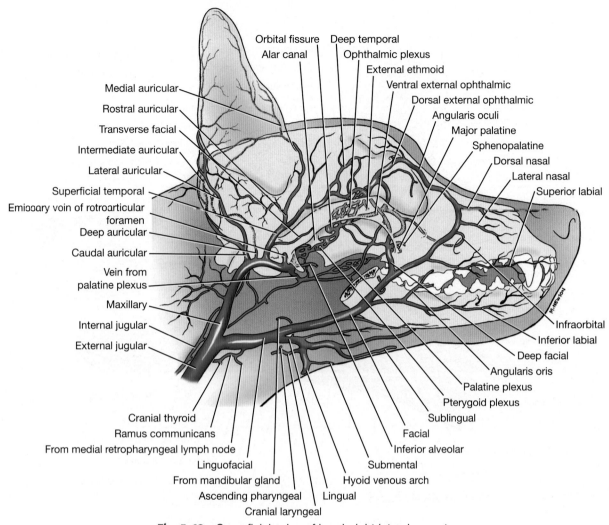

Fig. 5-42 Superficial veins of head, right lateral aspect.

field of the auriculopalpebral branch of the facial nerve. The auriculotemporal nerve emerges between the caudal border of the masseter muscle and the base of the external acoustic meatus below the zygomatic arch. It may be found deep to the origin of the auriculopalpebral nerve. The auriculotemporal nerve supplies sensory branches to the skin of the external ear and the temporal, zygomatic, and masseteric regions.

Cervical Structures

The **thyroid gland** (see Figs. 3-15, 5-44, 5-54) is dark-colored and usually consists of two separate lobes lying lateral to the first five tracheal rings. Occasionally, a connecting isthmus is present.

There are two **parathyroid glands** associated with each thyroid lobe. They are small, light-colored, spherical bodies. The **external parathyroid** most commonly lies in the fascia at the

cranial pole of the thyroid lobe. It may be entirely separate from the thyroid tissue or embedded in the cranial pole of the thyroid external to its capsule. The **internal parathyroid** lies deep to the thyroid capsule on the medial aspect of the lobe. Occasionally, it is embedded in the parenchyma of the thyroid and is difficult to locate. The location of these glands is subject to variation.

The **cervical portion of the esophagus** extends from the laryngopharynx to the thoracic portion of the esophagus at the thoracic inlet. It begins opposite the middle of the axis dorsally and opposite the caudal border of the cricoid cartilage ventrally. A plicated ridge of mucosa, the **pharyngoesophageal limen,** marks the boundary between the laryngopharynx and the esophagus (see Fig. 5-25). The esophagus inclines to the left, so that at the thoracic inlet it usually lies to the left of the trachea (see Fig. 3-15).

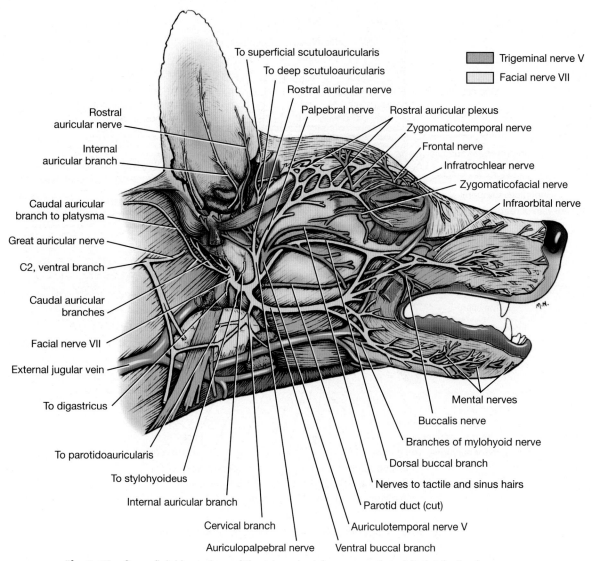

Trigeminal nerve V

Facial nerve VII

Fig. 5-43 Superficial branches of the trigeminal *(orange-red)* and facial *(yellow)* nerves.

The **trachea** extends from a transverse plane through the middle of the axis to a plane between the fourth and fifth thoracic vertebrae. It is composed of approximately 35 C-shaped **tracheal cartilages**. They are open dorsally, and the space is bridged by the tracheal muscle.

Common Carotid Artery

Common carotid a.
   Caudal thyroid a.
   Cranial thyroid a.
   Internal carotid a.
   External carotid a.
      Occipital a.
      Cranial laryngeal a.
      Lingual a.
      Facial a.

      Sublingual a.
   Caudal auricular a.
   Superficial temporal a.
   Maxillary a.

On the right side, expose the **common carotid artery** in the carotid sheath and observe the following branches.

1. The **caudal thyroid artery** (see Figs. 3-14, 3-16) has a variable origin from the major arterial branches in the thoracic inlet. It passes cranially on the trachea supplying the trachea, esophagus, and thyroid gland.

2. The **cranial thyroid artery** (see Figs. 5-45, 5-47) arises from the ventral surface of the common carotid at the level of the larynx. It supplies the thyroid and parathyroid glands, the pharyngeal muscles, the laryngeal muscles and mucosa, the

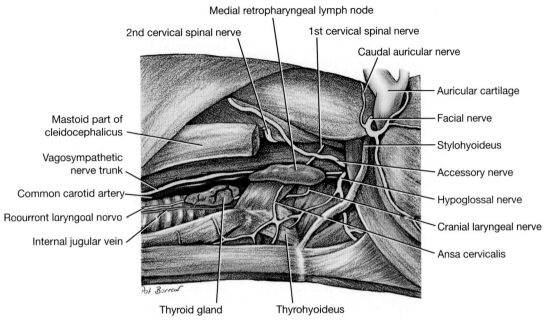

Medial retropharyngeal lymph node

2nd cervical spinal nerve

1st cervical spinal nerve

Caudal auricular nerve

Mastoid part of cleidocephalicus

Auricular cartilage

Facial nerve

Stylohyoideus

Vagosympathetic nerve trunk

Accessory nerve

Common carotid artery

Hypoglossal nerve

Reourrent laryngeal norve

Cranial laryngeal nerve

Internal jugular vein

Ansa cervicalis

Thyroid gland

Thyrohyoideus

Fig. 5-44 Retropharyngeal lymph node and thyroid gland, lateral aspect of the neck.

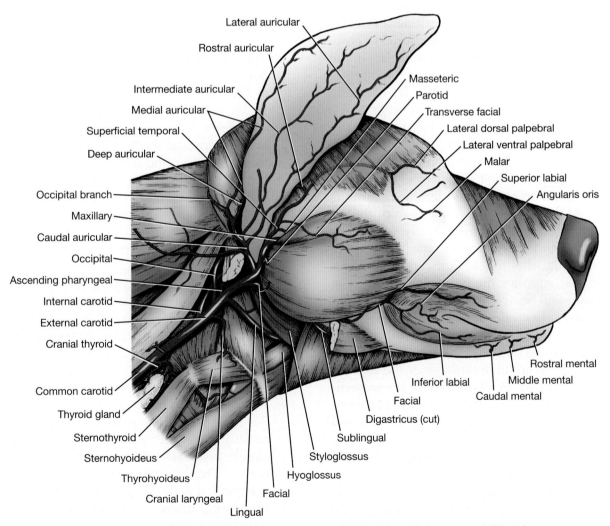

Lateral auricular

Rostral auricular

Intermediate auricular

Medial auricular

Superficial temporal

Deep auricular

Occipital branch

Maxillary

Caudal auricular

Occipital

Ascending pharyngeal

Internal carotid

External carotid

Cranial thyroid

Common carotid

Thyroid gland

Sternothyroid

Sternohyoideus

Thyrohyoideus

Cranial laryngeal

Lingual

Facial

Hyoglossus

Styloglossus

Sublingual

Digastricus (cut)

Facial

Inferior labial

Masseteric

Parotid

Transverse facial

Lateral dorsal palpebral

Lateral ventral palpebral

Malar

Superior labial

Angularis oris

Rostral mental

Middle mental

Caudal mental

Fig. 5-45 Branches of common carotid artery, superficial lateral view, part of digastricus removed.

cervical parts of the trachea and esophagus, and the adjacent portions of the sternocephalicus and the mastoid part of the cleidocephalicus. Clean the origin of this vessel.

The large **medial retropharyngeal lymph node** (see Figs. 2-12, 5-44) is dorsal to the common carotid artery at the larynx and ventral to the wing of the atlas. Afferent vessels arise from the tongue, the nasal cavity, the pharynx, the salivary glands, the external ear, the larynx, and the esophagus. The tracheal trunk of each side arises from this lymph node.

Identify the internal and external carotid arteries, which are the terminal branches of the common carotid artery.

3. The **internal carotid artery** (see Figs. 5-45, 5-47) is closely associated with the occipital artery, the first branch of the external carotid. A bulbous enlargement at the origin of the internal carotid artery is the **carotid sinus,** a baroreceptor. (The carotid body, a chemoreceptor, lies at the bifurcation of the carotid arteries.) Beyond this the internal carotid artery ascends across the lateral surface of the pharynx medial to the occipital artery. No branches leave the internal carotid in its extracranial course. It enters the carotid canal deep in the tympano-occipital fissure. The internal carotid passes rostrally through this canal and emerges at the foramen lacerum, where it loops back on itself to reenter the canal. It passes on to the floor of the cranial cavity and turns rostrally within the cavernous sinus. At the level of the attachment of the pituitary, it leaves the sinus dorsally, penetrates the dura, and enters the subarachnoid space where it branches to form the cerebral arterial circle that supplies the brain. Its branches to the brain will be dissected later.

4. The **external carotid artery** (see Figs. 5-45 to 5-47) passes cranially, medial to the digastricus.

At the caudal border of the mandible, rostroventral to the annular cartilage of the ear, the vessel terminates by dividing into the **superficial temporal** and **maxillary arteries**. The maxillary is the direct continuation of the external carotid. Dissect the following branches of the external carotid. Transect the digastricus muscle and remove the caudal portion.

a. The **occipital artery** (see Figs. 5-47, 5-54) leaves the external carotid adjacent to the internal carotid and passes dorsally to supply the muscles on the caudal aspect of the skull and the meninges. Do not trace this artery.

b. The **cranial laryngeal artery** (Figs. 5-45, 5-54) is a ventral branch that supplies the adjacent sternomastoideus and pharyngeal muscles. It enters the larynx between the thyrohyoid bone and the thyroid cartilage to supply the mucosa and laryngeal muscles.

c. The **lingual artery** (see Figs. 5-41, 5-54) leaves the ventral surface of the external carotid and passes rostrally to supply the tonsil and tongue. On its course to the tongue it is accompanied by the hypoglossal nerve.

d. The **facial artery** (see Fig. 5-41) leaves the external carotid beyond the lingual, medial to the digastricus. A branch, the **sublingual artery,** continues medial to the digastric muscle and is accompanied by the mylohyoid nerve. It runs rostrally into the tongue. The facial artery courses rostrolaterally between the digastric and masseter muscles to reach the cheek lateral to the mandible, where it supplies the lips and nose.

e. The **caudal auricular artery** (see Figs. 5-45, 5-46) usually arises from the external carotid at the base of the ear and courses dorsally under the caudal auricular muscles. Reflect the caudal limb of the parotid gland to expose the caudal auricular and its branches, which need not be dissected. Lateral, intermediate, and medial auricular branches course distally on the convex caudal surface of the ear. Occasionally, this artery arises closer to the origin of the external carotid.

f. The external carotid artery terminates in the superficial temporal and maxillary artery. The **superficial temporal artery** (see Figs. 5-45, 5-46) arises rostral to the base of the auricular cartilage at the caudodorsal border of the mandible and courses dorsally. It supplies the parotid gland, the masseter and temporal muscles, the rostral auricular muscles, and the eyelids.

g. The **maxillary artery** (see Figs. 5-46, 5-47) is the larger terminal branch of the external carotid artery. It is deeply placed and is closely associated with a number of cranial nerves. From its origin with the superficial temporal, it passes rostromedially ventral to the temporomandibular joint medial to the retroarticular process in its course to the alar canal.

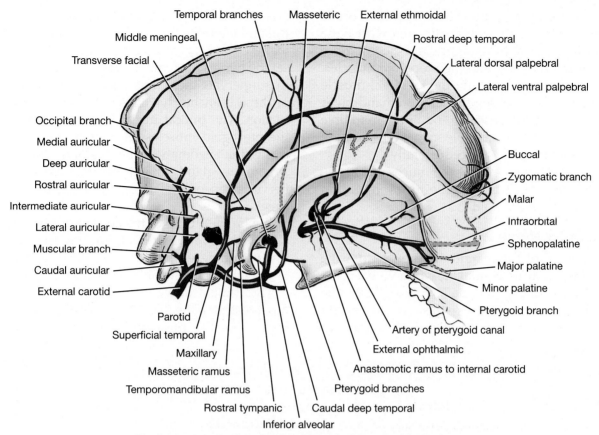

Fig. 5-46 Arteries of head in relation to lateral aspect of skull.

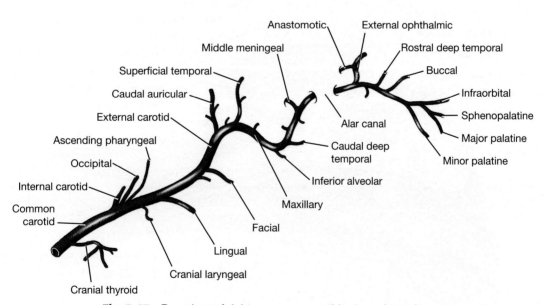

Fig. 5-47 Branches of right common carotid artery, deep view.

Remove the auricular muscles and reflect the ear caudally. Repeat the dissection that was done on the left side to expose the orbital structures. Cut through the origin of the temporal muscle along its margin. With a blunt instrument, remove it from the temporal fossa. Cut the attachments of the temporal and masseter muscles to both sides of the zygomatic arch. Sever the orbital ligament at the arch. With bone cutters or Stryker saw, detach each end of the zygomatic arch and remove all of it. Transect the temporal muscle as close to its insertion on the coronoid process as possible.

Cut off the coronoid process below the level of the ventral border of the zygomatic arch with bone cutters. Remove all the temporal muscle to expose the periorbital tissues and the pterygoid muscles. Vessels and nerves entering the temporal muscle must be severed. Loosen the temporomandibular joint by forcing the articular end of the mandible medially. Rotate the mandible so that the stump of the coronoid process is forced laterally.

In the oral cavity, reflect the mucosa from the level of the root of the tongue to the frenulum along the sublingual fold.

Mandibular Nerve

The branches of the mandibular nerve from the **trigeminal** or **fifth cranial nerve** have been exposed by this dissection (see Figs. 5-43, 5-48). The mandibular nerve leaves the cranial cavity through the oval foramen (Fig. 5-49). Branches arise on the surface of the pterygoid muscles ventral and lateral to the apex of the periorbita. These include the pterygoid, deep temporal, and masseteric nerves that contain somatic motor neurons that innervate these muscles of mastication. Most of these branches have been severed by the dissection. The **buccal nerve** (see Fig 5-48) crosses the pterygoid muscles and enters the cheek lateral to the zygomatic salivary gland. Remove the zygomatic gland to get better exposure. This nerve is sensory to the mucosa and skin of the cheek.

Rotate the stump of the coronoid process laterally to observe the lingual, inferior alveolar, and mylohyoid nerves, which cross the dorsal surface of the medial pterygoid muscle (see Fig. 5-48).

The **lingual nerve** (sensory) is the largest and most rostral of the three. It can be observed coursing across the pterygoid muscles and passing

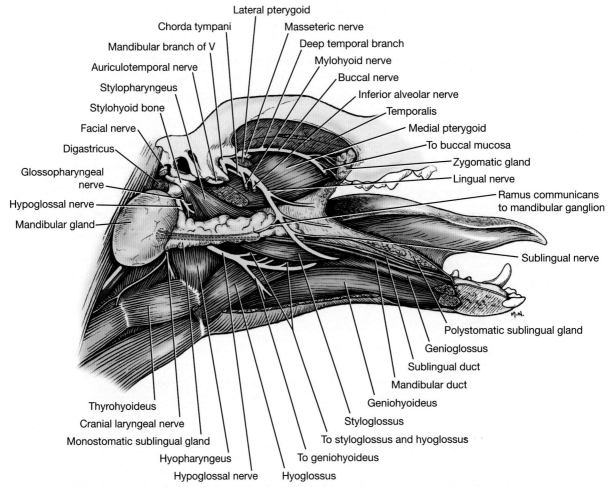

Fig. 5-48 Muscles, nerves, and salivary glands medial to right mandible, lateral view, dorsally. It supplies the parotid gland, the masseter and temporal muscles, the rostral auricular muscles, and the eyelids.

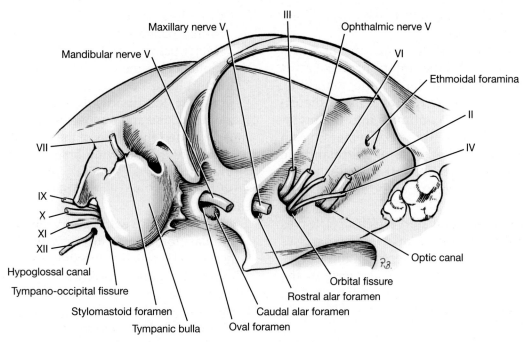

Fig. 5-49 Cranial nerves leaving skull, ventrolateral view.

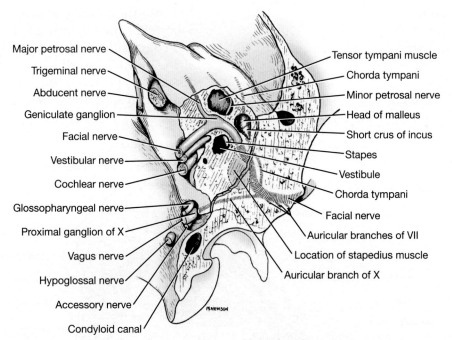

Fig. 5-50 Petrous part of temporal bone sculptured to show path of facial nerve, dorsal aspect.

between the styloglossus and mylohyoideus. On the medial side of the specimen, pull the tongue medially and observe the nerve between these muscles and the place where it crosses the lateral side of the mandibular and sublingual ducts and enters the tongue. It is sensory to the rostral two thirds of the tongue. Taste (SVA) is

via the chorda tympani, a branch of cranial nerve VII.

The **inferior alveolar nerve** (sensory) enters the mandibular foramen on the medial side of the ramus of the mandible. It courses through the mandibular canal, supplying sensory nerves to the teeth. The mental nerves that emerge through the mental foramina and supply the lower lip are branches from this nerve.

The **mylohyoid nerve** (motor and sensory) is a caudal branch of the inferior alveolar. It reaches the ventral border of the mandible, supplies a branch to the rostral belly of the digastricus muscle, and continues into the mylohyoid muscle. Observe this nerve emerging on the medial side of the angle of the mandible lateral to the mylohyoideus. It is motor to the mylohyoideus and sensory to the skin between the mandibles.

The **auriculotemporal nerve** (sensory) leaves the mandibular nerve at the oval foramen, passes caudal to the retroarticular process of the temporal bone, and emerges between the base of the auricular cartilage and the masseter muscle, where it was previously seen.

Maxillary Artery

Maxillary artery
    Inferior alveolar a.
    Caudal deep temporal a.
    Middle meningeal a.
    External ophthalmic a.
        Anastomotic rami
        Muscular rami
        External ethmoidal a.

Descending palatine
    Minor palatine a.
    Major palatine a.
    Sphenopalatine a.
Infraorbital a.

Complete the disarticulation of the temporomandibular joint and remove the lateral pterygoid muscle. Reflect the ramus of the mandible laterally and identify the following branches of the maxillary artery (see Figs. 5-46, 5-47, 5-51). The first three arise before the maxillary artery enters the alar canal.

1. The **inferior alveolar artery** enters the mandibular foramen with the inferior alveolar nerve and courses through the mandibular canal. It supplies branches to the roots of the teeth in the lower jaw. Mental branches supply the skin (see Fig. 5-45).

2. The **caudal deep temporal artery** arises near the inferior alveolar artery and enters the temporal muscle. Only the origin of this artery may be seen.

3. The **middle meningeal artery** (see Figs. 5-46, 5-47, 5-52) passes through the oval foramen and courses dorsally in a groove on the inside of the calvaria. It will be followed in a later dissection to the dura over the cerebral hemispheres. Do not dissect its origin.

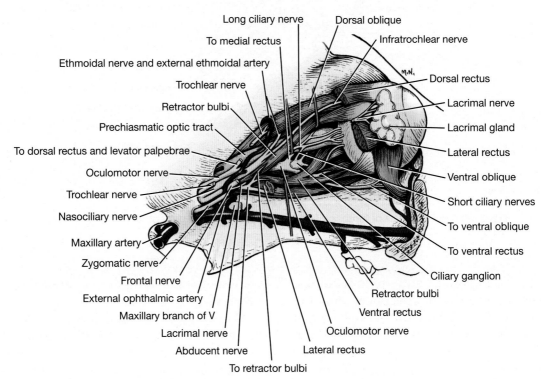

Fig. 5-51 Nerves and muscles of eyeball, lateral view.

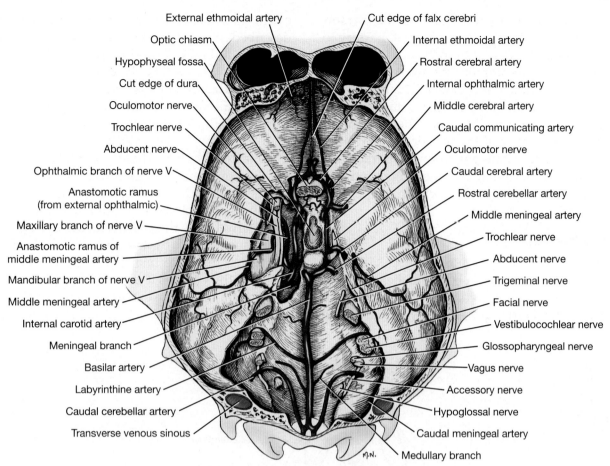

External ethmoidal artery
Optic chiasm
Hypophyseal fossa
Cut edge of dura
Oculomotor nerve
Trochlear nerve
Abducent nerve
Ophthalmic branch of nerve V
Anastomotic ramus (from external ophthalmic)
Maxillary branch of nerve V
Anastomotic ramus of middle meningeal artery
Mandibular branch of nerve V
Middle meningeal artery
Internal carotid artery
Meningeal branch
Basilar artery
Labyrinthine artery
Caudal cerebellar artery
Transverse venous sinous

Cut edge of falx cerebri
Internal ethmoidal artery
Rostral cerebral artery
Internal ophthalmic artery
Middle cerebral artery
Caudal communicating artery
Oculomotor nerve
Caudal cerebral artery
Rostral cerebellar artery
Middle meningeal artery
Trochlear nerve
Abducent nerve
Trigeminal nerve
Facial nerve
Vestibulocochlear nerve
Glossopharyngeal nerve
Vagus nerve
Accessory nerve
Hypoglossal nerve
Caudal meningeal artery
Medullary branch

Fig. 5-52   Dorsal aspect of base of the skull showing arteries and nerves.

4. The **external ophthalmic artery** (see Figs. 5-46, 5-47, 5-51) arises from the maxillary on its emergence from the alar canal and penetrates the apex of the periorbita adjacent to the orbital fissure. The external ophthalmic artery gives rise to the vessels that supply the structures within the periorbita. Incise the periorbita longitudinally along its dorsolateral border and reflect it.

The branches of the external ophthalmic artery need not be dissected. One anastomotic branch passes caudally through the orbital fissure to join the internal carotid and middle meningeal arteries within the cranial cavity. Another anastomotic branch joins the internal ophthalmic artery emerging from the optic canal on the prechiasmatic optic tract. From this anastomosis posterior ciliary arteries are supplied to the eyeball. Branches of the external ophthalmic artery supply the extrinsic muscles of the eyeball and the lacrimal gland. The **external ethmoidal artery** passes dorsal to the extraocular muscles and enters an ethmoidal foramen. Within the cranial cavity it joins with the internal ethmoidal

artery and passes through the cribriform plate to the ethmoid labyrinth and the nasal septum.

5. Among the terminal branches of the maxillary artery are the minor and major palatine and sphenopalatine arteries (see Figs. 5-46, 5-47). The latter two usually arise from the **descending palatine artery** as it courses rostroventrally over the medial pterygoid muscle. Only the origins of these vessels need be observed. Their origins can be seen at the rostral border of the medial pterygoid muscle deep to the zygomatic salivary gland, which should be removed.

The **minor palatine artery** passes ventrally, caudal to the hard palate, and is distributed to the adjacent soft and hard palates. Clean the mucosa from the palate just medial to the last molar and see the branches of this vessel.

The **major palatine artery** enters the caudal palatine foramen and passes through the major palatine canal to supply the hard palate.

The **sphenopalatine artery** passes through the sphenopalatine foramen to the interior of the nasal cavity.

6. The maxillary artery terminates as the **infraorbital artery,** which supplies the malar artery to the eyelids and dental branches to the caudal cheek teeth. The infraorbital artery enters the maxillary foramen and passes through the infraorbital canal. Within the canal, dental branches arise. These supply the premolars, the canine teeth, and the incisor teeth. The infraorbital artery emerges from the infraorbital foramen and terminates as the lateral and rostral dorsal nasal arteries, which supply the nose and the superior lip.

Cranial Nerves

There are 12 pairs of cranial nerves (see Figs. 5-48 through 5-56). Each pair is both numbered with a Roman numeral and named. The numbers indicate the rostrocaudal order in which they arise from the brain; their names are descriptive. As previously described, the optic nerve is now considered to be a tract of the brain. Some of these have already been dissected; others will be dissected now.

I. The **olfactory,** or **first cranial, nerve** consists of numerous axons that arise in the olfactory epithelium of the caudal nasal mucosa and pass through the cribriform foramina to the olfactory bulbs. These include axons from the vomeronasal organ that course along the nasal septum. No dissection is necessary.

II. The **optic,** or **second cranial, nerve** is now referred to as the **prechiasmatic optic tract.** It is surrounded by the retractor bulbi muscle within the periorbita. Observe the tract in the periorbita and as it enters the optic canal. It is surrounded by an extension of meninges from the cranial cavity.

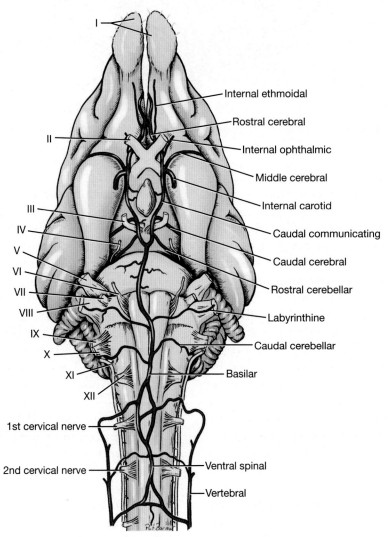

Fig. 5-53 Arteries and nerves of brain and first two cervical spinal cord segments, ventral view.

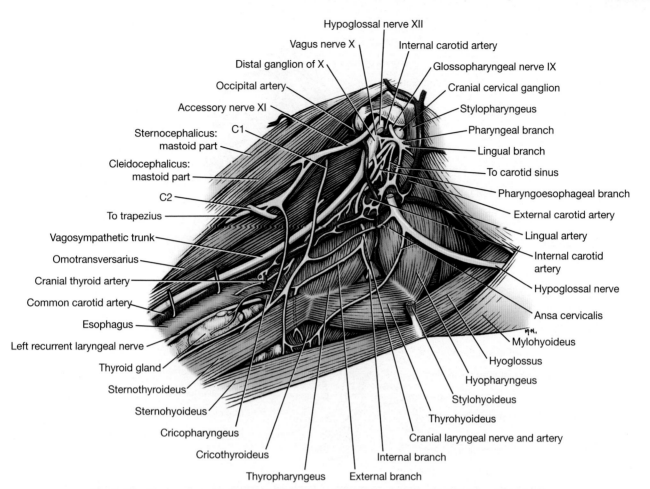

Fig. 5-54 Nerves emerging from tympano-occipital fissure, right lateral view. The digastricus muscle and the medial retropharyngeal lymph node were removed.

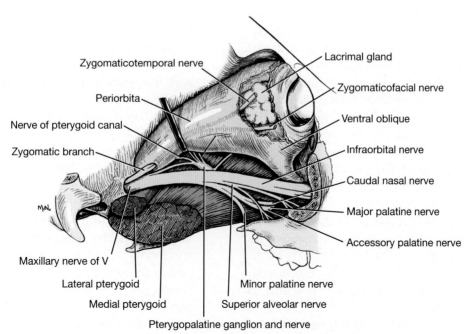

Fig. 5-55 Maxillary branch of trigeminal nerve, lateral aspect.

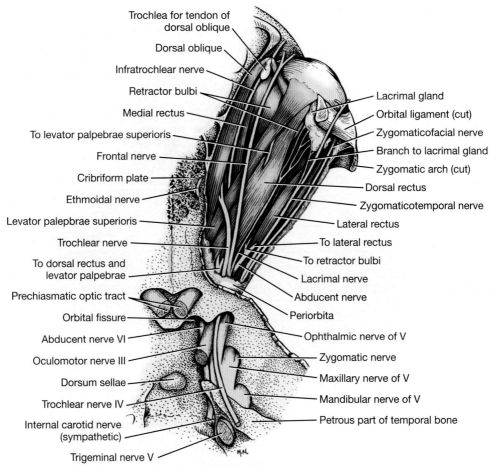

Trochlea for tendon of dorsal oblique
Dorsal oblique
Infratrochlear nerve
Retractor bulbi
Medial rectus
To levator palpebrae superioris
Frontal nerve
Cribriform plate
Ethmoidal nerve
Levator palepbrae superioris
Trochlear nerve
To dorsal rectus and levator palpebrae
Prechiasmatic optic tract
Orbital fissure
Abducent nerve VI
Oculomotor nerve III
Dorsum sellae
Trochlear nerve IV
Internal carotid nerve (sympathetic)
Trigeminal nerve V

Lacrimal gland
Orbital ligament (cut)
Zygomaticofacial nerve
Branch to lacrimal gland
Zygomatic arch (cut)
Dorsal rectus
Zygomaticotemporal nerve
Lateral rectus
To lateral rectus
To retractor bulbi
Lacrimal nerve
Abducent nerve
Periorbita
Ophthalmic nerve of V
Zygomatic nerve
Maxillary nerve of V
Mandibular nerve of V
Petrous part of temporal bone

Fig. 5-56 Schema of optic, oculomotor, trochlear, trigeminal, and abducent nerves, dorsal aspect.

III. The **oculomotor,** or **third cranial, nerve** passes through the orbital fissure and enters the periorbita with the prechiasmatic optic tract. Expose the proximal half of the prechiasmatic optic tract. Lift it gently and observe the oculomotor nerve on its lateroventral aspect. Do not dissect its individual branches. The oculomotor nerve innervates the dorsal, medial, and ventral recti; the ventral oblique; and the levator palpebrae superioris. The **ciliary ganglion** is an irregular enlargement at the termination of the oculomotor nerve on the ventral surface of the middle of the optic nerve. This ganglion contains parasympathetic cell bodies of postganglionic axons that innervate the sphincter pupillae of the iris. It functions to regulate the size of the pupil in response to the amount of light entering the eye and in accommodation.

IV. The **trochlear,** or **fourth cranial, nerve** enters the periorbita through the orbital fissure. It

innervates the dorsal oblique; it need not be dissected.

V. The **trigeminal,** or **fifth cranial, nerve** divides into three nerves as it emerges from the trigeminal canal in the petrosal part of the temporal bone: the ophthalmic, the maxillary, and the mandibular. The mandibular nerve has been dissected.

The **ophthalmic nerve** (sensory) passes through the orbital fissure and supplies sensory nerves that enter the periorbita. These need not be dissected. The **frontal** and **infratrochlear nerves** pass rostrally between the dorsal oblique and dorsal rectus muscles to innervate the medial aspect of the superior and inferior eyelids. Long **ciliary nerves** follow the optic nerve and innervate the eyeball. The **ethmoidal nerve** passes through an ethmoidal foramen and the cribriform plate to innervate the nasal mucosa and skin of the nose.

The **maxillary nerve** (sensory) enters the alar canal through the round foramen. It emerges from the rostral alar foramen and crosses the pterygopalatine fossa dorsal to the pterygoid muscles and ventral to the periorbita, accompanied by the maxillary artery.

a. The **zygomatic nerve** (sensory) here enters the periorbita and divides into two branches that pass rostrally on the inner surface of the lateral part of the periorbita to innervate the lacrimal gland and the lateral portion of the superior and inferior eyelids.

b. The **pterygopalatine ganglion** is dorsal to the maxillary nerve on the surface of the medial pterygoid muscle. It contains cell bodies of postganglionic parasympathetic axons that supply the lacrimal, nasal, and palatine glands. The postganglionic axons course with the branches of the maxillary nerve to their terminations. Reflect the periorbita dorsally and the maxillary nerve ventrally to see this small, flat ganglion on the pterygoid muscle.

c. The **pterygopalatine nerve** arises beyond the level of the pterygopalatine ganglion from the ventral surface of the maxillary nerve and divides into three nerves: the **minor** and **major palatine nerves** of the palate and the **caudal nasal nerve** of the nasal mucosa. Dissect their origin only.

d. The **infraorbital nerve** (sensory) is the continuation of the maxillary nerve in the pterygopalatine fossa. It enters the infraorbital canal through the maxillary foramen. Along its course through the infraorbital canal, it gives off **superior alveolar branches,** which supply the roots of the teeth of the superior arcade via the alveolar canals. As the infraorbital nerve emerges from the infraorbital foramen, it divides into a number of fasciculi, which are distributed to the skin and adjacent structures of the superior lip and nose. Dissect these branches as they emerge from the infraorbital foramen.

VI. The **abducent,** or **sixth cranial, nerve** passes through the orbital fissure and enters the periorbita. It innervates the retractor bulbi and the lateral rectus. Observe this small nerve entering the dorsal border of the lateral rectus near its origin.

VII. The **facial,** or **seventh cranial, nerve** enters the internal acoustic meatus of the petrosal part of the temporal bone. It courses through the facial canal and emerges through the stylomastoid foramen, where its motor branches to the facial muscles have been dissected.

VIII. The **vestibulocochlear, or eighth cranial, nerve** enters the internal acoustic meatus and terminates in the membranous labyrinth of the inner ear. It is the nerve involved in balance and hearing. It will be dissected with the brain.

Observation of the ninth, tenth, and eleventh cranial nerves and the sympathetic trunk ganglion at the base of the skull is facilitated by removal of the origin of the digastricus muscle for a lateral view. Likewise, removal of the insertion of the longus capitis muscle provides a medial view. These neural structures are found just medial and ventral to the tympanic bulla near the tympano-occipital fissure.

Locate the sympathetic trunk where it is joined with the vagus. Follow it cranially to a level ventral and medial to the tympanic bulla, where the two nerves separate. The sympathetic trunk is ventral to the vagus. The **distal ganglion of the vagus** (sensory) is located dorsal to this separation and caudal to the **cranial cervical ganglion**. Trace the sympathetic trunk cranial to the separation and note an enlargement, the cranial cervical ganglion (visceral motor). This is the most cranial group of cell bodies of sympathetic postganglionic axons. These axons are distributed to the smooth muscles and glands of the head via blood vessels and other nerves. On the lateral side, observe the internal carotid artery coursing dorsocranially over the lateral surface of the cranial cervical ganglion. Notice the dense plexus that these nerves form in the immediate vicinity of the ganglion.

IX. The **glossopharyngeal,** or **ninth cranial, nerve** passes through the jugular foramen and the tympano-occipital fissure. Beyond the fissure the glossopharyngeal crosses the lateral surface of the cranial cervical ganglion and divides into pharyngeal and lingual branches that are sensory to the pharyngeal mucosa and motor to the stylopharyngeus and other pharyngeal muscles. In addition, some branches course to the carotid sinus and others contribute to the pharyngeal plexus along with branches of the vagus nerve. Observe the nerve where it crosses the ganglion.

X. The **vagus,** or **tenth cranial, nerve** passes through the jugular foramen and the tympano-occipital fissure. It courses along the common carotid artery in the neck with the sympathetic trunk and through the thorax on the esophagus to terminal branches in the thorax and abdomen (which have already been dissected).

There are two ganglia associated with this nerve. The **proximal ganglion** (see Fig. 5-50) of the vagus lies in the jugular foramen and cannot be seen. The **distal ganglion** (Fig. 5-57) of the vagus is found outside the tympano-occipital fissure, ventral and medial to the tympanic bulla

and caudal to the cranial cervical ganglion (see Fig. 5-54). These are sensory ganglia. Find the distal ganglion with the vagus nerve caudal to the cranial cervical ganglion on the sympathetic trunk. The distal ganglion contains the cell bodies of the visceral afferent neurons that are distributed to most of the viscera of the body. Caudal to the distal ganglion, the vagus joins the sympathetic trunk, with which it remains associated throughout its cervical course to the thoracic inlet. The following branches are distributed to cranial cervical structures.

Branches from the vagus and glossopharyngeal nerves and the cranial cervical ganglion form a **pharyngeal plexus,** which innervates the caudal pharyngeal muscles

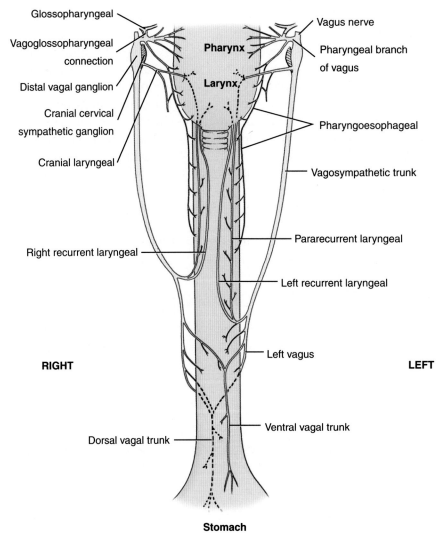

Fig. 5-57 Innervation of the esophagus. (After Watson AG: Some aspects of the vagal innervation of the canine esophagus: an anatomical study, Master's Thesis, New Zealand, 1974, Massey University.)

and the cranial esophagus. The **cranial laryngeal nerve** leaves the vagus nerve at the distal ganglion and passes ventrally to the larynx, where it supplies the cricothyroid muscle and the laryngeal mucosa. Identify this nerve. The origin of the recurrent laryngeal nerve was seen in the thoracic inlet. It innervates the cervical esophagus and trachea in its course up the neck and terminates as the **caudal laryngeal nerve**, which enters the larynx under the caudal edge of the cricopharyngeus muscle. It innervates all the muscles of the larynx except the cricothyroideus.

XI. The **accessory**, or **eleventh cranial, nerve** passes through the jugular foramen and the tympano-occipital fissure along with the ninth and tenth cranial nerves. It passes caudally and by a ventral branch innervates the mastoid part of the sternocephalicus and cleidocephalicus muscles. The dorsal branch supplies the cervical part of the cleidocephalicus and the trapezius.

XII. The **hypoglossal**, or **twelfth cranial, nerve** passes through the hypoglossal canal. It passes ventrorostrally, lateral to the vagosympathetic trunk and the carotid arteries. It lies medial to the mandibular salivary gland, digastricus, and mandible. The hypoglossal nerve is closely associated with the lingual artery. Deep to the mylohyoideus, it innervates the extrinsic and intrinsic muscles of the tongue. The **ansa cervicalis** (see Figs. 5-44, 5-54) consists of two branches that leave the hypoglossal nerve and join the ventral branch of the first cervical spinal nerve in the region of the hyoid muscles. This provides hypoglossal innervation to the sternothyroid and sternohyoid muscles.

LIVE DOG

Examine the lips and cheeks and the vestibule they border. Examine the teeth of both arcades. Evert the caudal part of the superior lip and find the opening of the parotid duct at the level of the fourth superior premolar. Try to feel the parotid duct through the platysma as the duct crosses the middle of the masseter muscle. Palpate the ventral portion of the external acoustic meatus. This is covered by the parotid salivary gland, but the gland is difficult to feel. Palpate the firm ovoid mandibular salivary gland ventral to the parotid.

The monostomatic sublingual gland is at the rostral end of the mandible but cannot be identified by palpation. Open the mouth and examine the oral cavity. Observe the frenulum of the tongue and the sublingual caruncle where the mandibular and sublingual salivary ducts open. Examine the surface of the body and apex of the tongue. Recognize and feel the filiform papillae. Observe the prominent lingual vein on the ventral surface. In the anesthetized dog, this vein can be used for intravenous injections. Pull the tongue to one side to see the palatoglossal arch where the oral cavity is continued by the oropharynx. Pull the tongue forward and see the root of the tongue in the floor of the oropharynx, the epiglottis caudal to it, the palatine tonsils partly covered by the semilunar folds on each side of the oropharynx, and the soft palate dorsally.

Observe the philtrum on the nose. Feel the cartilaginous parts of the nose rostral to the incisive and nasal bones. Palpate the infraorbital foramen where the infraorbital nerve can be anesthetized with a local nerve block. Touch the lateral angle of the eyelids and observe the reflex closure of the palpebral fissure: sensory V and motor VII.

Examine the eyelids and observe the caruncle at the medial commissure. Evert the eyelids slightly and look for the lacrimal puncta along their borders near the medial commissure. Consider lacrimal flow from its origin at the lacrimal gland, across the cornea and along the conjunctival sac, and through its collecting system to the ventral nasal meatus, where it is usually evaporated. Observe the margin of the third eyelid. Gently press the eyeball caudally into the periorbita in the orbit by pushing on it through the superior eyelid. Observe the passive protrusion of the third eyelid across the cornea. Recognize the palpebral and bulbar conjunctivae, the sclera, limbus, cornea, iris, pupil, and anterior chamber. Move the head side to side to stimulate the vestibular part of the vestibulocochlear nerve (VIII) and watch the involuntary quick horizontal movements of the eyeballs. The quick adduction toward the nose is a function of the medial rectus and its oculomotor (III) nerve innervation. The quick abduction away from the nose is a function of the lateral rectus and its abducent (VI) nerve innervation. You just elicited normal vestibular nystagmus. Palpate along the zygomatic arch and try to feel the palpebral branch of the auriculopalpebral (VII) nerve where it crosses the arch to innervate the orbicularis oculi.

Palpate the temporal and masseter muscles above and below the zygomatic arch, respectively. Palpate caudal and ventral to the masseter to feel the digastricus.

Palpate the scutiform cartilage in the auricular muscles medial to the external ear. Examine the external ear. Follow the helix and identify the cutaneous pouch laterally. At the opening into the external acoustic meatus, identify the crura of the helix medially, the pretragic incisure, the tragus rostrally, the intertragic incisure, and the antitragus laterally. Recognize the anthelix on the caudal wall of the external acoustic meatus opposite the tragus.

Palpate the trachea from the thoracic inlet to the larynx. Feel the cricoid and thyroid cartilages of the larynx. Palpate the basihyoid bone and try to feel the other hyoid bones. Normally, the thyroid gland and medial retropharyngeal lymph node cannot be palpated. Palpate the small flat subcutaneous mandibular lymph nodes at the angle of the mandible.

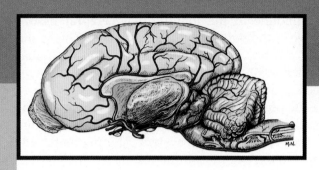
The Nervous System

CHAPTER OUTLINE

The nervous system may be divided into the **central nervous system,** consisting of the brain and spinal cord, and the **peripheral nervous system,** composed of cranial, spinal, and named nerves.

MENINGES

The brain and spinal cord are covered by three membranes of connective tissue, the **meninges** (see Figs. 6-1, 6-37, 6-39). The **dura mater,** or pachymeninx, is the thickest of these and the most external. Throughout most of the vertebral canal, the dura is separated from the periosteum of the bony canal by the loose connective tissue of the epidural space, which often contains fat.

As the spinal cord approaches the brain stem, the dura adheres to the periosteum in the first one or two cervical vertebrae and to the atlanto-occipital membrane. Inside the cranial cavity, the dura and periosteum are fused. Starting at the dorsal margin, free the hemisectioned brain from the skull of the sagittally split head. On one half of the head, a fold of dura will be found extending ventrally from the midline in the **longitudinal cerebral fissure** between the two cerebral hemispheres. This is the **falx cerebri,** which contains the dorsal sagittal sinus dorsally. Remove the falx cerebri to allow reflection of the cerebral hemisphere.

The **pia mater** and **arachnoid** (the **leptomeninges**) are the other two connective tissue coverings of the central nervous system. The pia mater adheres to the external surface of the nervous tissue. The arachnoid in the live animal is attached to the dura and sends delicate trabeculae to the pia. These trabeculae closely invest the blood vessels that course on the surface of the pia. The space between the pia and the arachnoid is the **subarachnoid space,** which is filled with cerebrospinal fluid that surrounds the entire central nervous system. After death, the arachnoid breaks free from the dura and collapses onto the pia of the central nervous system.

Subarachnoid cisterns occur in areas where the arachnoid and pia are more widely separated. The largest cistern is the **cerebellomedullary cistern,** located in the angle between the cerebellum and

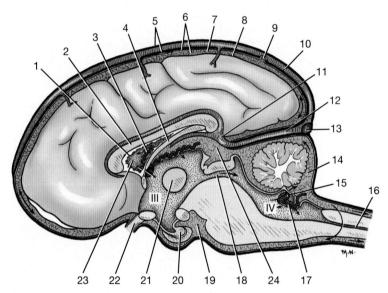

Fig. 6-1   Meninges and ventricles of brain, median plane. (*Arrows* indicate flow of cerebrospinal fluid.)

1. Cut edge of septum pellucidum
2. Corpus callosum
3. Choroid plexus, lateral ventricle
4. Fornix of hippocampus
5. Dura
6. Arachnoid membrane and trabeculae
7. Subarachnoid space
8. Pia
9. Arachnoid villus
10. Dorsal sagittal sinus
11. Great cerebral vein
12. Straight sinus
13. Transverse sinus
14. Cerebellomedullary cistern
15. Lateral aperture of fourth ventricle
16. Central canal
17. Choroid plexus, fourth ventricle
18. Mesencephalic aqueduct
19. Intercrural cistern
20. Neurohypophysis
21. Interthalamic adhesion
22. Prechiasmatic optic tract
23. Lateral ventricle over caudate nucleus
24. Quadrigeminal cistern

medulla. Cerebrospinal fluid may be obtained from this cistern (see Fig. 6-1) by means of a needle puncture through the atlanto-occipital membrane, dura, and arachnoid.

ARTERIES

Examine the arteries to the brain on the latex-injected specimen (see Figs. 5-52, 5-53, 6-2, 6-3). The arteries to the cerebrum and cerebellum are branches from the vessels on the ventral surface of the brain. These major arteries are not accompanied by veins. The **basilar artery** is formed by the terminal branches of the **vertebral arteries,** which enter the floor of the vertebral canal through the lateral vertebral foramina of the atlas.

It is continuous caudally with the **ventral spinal artery** of the spinal cord. The basilar artery courses along the midline of the ventral surface of the medulla and pons and then divides into two branches that form the caudal portion of the arterial circle of the brain.

The **internal carotid arteries** are the other main source of blood to the arterial circle of the brain. After traversing the carotid canal in the tympanic part of the temporal bone and forming a loop at the foramen lacerum, each internal carotid artery enters the middle cranial fossa ventral to the rostral end of the petrous temporal bone. It courses rostrally through the cavernous venous sinus beside the hypophyseal fossa and hypophysis. Between the hypophysis and the optic chiasm, it emerges

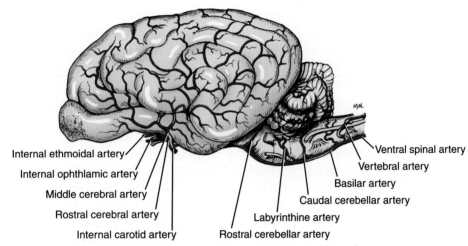

Fig. 6-2 Distribution of middle cerebral artery, lateral aspect.

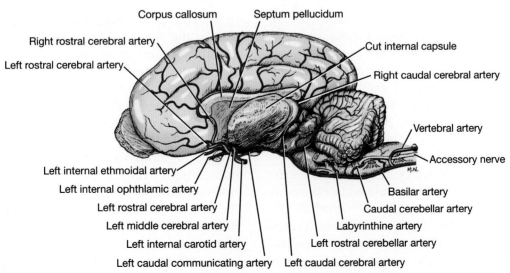

Fig. 6-3 Arteries of cerebellum and medial surface of cerebrum.

through the wall of the cavernous sinus and the dura that covers it and enters the subarachnoid space and divides into a middle cerebral, rostral cerebral, and caudal communicating artery. The small **caudal communicating arteries** from each internal carotid course caudally and join the terminal branches of the basilar artery. Rostrally, the two rostral cerebral arteries anastomose, completing the arterial circle on the ventral surface of the brain.

The **cerebral arterial circle** surrounds the pituitary gland, which receives small branches from the circle as well as directly from the internal carotid artery. Put the two halves of the latex-injected brain together to observe this arterial circle. Using the hemisectioned latex-injected brain, identify and trace the following vessels.

The **rostral cerebral artery** is a terminal branch of the internal carotid artery at the rostral aspect of the circle. It courses dorsally, lateral to the optic chiasm, and continues dorsally between the two cerebral hemispheres in the longitudinal cerebral fissure. It courses dorsally over the fibers that connect the two cerebral hemispheres (corpus callosum) and caudally along the dorsal surface of the corpus callosum adjacent to the cerebral gyri, which these vessels supply.

Internal ethmoidal and internal ophthalmic arteries branch from the rostral cerebral artery. The internal ethmoidal artery anastomoses with the external ethmoidal artery and leaves the cranial cavity through the cribriform plate of the ethmoid bone to supply structures in the nasal cavity. The internal ophthalmic artery anastomoses with a branch of the external ophthalmic on the optic nerve. This is the source of the long ciliary arteries that follow the optic nerve to the eyeball, which they supply. Do not dissect these arteries.

The **middle cerebral artery** arises from the arterial circle at the level of the rostral aspect of the pituitary gland. It courses laterally, rostral to the piriform lobe on the ventral surface of the olfactory peduncle. It continues dorsolaterally over the cerebral hemisphere, where it branches to supply the lateral surface.

The **caudal cerebral artery** arises from the caudal communicating artery at the level of the caudal aspect of the pituitary gland, rostral to the oculomotor nerve. The artery courses caudodorsally, following the optic tract over the lateral aspect of the thalamus to the longitudinal fissure. It passes rostrally on the corpus callosum to supply the medial surface of the caudal portion of the cerebral hemisphere. It also supplies the diencephalon and the rostral mesencephalon.

The **rostral cerebellar artery** leaves the caudal third of the arterial circle caudal to the oculomotor nerve and courses dorsocaudally along the pons and the middle cerebellar peduncle to the cerebellar hemisphere. It supplies the caudal midbrain and the rostral half of the cerebellum.

The **caudal cerebellar artery** is a branch of the basilar artery near the middle of the medulla. It courses dorsally to supply the caudal portion of the cerebellum.

VEINS

The **venous sinuses** (Figs. 6-4 through 6-6) of the cranial dura mater are large venous passageways located within the dura or within bony canals in the skull unaccompanied by arteries. These sinuses receive the veins draining the brain and the bones of the skull. They convey venous blood to the paired maxillary, internal jugular, and vertebral veins and to the ventral internal vertebral venous plexuses (see Fig. 6-4). The following venous sinuses should be located.

The **dorsal sagittal sinus** is located in the attached edge of the falx cerebri, which is a fold of dura extending ventrally into the longitudinal fissure between the two cerebral hemispheres. Caudally, this sinus enters the foramen for the dorsal sagittal sinus in the occipital bone dorsal to where the tentorium attaches. There it joins the right and left transverse sinuses.

Each **transverse sinus** runs laterally through the transverse canal and sulcus. At the distal end of the sulcus, at the dorsal border of the petrosal part of the temporal bone, the sinus divides into a temporal and a sigmoid sinus. Coursing caudolateral to the petrosal part of the temporal bone, the **temporal sinus** extends to the retroarticular foramen, where it emerges as the emissary vein of the retroarticular foramen and joins the maxillary vein.

Each **sigmoid sinus** forms an S-shaped curve as it courses over the dorsomedial side of the petrous part of the temporal bone. It passes through the jugular foramen into the tympano-occipital fissure. Within the fissure the **ventral petrosal sinus** enters rostrally from the petro-occipital canal and joins the sigmoid sinus. From this anastomosis the vertebral and internal jugular veins

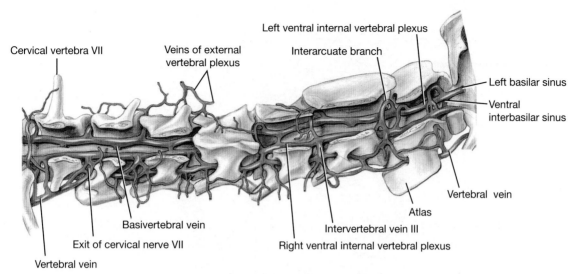

Left ventral internal vertebral plexus

Cervical vertebra VII

Veins of external vertebral plexus

Interarcuate branch

Left basilar sinus

Ventral interbasilar sinus

Vertebral vein

Atlas

Intervertebral vein III

Basivertebral vein

Exit of cervical nerve VII

Right ventral internal vertebral plexus

Vertebral vein

Fig. 6-4 Cervical vertebral veins, right lateral aspect. (From Reinhard K, Miller M, Evans H: The craniovertebral veins and sinuses of the dog, *Am J Anat* 11:67-87, 1962. Copyright © 1962 Wiley-Liss. Reprinted by permission of Wiley-Liss, Inc., a subsidiary of John Wiley & Sons, Inc.)

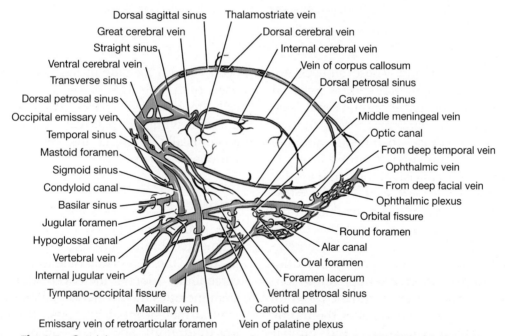

Dorsal sagittal sinus

Thalamostriate vein

Great cerebral vein

Dorsal cerebral vein

Straight sinus

Internal cerebral vein

Ventral cerebral vein

Vein of corpus callosum

Transverse sinus

Dorsal petrosal sinus

Dorsal petrosal sinus

Cavernous sinus

Occipital emissary vein

Middle meningeal vein

Temporal sinus

Optic canal

Mastoid foramen

From deep temporal vein

Sigmoid sinus

Ophthalmic vein

Condyloid canal

From deep facial vein

Basilar sinus

Ophthalmic plexus

Jugular foramen

Orbital fissure

Hypoglossal canal

Round foramen

Vertebral vein

Alar canal

Internal jugular vein

Oval foramen

Tympano-occipital fissure

Foramen lacerum

Maxillary vein

Ventral petrosal sinus

Emissary vein of retroarticular foramen

Carotid canal

Vein of palatine plexus

Fig. 6-5 Cranial venous sinuses, right lateral aspect. (From Reinhard K, Miller M, Evans H: The craniovertebral veins and sinuses of the dog, *Am J Anat* 11:67-87, 1962. Copyright © 1962 Wiley-Liss. Reprinted by permission of Wiley-Liss, Inc., a subsidiary of John Wiley & Sons, Inc.)

arise and leave the tympano-occipital fissure and course caudally. The vertebral vein descends the neck through the transverse foramina of the cervical vertebrae. The internal jugular vein was seen previously in the carotid sheath. The **basilar sinus** is a branch of the sigmoid sinus that continues caudally through the condyloid canal to the ventral internal vertebral venous plexus in the vertebral canal.

The **cavernous sinus** (see Fig. 6-6) lies on each side of the floor of the middle cranial fossa from the orbital fissure to the petro-occipital canal. Emissary veins connect each cavernous sinus with the ophthalmic plexus of veins rostrally and with

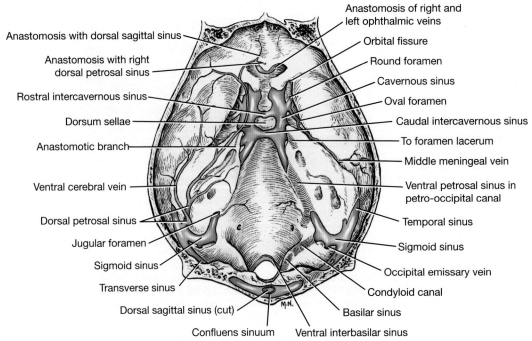

Fig. 6-6 Cranial venous sinuses, dorsal aspect, calvaria removed. (From Reinhard K, Miller M, Evans H: The craniovertebral veins and sinuses of the dog, *Am J Anat* 11:67-87, 1962.)

the maxillary vein laterally. These sinuses are each continued caudally by the **ventral petrosal sinus,** which lies in the petro-occipital canal. Two or three intercavernous sinuses connect the left and right cavernous sinuses rostral and caudal to the pituitary gland. The internal carotid artery is seen coursing through the cavernous sinus.

The **ventral internal vertebral venous plexuses** are paired vessels that lie on the floor of the vertebral canal in the epidural connective tissue. They extend from the venous sinuses of the cranium throughout the vertebral canal. At each intervertebral foramen, **intervertebral veins** connect the vertebral venous plexus with the vertebral veins of the neck, intercostal veins of the thorax (azygos and costocervical veins), and lumbar veins (caudal vena cava) in the abdomen. This plexus will be seen later when the spinal cord is removed from the vertebral canal.

There is a continuous venous pathway from the **angularis oculi vein** (see Fig. 5-42); through the external ophthalmic vein, ophthalmic plexus, cavernous sinus, ventral petrosal sinus, sigmoid sinus, and the basilar sinus in the condyloid canal; to the ventral internal vertebral venous plexus. This pathway can be demonstrated radiographically by compressing the external jugular veins and injecting a radiopaque solution into the angularis

oculi vein on the side of the face near the medial angle of the eye. This procedure can be used clinically to diagnose space-occupying lesions that interfere with this pathway. It can also be used anatomically to inject the venous system with various materials.

BRAIN

The brain is composed of the embryologically segmented brain stem and two suprasegmental portions, the cerebrum (telencephalon) and the cerebellum (dorsal metencephalon). The brain stem includes the myelencephalon (medulla), the ventral metencephalon (pons), the mesencephalon (midbrain), and the diencephalon (epithalamus, thalamus, and hypothalamus).

Dissect and identify the following structures on the intact brain that has been provided.

Cerebrum—Surface Structures

The cerebrum is divided into two cerebral hemispheres by the **longitudinal fissure**. Each cerebral hemisphere has outward folds (convolutions) called **gyri** separated by inward folds called **sulci**. Identify the following gyri and sulci (Figs. 6-7, 6-8): the rostral and caudal parts of the lateral rhinal sulcus, the pseudosylvian fissure,

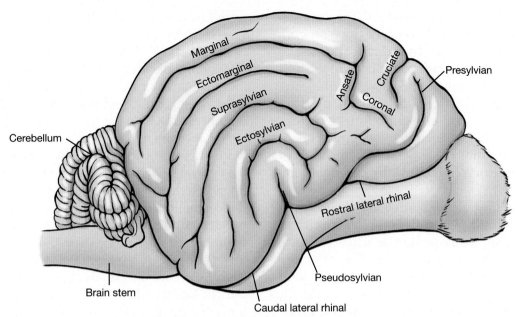

Fig. 6-7 Sulci of brain, right lateral view.

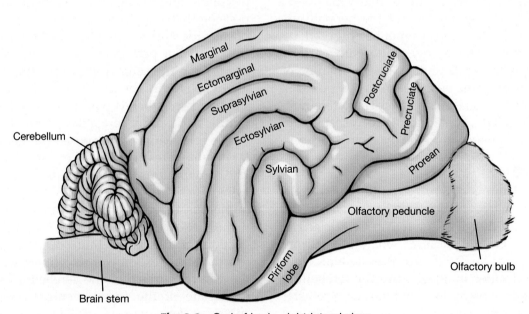

Fig. 6-8 Gyri of brain, right lateral view.

the rostral and caudal sylvian gyri, the ectosylvian sulcus and gyrus, the suprasylvian sulcus and gyrus, the cruciate sulcus, the postcruciate and precruciate gyri, the coronal sulcus, the ectomarginal sulcus and gyrus, and the marginal sulcus and gyrus.

Each cerebral hemisphere may be divided into lobes named for that portion of the calvaria that covers them. The relationship is not precise and varies among species.

The **frontal lobe** is that portion of each cerebral hemisphere rostral to the cruciate sulcus. The precruciate gyrus is part of this lobe and functions as part of the motor cortex. The **parietal lobe** is caudal to the cruciate sulcus and dorsal to the sylvian gyri. It extends caudally to approximately the caudal third of the cerebral hemisphere. The postcruciate and rostral suprasylvian gyri are found in this lobe and function as part of the motor and somesthetic sensory cerebral cortex. The **occipital** lobe includes the caudal third of the cerebral hemisphere. Caudal portions of this lobe on both medial and lateral sides function as the visual cortex. The **temporal lobe** is composed of the gyri and sulci on the ventrolateral aspect of the cerebral hemisphere. Parts of the sylvian gyri are located here and function as the auditory cortex.

The **rhinal sulcus** separates the phylogenetically new cerebrum or neopallium, above, from the older olfactory cerebrum, the paleopallium, below.

Portions of the paleopallium that are visible are the **olfactory bulb,** which rests on the cribriform plate, and the **olfactory peduncle,** which joins the bulb to the cerebral hemisphere. The **olfactory peduncle** (see Figs. 6-8, 6-9) courses caudally with a band of fibers on its ventral surface. Caudally, this band divides into **lateral** and **medial olfactory tracts.** Observe the lateral olfactory tract passing caudally to the **piriform lobe,** which forms a ventral bulge just lateral to the pituitary gland and medial to the temporal lobe of the neopallium. The medial olfactory tract cannot be observed.

Each gyrus contains gray matter superficially and white matter in its center. The gray matter, or **cerebral cortex** of the neopallium, is composed of six layers of neuronal cell bodies. The white matter, **corona radiata,** contains the processes of neurons coursing to and from the overlying cortex.

Cerebellum

The **cerebellum** is derived from the dorsal portion of the metencephalon and lies caudal to the cerebrum and dorsal to the fourth ventricle. The **transverse cerebral fissure** separates it from the cerebrum. The dural and osseous **tentorium cerebelli** is located in this fissure. The cerebellum is connected to the brain stem by three cerebellar peduncles on each side of the fourth ventricle and by portions of the roof of the fourth ventricle.

The **choroid plexus** (see Fig. 6-1) is a compact mass of pia, blood vessels, and ependyma. A choroid plexus develops where neural tube neuroepithelium did not proliferate to form parenchyma but remained as a single layer of the neuroepithelial cells, a roof plate. These areas are found in the medulla (roof plate of the fourth ventricle), the diencephalon (roof plate of the third ventricle), and each telencephalon (roof plate of the lateral ventricles). At these sites the vessels in the pia covering the single layer of neuroepithelial cells proliferate to form a dense plexus of capillaries intimately related to the neuroepithelial cells. These cells and blood vessels are involved in passive and active secretion of cerebrospinal fluid into the ventricular system. The choroid plexus of the fourth ventricle protrudes into the lumen of the fourth ventricle and is visible caudolateral to the cerebellum on the dorsal surface of the medulla where it protrudes through the lateral aperture.

Identify the **transverse fibers of the pons** on the ventral surface of the brain stem. Follow these fibers laterally as they course dorsocaudally into the cerebellum on each side as the **middle cerebellar peduncle** (see Figs. 6-9, 6-10, 6-34). At the point where they merge into the cerebellum, cut this peduncle with a scalpel. Continue the cut slightly rostral to cut the rostral cerebellar peduncle. Gently lift the caudal part of the cerebellum from the medulla. Remove the choroid plexus so you can see the **caudal cerebellar peduncle** connecting the medulla and cerebellum. Cut this peduncle and detach the cerebellum from the pons on that side. Cut these peduncles on the opposite side and remove the cerebellum. The rostral cerebellar peduncle contains mainly efferent axons from the cerebellum to the brain stem. Afferent axons to the cerebellum from the brain stem and spinal cord pass primarily through the middle and caudal cerebellar peduncles.

The cerebellum is composed of lateral **cerebellar hemispheres** and a middle portion, the **vermis.** The convolutions of the cerebellum are known as **folia.** These are grouped into three lobes and numerous cerebellar lobules that have specific names. The vermis comprises the entire middle portion of the cerebellum directly above the fourth ventricle. Some of its lobules are found on the ventral surface of the cerebellum facing the roof plate of the fourth ventricle. Each hemisphere projects over the cerebellar peduncles and the adjacent brain stem. A lateral component lies in the cerebellar fossa of the petrosal part of the temporal bone.

Make a median incision through the vermis, hemisectioning the cerebellum. Examine the cut surface. Note the pattern of white matter as it branches and arborizes from the medulla of the cerebellum into the folia (see Figs. 6-15, 6-34, 6-36). The **medulla of the cerebellum** is the white matter in its central portion that contains the **cerebellar nuclei** and connects with all the folia and the **cerebellar peduncles.** Observe the laminae of foliate white matter and the cerebellar cortex.

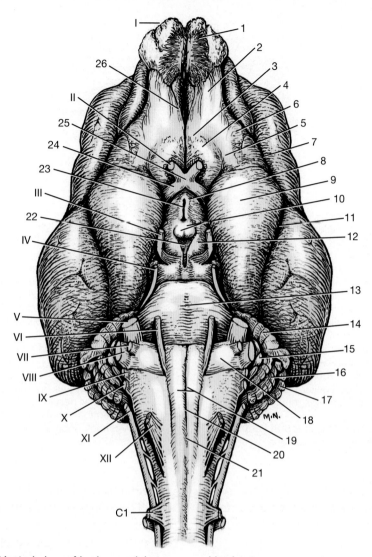

Fig. 6-9 Ventral view of brain, cranial nerves, and brain stem.

1. Olfactory bulb
2. Olfactory peduncle
3. Medial olfactory tract
4. Rostral perforated substance
5. Lateral olfactory tract
6. Lateral olfactory gyrus
7. Rostral rhinal sulcus
8. Tuber cinereum
9. Piriform lobe
10. Mamillary bodies
11. Caudal rhinal sulcus
12. Crus cerebri
13. Pons, transverse fibers
14. Ventral paraflocculus
15. Flocculus
16. Dorsal paraflocculus
17. Ansiform lobule
18. Trapezoid body
19. Pyramids
20. Ventral median fissure
21. Decussation of pyramids
22. Caudal perforated substance in inter-
    peduncular fossa
23. Infundibulum
24. Postchiasmatic optic tract
25. Optic chiasm
26. Medial rhinal sulcus
   II. Prechiasmatic optic tract
  III. Oculomotor nerve
   IV. Trochlear nerve
    V. Trigeminal nerve
   VI. Abducent nerve
  VII. Facial nerve
 VIII. Vestibulocochlear nerve
   IX. Glossopharyngeal nerve
    X. Vagus nerve
   XI. Accessory nerve
  XII. Hypoglossal nerve
  C1. First cervical spinal nerve

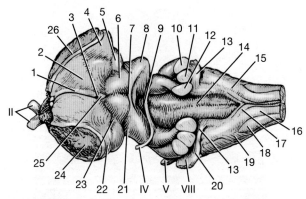

Fig. 6-10   Dorsal view of brain stem.

1. Stria habenularis thalami
2. Thalamus
3. Habenular commissure
4. Lateral geniculate nucleus
5. Medial geniculate nucleus
6. Rostral colliculus
7. Commissure of caudal colliculus
8. Caudal colliculus
9. Crossing of trochlear nerve fibers in rostral medullary velum
10. Middle cerebellar peduncle
11. Caudal cerebellar peduncle
12. Rostral cerebellar peduncle
13. Dorsal cochlear nucleus in acoustic stria
14. Median sulcus in fourth ventricle
15. Lateral cuneate nucleus
16. Fasciculus cuneatus
17. Nucleus gracilis
18. Spinal tract of trigeminal nerve
19. Superficial arcuate fibers
20. Left ventral cochlear nucleus
21. Brachium of caudal colliculus
22. Postchiasmatic optic tract
23. Brachium of rostral colliculus
24. Cut internal capsule between cerebral hemisphere and brain stem
25. Pineal body
26. Stria terminalis
II. Prechiasmatic optic tract
IV. Trochlear nerve
V. Trigeminal nerve
VIII. Vestibulocochlear nerve

Make a transverse section of one half of the cerebellum through its medulla to observe the lateral extent of the medullary white matter and its nuclei (see Fig. 6-15).

Brain Stem—Surface Structures

To expose the dorsal surface structures of the brain stem, the left cerebral hemisphere will be removed by the following dissection.

Gently separate the two cerebral hemispheres at the longitudinal fissure. Expose the band of fibers that course transversely from one hemisphere to the other in the depth of the fissure. This structure is the corpus callosum. Completely divide the corpus callosum longitudinally along the median plane in the depth of the longitudinal fissure. Cut deep enough to include the hippocampal commissure and body of the fornix, but do not cut into the thalamus (see Figs. 6-11, 6-12, 6-34). Continue the cut rostrally and ventrally through the rostral commissure just dorsal to the optic chiasm and rostral to the thalamus. On the ventral surface, follow the postchiasmatic optic tract in a dorsocaudal direction from the optic chiasm and cut the fibers of the internal capsule

rostral and medial to this tract. This is an oblique cut. The fibers of the internal capsule attach the cerebral hemisphere to the brain stem. Gently lift the medial side of the cerebrum off the thalamus and continue this separation over the dorsal aspect of the diencephalon. Cut any remaining attachments, and remove the cerebral hemisphere from the diencephalon.

Examine Fig. 6-12 and recognize the structures you have cut to remove the cerebral hemisphere. The internal capsule is the only structure connecting the cerebral hemisphere with the brain stem. It consists of neuronal processes projecting from the cerebral hemisphere to the brain stem and neuronal processes projecting from the thalamus to the cerebral hemisphere. This will be dissected further later.

Examine the surface of the brain stem and locate the following structures (see Figs. 6-9, 6-10).

Diencephalon

The **diencephalon** consists of a large, centrally located **thalamus;** a smaller **hypothalamus** below; and a very small **epithalamus** on the dorsal midline. It is the most rostral part of the brain stem.

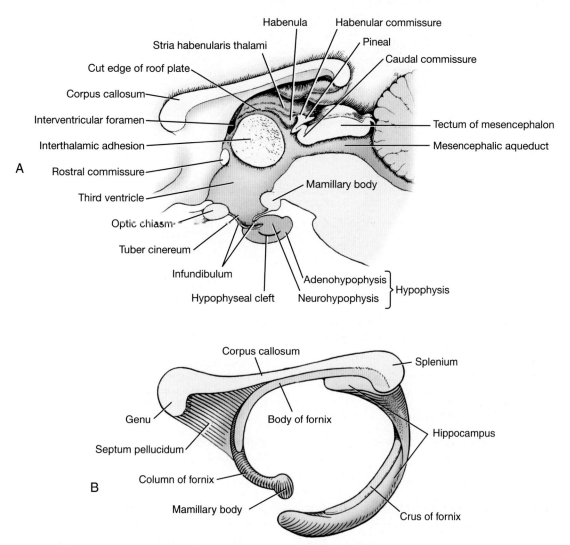

Fig. 6-11 **A,** Median section of diencephalon. **B,** Hippocampal complex dissected out.

The prechiasmatic optic tract (formerly optic nerve or second cranial nerve) form the **optic chiasm** of the diencephalon rostral to the hypophysis or pituitary gland (see Figs. 6-9, 6-10). The **postchiasmatic optic tracts** course laterally and dorsocaudally from the chiasm, pass over the lateral surface of the diencephalon, and enter the lateral geniculate nucleus of the thalamus. In this pathway, each tract curves around the caudal edge of the internal capsule (see Figs. 6-12, 6-34, 6-36).

Caudal to the optic chiasm on the median plane is the **hypophysis (pituitary gland),** which is attached by the **infundibulum** to the **tuber cinereum** of the hypothalamus. If the gland is missing, the lumen of the infundibulum will be evident. This lumen communicates with the overlying third ventricle of the diencephalon.

The **mamillary bodies** of the hypothalamus bulge ventrally caudal to the tuber cinereum.

They demarcate the most caudal extent of the hypothalamus on the ventral surface of the diencephalon.

The internal capsule bounds the diencephalon laterally and was cut when the left cerebral hemisphere was removed. The thalamus and epithalamus can be seen on the dorsal aspect of the diencephalon (see Figs. 6-10, 6-11).

Three structures compose the **epithalamus**. They all are located adjacent to the median plane. The **stria habenularis** lies on either side of the midline, coursing dorsally and caudally from the rostroventral aspect of the hypothalamus over the thalamus to the dorsocaudal aspect of the diencephalon. Here the stria enters the **habenular nucleus**. The habenula nuclei on each side are connected by a small commissure. Caudal to the habenular nucleus is the small, unpaired **pineal body**. This caudal

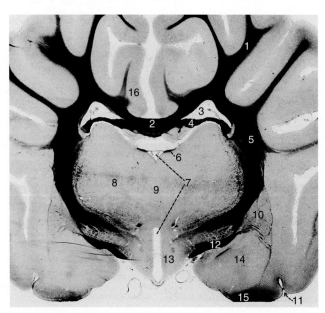

Fig. 6-12   Diencephalon and cerebral hemispheres. (In this and the following transverse sections, the white matter is stained with iron hematoxylin and appears black in the photographs.)

1. Corona radiata
2. Corpus callosum
3. Lateral ventricle
4. Crus of fornix
5. Internal capsule
6. Stria habenularis
7. Third ventricle
8. Thalamus
9. Interthalamic adhesion
10. Lentiform nucleus
11. Lateral rhinal sulcus
12. Postchiasmatic optic tract
13. Hypothalamus
14. Amygdala
15. Piriform lobe
16. Cingulate gyrus

projection from the diencephalon is small in the dog but very prominent in larger domestic animals.

A space is located between the stria habenularis of each side. This is the dorsal part of the **third ventricle** (see Figs. 6-10 through 6-12). It is covered by a thin remnant of the roof plate of the neural tube, a layer of ependyma that extends from one stria habenularis to the other. Branches of the caudal cerebral artery course over the diencephalon and with this ependyma form the **choroid plexus of the third ventricle**. This is usually pulled out when the calvaria is removed to expose the brain. Rostrally, the choroid plexus of the third ventricle is continuous with the choroid plexus of the lateral ventricle at the **interventricular foramen**. This foramen is caudal to the column of the fornix at the level of the rostral commissure. These structures will be seen in the dissection of the telencephalon.

The **thalamus** lies between the internal capsule on each side and dorsal to the hypothalamus. It is covered by pia, arachnoid trabeculations, and the subarachnoid space. It consists of two bilaterally symmetrical collections of nuclei that primarily project axons to the ipsilateral cerebral hemisphere. These two collections are separated by the third ventricle. Two of these nuclei are prominent and readily recognized on the caudal surface. These are the geniculate nuclei, which comprise the metathalamus. A lateral eminence on the caudodorsal surface of the thalamus is the **lateral geniculate nucleus,** which receives fibers of the optic tract and functions in the visual system. The lateral geniculate nucleus is connected with the rostral colliculus of the midbrain. Caudoventral to the lateral geniculate nucleus is the **medial geniculate nucleus** of the thalamus. This nucleus functions in the auditory system and is connected to the caudal colliculus of the midbrain by the brachium of the caudal colliculus.

In the third ventricle, between the stria habenularis of each side, observe the **interthalamic adhesion** between the right and left sides of the thalamus. This area appears round on median section because the third ventricle encircles it (see Fig. 6-11). In transverse section the narrow, vertically oriented third ventricle appears as a perpendicular slit below the interthalamic adhesion (see Fig. 6-12). Its lateral and ventral walls are formed by the **hypothalamus**. The hypothalamic nuclei are symmetrically organized on both sides of the ventral portion of the third ventricle bordered laterally by the ventral portion of the internal capsule, the endopeduncular nucleus and the postchiasmatic optic tract. The dorsal portion of the third ventricle is small and tubular. It passes over the interthalamic adhesion, but its thin roof plate, which is attached on each side to the stria habenularis, cannot be observed grossly.

Mesencephalon

The **mesencephalon** (midbrain) is relatively short. It is nearly round on transverse section with a canal, the **mesencephalic aqueduct** (Figs. 6-13, 6-14), passing through it. The mesencephalon consists of a **tectum** or roof dorsal to the aqueduct, which is composed of four groups of neuronal cell bodies: the **colliculi**. That portion of the mesencephalon ventral to the aqueduct is the **cerebral peduncle,** which consists of a tegmentum (reticular formation), substantia nigra, and crus cerebri, from dorsal to ventral.

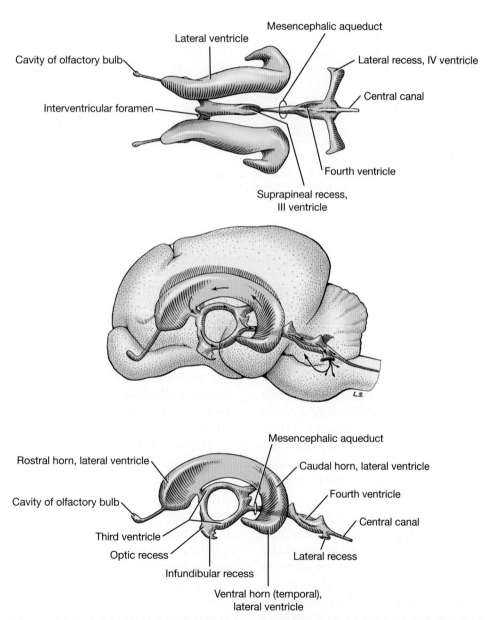

Fig. 6-13 Ventricles of brain. Direction of *arrows* indicates flow of cerebrospinal fluid. (From de Lahunta A: *Veterinary neuroanatomy and clinical neurology,* ed 3, St Louis, 2009, Elsevier.

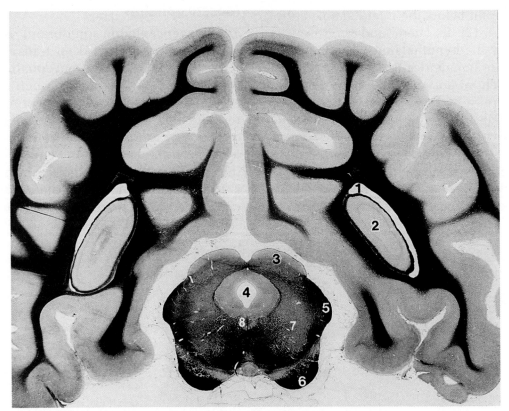

Fig. 6-14 Mesencephalon and cerebral hemispheres. (The white matter is stained with iron hematoxylin and appears black in the photograph.)

1. Lateral ventricle
2. Hippocampus
3. Rostral colliculus
4. Mesencephalic aqueduct

5. Brachium of caudal colliculus
6. Crus cerebri
7. Tegmentum (reticular formation)
8. Oculomotor nucleus

Between the mamillary bodies of the hypothalamus and the transverse fibers of the pons is the ventral surface of the **mesencephalon**. The transverse fibers of the pons cover part of the caudal mesencephalon ventrally. Caudally projecting tracts of projection processes that connect portions of the cerebral cortex with brain stem centers and the spinal cord course on the ventral surface of the midbrain. These are grouped together on each side as the **crus cerebri** (see Figs. 6-9, 6-14). The **oculomotor,** or third cranial, nerve leaves the midbrain medial to the crus (see Fig. 6-9).

The mesencephalic structures dorsal to the mesencephalic aqueduct compose the tectum of the midbrain (see Fig. 6-11). The **mesencephalic aqueduct** is a short, narrow tube, derived from the neural canal in the midbrain, that connects the third ventricle rostrally with the fourth ventricle caudally. Four dorsal bulges, the **corpora quadrigemina,** are evident on the dorsal side. The rostral pair are the **rostral colliculi,** which

function with the visual system. The smaller caudal pair are the **caudal colliculi,** which function in the **auditory system** (see Fig. 6-10).

The **trochlear,** or fourth cranial, nerve courses laterally out of the roof of the fourth ventricle, the **rostral medullary velum,** adjacent to the caudal colliculus (see Fig. 6-10). It continues rostroventrally on the lateral surface of the midbrain.

The **lateral lemniscus** (see Figs. 6-34, 6-36) is a band of auditory system axons on the lateral side of the midbrain. It courses rostrodorsally from the level of the cochlear nucleus to the caudal colliculus and emerges medial to the middle cerebellar peduncle. Many of these fibers arise from the cochlear nucleus. The **brachium of the caudal colliculus** (see Figs. 6-10, 6-34, 6-36) runs rostroventrally from the caudal colliculus to the medial geniculate nucleus of the thalamus. On the dorsal surface the **commissure of the caudal colliculi** (see Fig. 6-10) can be seen crossing between these two structures. The rostral colliculus is connected to the lateral geniculate nucleus of the thalamus by a short **brachium of the rostral colliculus** (see Fig. 6-10).

Ventral Metencephalon

The metencephalic portion of the rhombencephalon includes a segment of the brain stem, the **pons,** and the dorsal development, the **cerebellum**. The ventral surface of the pons includes the **transverse fibers of the pons** (see Fig. 6-9), which course laterally into the **middle cerebellar peduncles.** This large band of transverse fibers borders the trapezoid body of the medulla caudally. Its rostral border covers part of the ventral surface of the midbrain. The **trigeminal nerve** is associated with the pons and can be found entering the pons along the caudolateral aspect of the transverse fibers (see Figs. 6-9, 6-34). The caudally projecting fibers of the crus cerebri enter the pons dorsal to the transverse fibers, where they are called the **longitudinal fibers of the pons**. These longitudinal fibers are covered ventrally by the transverse fibers. The longitudinal fibers that do not terminate in pontine nuclei continue caudally on the ventral surface of the trapezoid body of the medulla as the pyramids. Many of the axons in the crus cerebri and the longitudinal fibers of the pons, and most of those in the transverse fibers of the pons, make up a large cerebropontocerebellar pathway. Synapse occurs in the pontine nuclei that are covered by the transverse fibers, and crossing occurs through the transverse fibers to enter the cerebellum through the contralateral middle cerebellar peduncle. Therefore impulses that arise in the left cerebrum are projected to the right cerebellar hemisphere.

The **rostral medullary velum** forms the roof of the fourth ventricle between the caudal colliculi of the mesencephalon rostrally and the midventral surface of the cerebellum caudally. The crossing fibers of the trochlear nerves course through this velum (see Fig. 6-10). The velum in the preserved specimen lies on the floor of the fourth ventricle and covers the caudal opening of the mesencephalic aqueduct. Insert a probe into the slitlike fourth ventricle under the caudal cut edge of this velum and raise the velum to demonstrate its attachments and the continuity of the fourth ventricle with the aqueduct. This velum lies between the fourth ventricle, which it covers, and the rostral cerebellar vermis. Between the velum and the vermis is subarachnoid space.

Myelencephalon (Medulla)

The **myelencephalon,** or medulla, extends from the transverse fibers of the pons to the level of the ventral rootlets of the first cervical spinal nerve. The **trapezoid body** is the transverse band of fibers rostrally that course parallel but caudal to the transverse pontine fibers (see Figs. 6-9, 6-34, 6-36). It is continuous with the vestibulocochlear nerve and cochlear nuclei laterally on the side of the medulla and functions in the auditory system. The **pyramids** are a pair of longitudinally coursing fiber bundles on either side of the ventral median plane. They emerge from the transverse fibers as the caudal continuations of axons from the longitudinal fibers of the pons that did not terminate in pontine nuclei. They course caudally across the trapezoid body to continue on the ventral surface of the medulla. They are separated by the **ventral median fissure**. This fissure can be followed caudally until it is obliterated over a short distance by the **decussation of the pyramids** located at the level of the emerging hypoglossal nerve fibers. The decussation itself is difficult to see because it occurs as the pyramidal fibers are passing dorsally into the parenchyma of the medulla. Pyramidal axons continue in the spinal cord as the corticospinal tracts. These are cerebral projection processes that project to the spinal cord.

The **abducent,** or sixth cranial, nerve leaves the medulla through the trapezoid body on the lateral border of each pyramid.

Cranial nerve VII, the **facial nerve** (see Fig. 6-9), is smaller and leaves the lateral surface of the medulla through the trapezoid body caudal to the trigeminal nerve and rostroventral to the eighth cranial nerve.

Cranial nerve VIII, the **vestibulocochlear nerve** (see Figs. 6-9, 6-10, 6-21), is on the lateral side of the medulla at the most lateral extent of the trapezoid body just dorsal to the facial nerve. The **cochlear nuclei** are located in this nerve where it attaches to the medulla (see Figs. 6-10, 6-15, 6-34). All cochlear neurons in the vestibulocochlear nerve synapse in cochlear nuclei. The axons of these cell bodies in the cochlear nuclei continue into the medulla by one of two pathways. Some continue as the **acoustic stria** (see Fig. 6-10) and pass over the dorsolateral surface of the medulla and caudal cerebellar peduncle to enter the medulla. Others pass on the ventral surface in the **trapezoid body** (see Figs. 6-9, 6-15). The vestibular

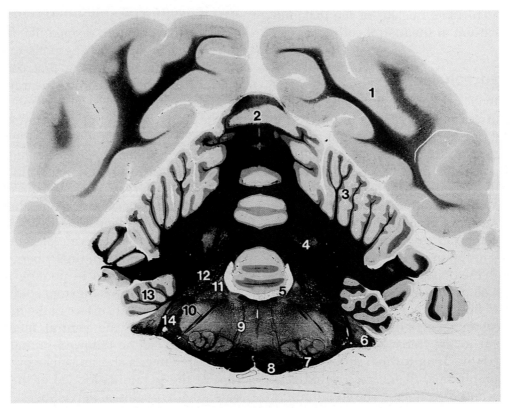

Fig. 6-15   Cerebellum and myelencephalon. (The white matter is stained with iron hematoxylin and appears black in the photographs.)

1. Occipital lobe
2. Cerebellar vermis
3. Cerebellar hemisphere
4. Cerebellar nucleus
5. Fourth ventricle
6. Cochlear nuclei and vestibulocochlear nerve
7. Trapezoid body
8. Pyramid
9. Abducent nerve fibers
10. Descending facial nerve fibers
11. Vestibular nuclei
12. Caudal cerebellar peduncle
13. Flocculus
14. Spinal tract of trigeminal nerve

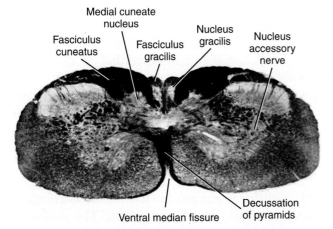

Fig. 6-16   Caudal myelencephalon. Figs. 6-16 through 6-32 are transverse sections from *The Brain of the Dog in Section* by Marcus Singer, 1962, with selected structures labeled. The white matter is stained with iron hematozylin, which gives it a black color. The plates are in sequence from caudal to rostral but at varying intervals. (From Singer M: *The brain of the dog in section*, Philadelphia, 1962, Saunders.)

neurons in the vestibulocochlear nerve pass directly into the medulla, where most of them synapse in a vestibular nucleus (see Fig. 6-15).

The **hypoglossal nerve,** cranial nerve XII (see Fig. 6-9), emerges as a number of fine rootlets from the ventrolateral surface of the myelencephalon caudal to the trapezoid body, lateral to the caudal portion of the pyramid. The junction of the myelencephalon and the spinal cord is between the hypoglossal fibers and the ventral rootlets of the first cervical spinal nerve. The hypoglossal nerve outside the skull is much larger, owing to the addition of connective tissue components.

Dorsolateral to the emergence of the hypoglossal fibers and the fibers of the ventral root of the first cervical spinal nerve, a nerve runs lengthwise along the lateral surface of the spinal cord. This is the eleventh cranial nerve, the **accessory nerve** (see Figs. 6-9, 6-37). Its spinal rootlets emerge from the lateral surface of the spinal cord as far caudally as the seventh cervical segment. They

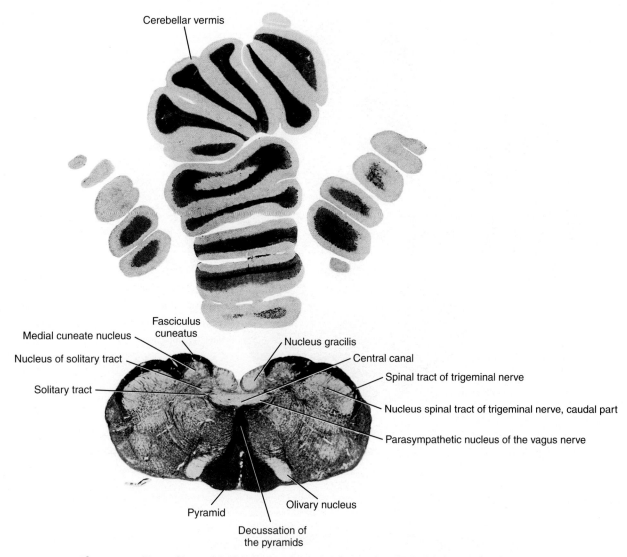

Cerebellar vermis

Fasciculus cuneatus

Medial cuneate nucleus

Nucleus of solitary tract

Nucleus gracilis

Solitary tract

Central canal

Spinal tract of trigeminal nerve

Nucleus spinal tract of trigeminal nerve, caudal part

Parasympathetic nucleus of the vagus nerve

Pyramid

Olivary nucleus

Decussation of the pyramids

Fig. 6-17   (From Singer M: *The brain of the dog in section*, Philadelphia, 1962, Saunders.)

emerge between the level of the dorsal and ventral rootlets of the cervical spinal nerves and course cranially within the subarachnoid space through the vertebral canal and foramen magnum. A few cranial rootlets emerge from the lateral side of the medulla caudal to the tenth cranial nerve and join the accessory nerve as it courses by the medulla (see Fig. 6-9). These are usually torn off the medulla in removing the brain for dissection. The accessory nerve leaves the cranial cavity through the jugular foramen and tympano-occipital fissure along with the ninth and tenth cranial nerves.

Cranial nerves IX and X, the **glossopharyngeal** and **vagal nerves**, respectively, leave the lateral side of the myelencephalon caudal to the eighth cranial nerve and rostral to the accessory nerve. These rootlets are small and are rarely preserved on the brain when it is removed.

Examine the dorsal surface of the pons and medulla. On either side of the fourth ventricle are the cut ends of the three cerebellar peduncles. The **rostral cerebellar peduncle** is medial and courses rostrally into the mesencephalon; the **middle cerebellar peduncle** is lateral and arises from the transverse fibers on the lateral side of the pons; and the **caudal cerebellar peduncle** is in the middle, entering from the myelencephalon after passing beneath the acoustic stria.

The groove in the center of the floor of the fourth ventricle is the **median sulcus**. On the lateral wall the longitudinal groove is the **sulcus limitans**. Just lateral to this latter groove, at the level of the acoustic stria, there is a slight dorsal bulge of the medulla. This demarcates the location of the **vestibular nuclei**. Most of the vestibular neurons in the vestibulocochlear nerve terminate here.

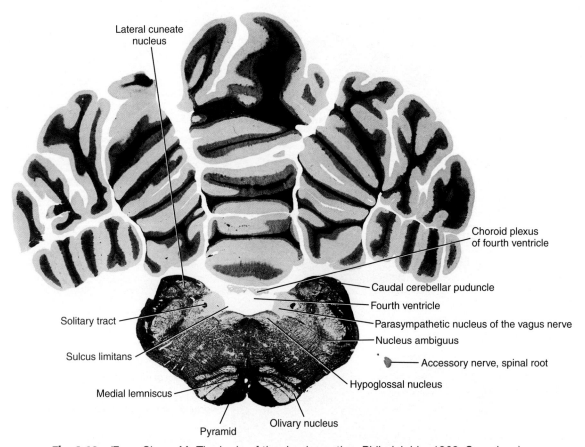

Lateral cuneate nucleus

Choroid plexus of fourth ventricle

Caudal cerebellar puduncle

Fourth ventricle

Solitary tract

Parasympathetic nucleus of the vagus nerve

Sulcus limitans

Nucleus ambiguus

Accessory nerve, spinal root

Medial lemniscus

Hypoglossal nucleus

Pyramid

Olivary nucleus

Fig. 6-18   (From Singer M: *The brain of the dog in section,* Philadelphia, 1962, Saunders.)

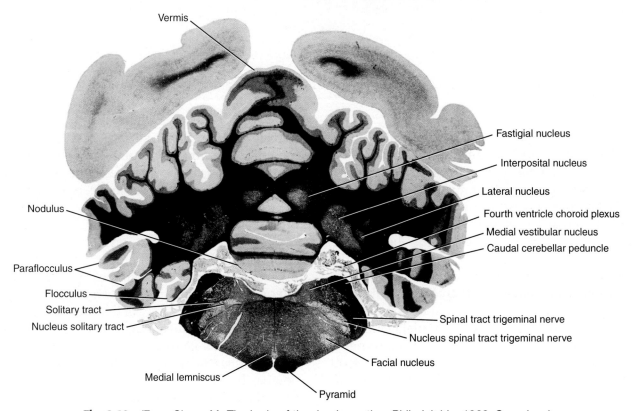

Vermis

Fastigial nucleus

Interposital nucleus

Lateral nucleus

Nodulus

Fourth ventricle choroid plexus

Medial vestibular nucleus

Caudal cerebellar peduncle

Paraflocculus

Flocculus

Solitary tract

Spinal tract trigeminal nerve

Nucleus solitary tract

Nucleus spinal tract trigeminal nerve

Facial nucleus

Medial lemniscus

Pyramid

Fig. 6-19   (From Singer M: *The brain of the dog in section,* Philadelphia, 1962, Saunders.)

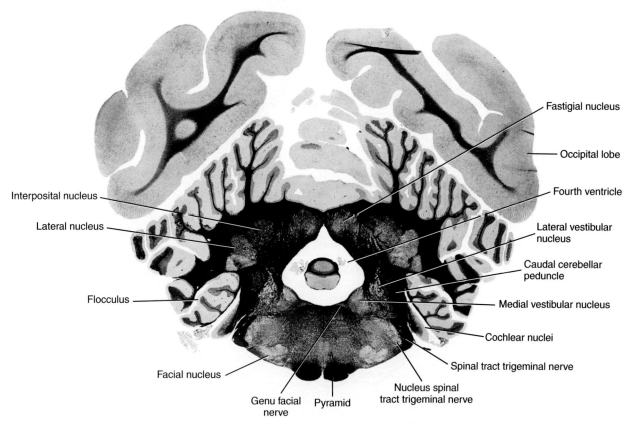

Fastigial nucleus

Occipital lobe

Fourth ventricle

Interposital nucleus

Lateral vestibular nucleus

Lateral nucleus

Caudal cerebellar peduncle

Medial vestibular nucleus

Flocculus

Cochlear nuclei

Spinal tract trigeminal nerve

Facial nucleus

Nucleus spinal tract trigeminal nerve

Genu facial nerve   Pyramid

Fig. 6-20   (From Singer M: *The brain of the dog in section,* Philadelphia, 1962, Saunders.)

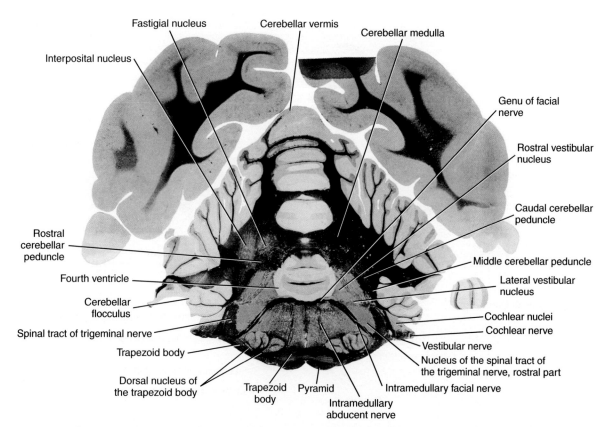

Fastigial nucleus   Cerebellar vermis

Cerebellar medulla

Interposital nucleus

Genu of facial nerve

Rostral vestibular nucleus

Caudal cerebellar peduncle

Rostral cerebellar peduncle

Middle cerebellar peduncle

Fourth ventricle

Lateral vestibular nucleus

Cerebellar flocculus

Cochlear nuclei

Spinal tract of trigeminal nerve

Cochlear nerve

Vestibular nerve

Trapezoid body

Nucleus of the spinal tract of the trigeminal nerve, rostral part

Dorsal nucleus of the trapezoid body

Trapezoid body   Pyramid

Intramedullary facial nerve

Intramedullary abducent nerve

Fig. 6-21   (From Singer M: *The brain of the dog in section,* Philadelphia, 1962, Saunders.)

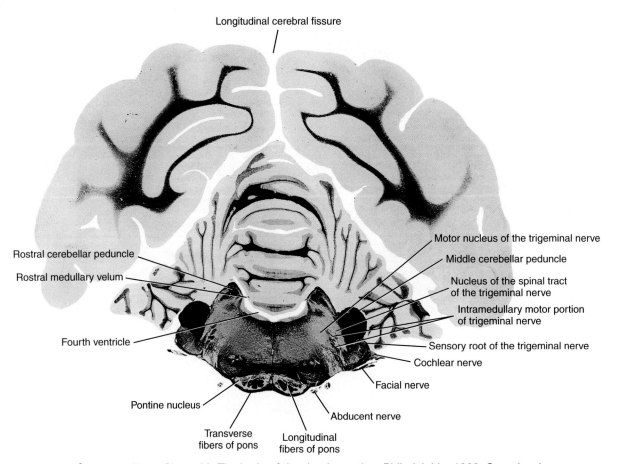

Longitudinal cerebral fissure

Rostral cerebellar peduncle

Rostral medullary velum

Fourth ventricle

Pontine nucleus

Transverse fibers of pons

Longitudinal fibers of pons

Motor nucleus of the trigeminal nerve

Middle cerebellar peduncle

Nucleus of the spinal tract of the trigeminal nerve

Intramedullary motor portion of trigeminal nerve

Sensory root of the trigeminal nerve

Cochlear nerve

Facial nerve

Abducent nerve

Fig. 6-22   (From Singer M: *The brain of the dog in section,* Philadelphia, 1962, Saunders.)

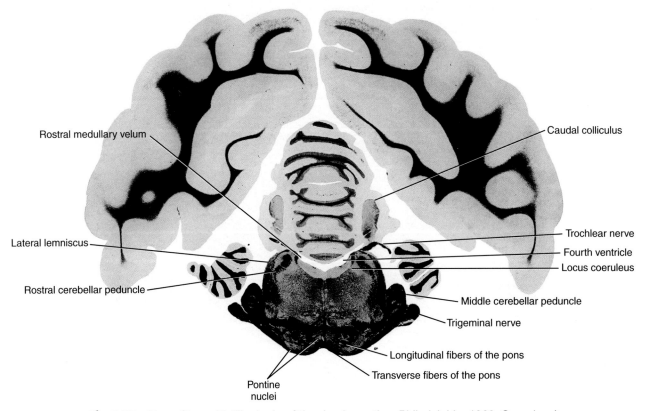

Rostral medullary velum

Lateral lemniscus

Rostral cerebellar peduncle

Pontine nuclei

Caudal colliculus

Trochlear nerve

Fourth ventricle

Locus coeruleus

Middle cerebellar peduncle

Trigeminal nerve

Longitudinal fibers of the pons

Transverse fibers of the pons

Fig. 6-23   (From Singer M: *The brain of the dog in section,* Philadelphia, 1962, Saunders.)

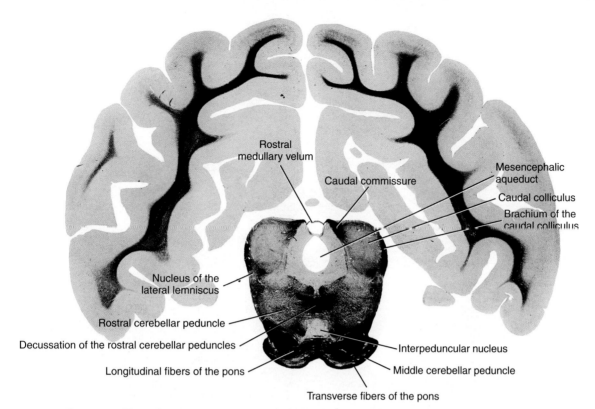

Fig. 6-24 (From Singer M: *The brain of the dog in section,* Philadelphia, 1962, Saunders.)

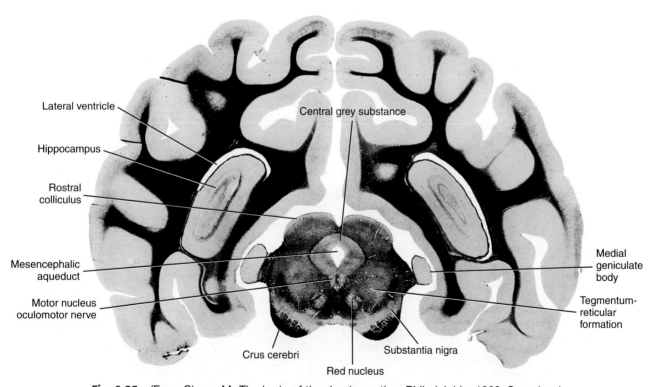

Fig. 6-25 (From Singer M: *The brain of the dog in section,* Philadelphia, 1962, Saunders.)

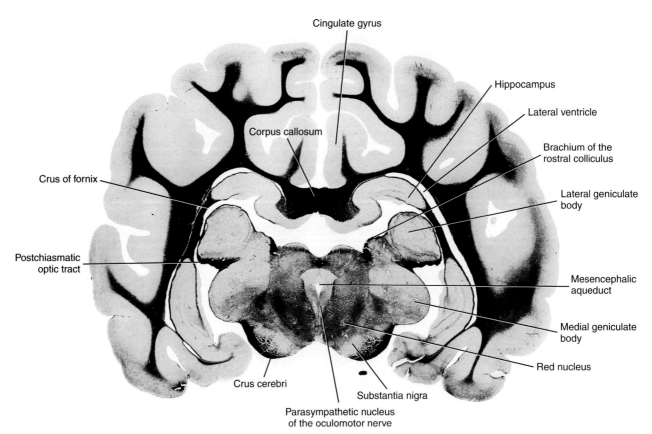

Cingulate gyrus

Hippocampus

Lateral ventricle

Corpus callosum

Brachium of the rostral colliculus

Lateral geniculate body

Crus of fornix

Postchiasmatic optic tract

Mesencephalic aqueduct

Medial geniculate body

Red nucleus

Crus cerebri

Substantia nigra

Parasympathetic nucleus of the oculomotor nerve

Fig. 6-26   (From Singer M: *The brain of the dog in section,* Philadelphia, 1962, Saunders.)

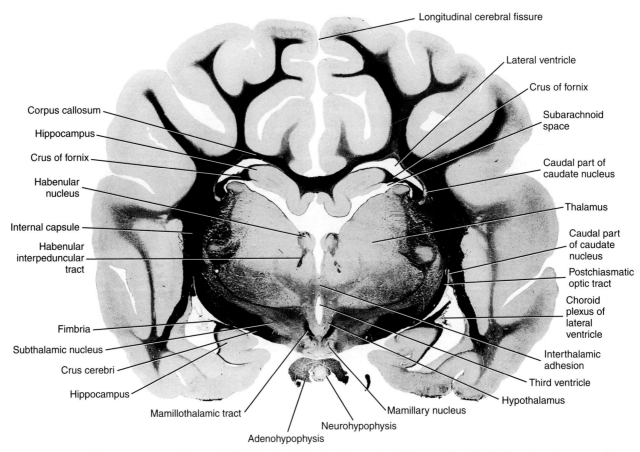

Longitudinal cerebral fissure

Lateral ventricle

Crus of fornix

Corpus callosum

Subarachnoid space

Hippocampus

Crus of fornix

Caudal part of caudate nucleus

Habenular nucleus

Thalamus

Internal capsule

Caudal part of caudate nucleus

Habenular interpeduncular tract

Postchiasmatic optic tract

Choroid plexus of lateral ventricle

Fimbria

Subthalamic nucleus

Interthalamic adhesion

Crus cerebri

Third ventricle

Hippocampus

Hypothalamus

Mamillothalamic tract

Mamillary nucleus

Neurohypophysis

Adenohypophysis

Fig. 6-27   (From Singer M: *The brain of the dog in section,* Philadelphia, 1962, Saunders.)

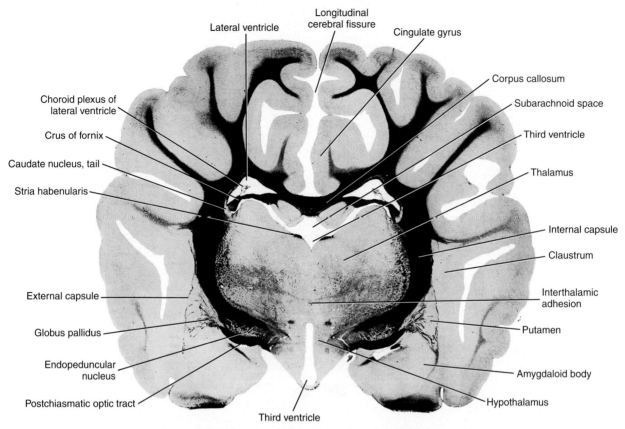

Lateral ventricle

Longitudinal cerebral fissure

Cingulate gyrus

Corpus callosum

Subarachnoid space

Third ventricle

Thalamus

Internal capsule

Claustrum

Interthalamic adhesion

Putamen

Amygdaloid body

Hypothalamus

Choroid plexus of lateral ventricle

Crus of fornix

Caudate nucleus, tail

Stria habenularis

External capsule

Globus pallidus

Endopeduncular nucleus

Postchiasmatic optic tract

Third ventricle

Fig. 6-28 (From Singer M: *The brain of the dog in section,* Philadelphia, 1962, Saunders.)

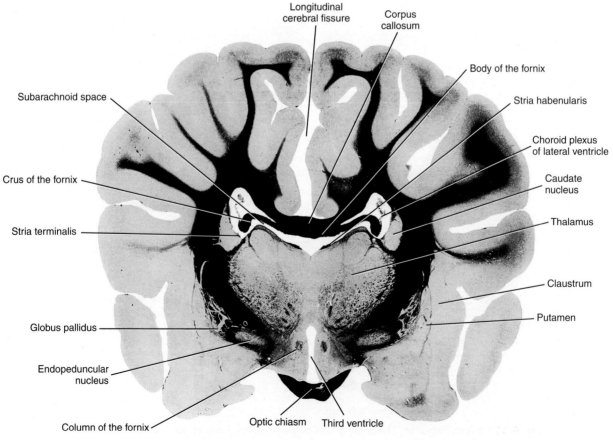

Longitudinal cerebral fissure

Corpus callosum

Body of the fornix

Stria habenularis

Choroid plexus of lateral ventricle

Caudate nucleus

Thalamus

Claustrum

Putamen

Subarachnoid space

Crus of the fornix

Stria terminalis

Globus pallidus

Endopeduncular nucleus

Column of the fornix

Optic chiasm

Third ventricle

Fig. 6-29 (From Singer M: *The brain of the dog in section,* Philadelphia, 1962, Saunders.)

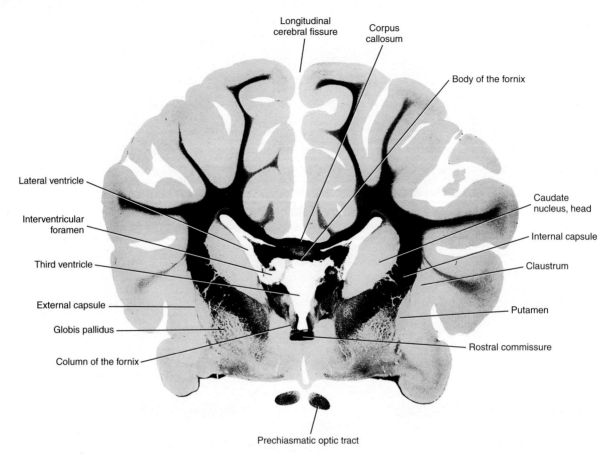

Fig. 6-30 (From Singer M: *The brain of the dog in section,* Philadelphia, 1962, Saunders.)

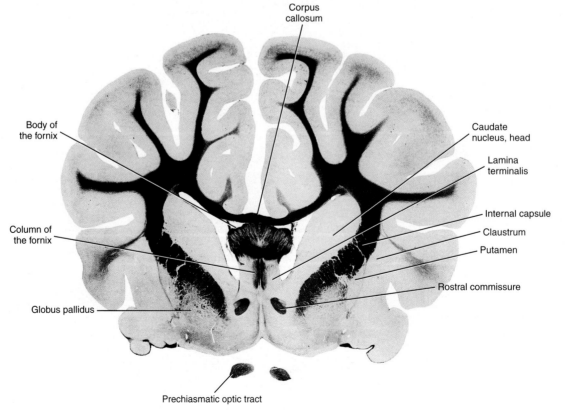

Fig. 6-31 (From Singer M: *The brain of the dog in section,* Philadelphia, 1962, Saunders.)

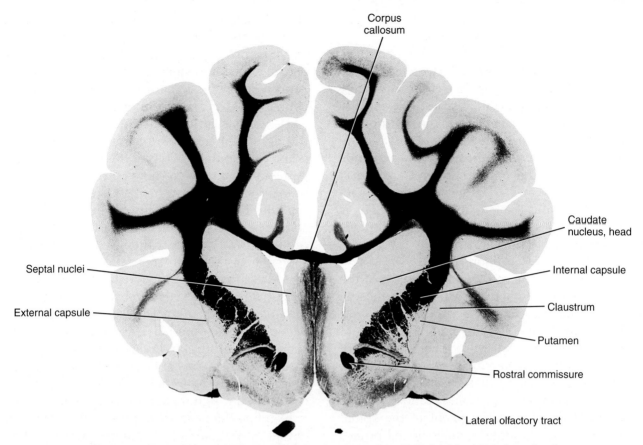

Corpus
callosum

Caudate
nucleus, head

Septal nuclei

Internal capsule

Claustrum

External capsule

Putamen

Rostral commissure

Lateral olfactory tract

Fig. 6-32   (From Singer M: *The brain of the dog in section,* Philadelphia, 1962, Saunders.)

The roof of the fourth ventricle caudal to the cerebellum is the **caudal medullary velum**. It is a thin layer composed of ependyma lining the ventricle and a supporting layer of vascularized pia. It attaches to the cerebellum rostrally. This attachment is in the midventral portion of the cerebellum between the rostral and caudal ventral portions of the vermis. This velum attaches to the caudal cerebellar peduncle and the fasciculus gracilis laterally and caudally. Its attachment caudally at the apex is known as the **obex**. At this level the fourth ventricle is continuous with the central canal of the spinal cord.

At the level of the eighth cranial nerve, dorsal to the acoustic stria, there is an opening in the caudal medullary velum known as the **lateral aperture** of the fourth ventricle (see Fig. 6-1). The cerebrospinal fluid produced in the ventricular system communicates with the subarachnoid space of the meninges via this aperture. It then courses through the subarachnoid space over the entire surface of the brain and spinal cord and is absorbed into the venous system. Most of this absorption occurs where the arachnoid is in close apposition to the cerebral venous sinuses and

where it has formed specialized structures known as *arachnoid villi.* Cerebrospinal fluid is also absorbed from the subarachnoid space, where the spinal nerves leave the vertebral canal through the intervertebral foramina, and along the olfactory and prechiasmatic optic tracts.

The choroid plexus of the fourth ventricle bulges into the lumen of the ventricle on each side of the dorsal midline. Each plexus extends outward through the lateral recess and aperture, where it was seen caudal to the cerebellum before the latter was removed.

Examine the dorsal surface of the myelencephalon caudal to the fourth ventricle. The structures to be observed can be more easily recognized if the pia arachnoid is removed and the medulla is examined under a dissecting microscope. The median groove is the **dorsal median sulcus**. The narrow longitudinal bulge flanking the sulcus is the **fasciculus gracilis** (see Fig. 6-10). This longitudinal tract courses cranially the entire length of the spinal cord in this position. At the caudal end of the myelencephalon, it ends at the **nucleus gracilis**.

This nucleus is located at the caudal end of the fourth ventricle, where the fasciculus widens and ends. This fasciculus and nucleus function primarily in pelvic limb proprioception.

The groove lateral to the fasciculus gracilis is the **dorsal intermediate sulcus**. The longitudinal bulge lateral to this is the **fasciculus cuneatus**. This tract also courses cranially on the dorsal aspect of the spinal cord, starting in the midthoracic region. The fasciculus cuneatus diverges laterally at the caudal end of the fourth ventricle and ends in a slight bulge. This bulge represents the **lateral cuneate nucleus** and is known as the **cuneate tubercle**. Rostrally, the lateral cuneate nucleus is continuous with the caudal cerebellar peduncle. This fasciculus and nucleus primarily function in thoracic limb proprioception.

The groove on the caudodorsal surface of the myelencephalon lateral to the fasciculus cuneatus is the **dorsolateral sulcus**.

The longitudinal bulge lateral to it is the **spinal tract of the trigeminal nerve** (see Figs. 6-10, 6-34). The axons in this tract are from sensory cell bodies in the trigeminal ganglion that supply the head. The trigeminal tract extends caudally to the level of the first cervical segment of the spinal cord because of the large number of cell bodies serving its extensive peripheral distribution in the head. This tract emerges on the lateral surface of the myelencephalon caudal to a band of obliquely ascending fibers, the **superficial arcuate** fibers. The arcuate fibers connect structures in the medulla with the caudal cerebellar peduncle.

The dorsal rootlets of the spinal cord enter through the dorsolateral sulcus along the spinal cord.

Telencephalon (Cerebrum)

The left cerebral hemisphere was previously removed (see Fig. 6-34) by cutting the rostral commissure, corpus callosum, and hippocampal commissure; separating the two halves of the body of the fornix on the median plane; and sectioning the internal capsule, which attached the cerebral hemisphere to the thalamus of the brain stem.

There are three commissural pathways crossing between the hemispheres, one for each phylogenetic division of the cerebrum. The corpus callosum connects the neopallial portion of each hemisphere and is the largest of the three pathways. The rostral commissure connects the paleopallial or olfactory components of each hemisphere. The hippocampal commissure is small and is located just caudal to the junction of the crus of each fornix. This connects the archipallial components of each hemisphere. The internal capsule consists of projection fibers that course between the brain stem and cerebral hemisphere. Association fibers remain within the hemisphere, coursing between adjacent or distant gyri.

The **corpus callosum** (see Figs. 6-11, 6-12, 6-33 through 6-35) consists of a rostral genu, middle body, and caudal splenium. It is the commissural pathway for axons crossing between the neopallium of each cerebral hemisphere. The **internal capsule** (Fig. 6-36) contains projection fibers that course between the telencephalon and the diencephalon and course caudally from the telencephalon to the brain stem and the spinal cord. The fibers that were previously seen in the mesencephalon as the crus cerebri descend through the internal capsule. The projection pathway of most sensory modalities to the cerebrum for conscious perception involves synapses in the thalamus. The axons of these thalamic cell bodies then enter the internal capsule to reach the cerebrum through thalamocortical fibers.

Examine the isolated left cerebral hemisphere. On its medial surface, locate the portions of the corpus callosum and note the thin vertical sheet of tissue ventral to the corpus callosum. This is the **septum pellucidum,** which is more developed rostrally where it extends from the genu to the rostral commissure. A thickening in the septum dorsal and rostral to the rostral commissure represents the **septal nuclei**. Caudal to the rostral commissure, the septum attaches the corpus callosum to a column of fibers that courses rostrally and then descends in a rostroventral curve caudal to the rostral commissure. These fibers are part of the **fornix**. They connect the hippocampus with the diencephalon and rostral cerebrum. The hippocampus is a specialized region of cerebral cortex that will be seen shortly. Cut the septum pellucidum to separate the corpus callosum from the fornix. The fornix begins caudally by the accumulation of fibers on the lateral side of the hippocampus. These form the **crus of the fornix**. The crura join rostral to the hippocampus and dorsal to the thalamus to form the **body of the fornix**.

The body of the fornix courses rostrally and then descends rostroventrally as the **column of the fornix**. At the rostral commissure, some fibers course dorsal and rostral to the rostral commissure, but most course caudal to the commissure and continue caudoventrally, lateral to the third

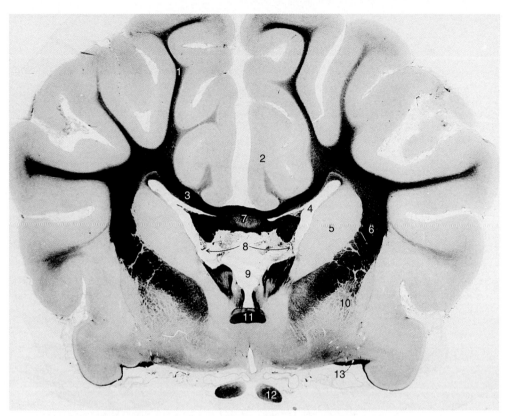

Fig. 6-33 Rostral telencephalon. (The white matter is stained with iron hematoxylin and appears black in the photograph.)

1. Corona radiata
2. Cingulate gyrus
3. Corpus callosum
4. Lateral ventricle
5. Caudate nucleus
6. Internal capsule
7. Body of fornix
8. Interventricular foramen
9. Third ventricle
10. Lentiform nucleus
11. Rostral commissure
12. Prechiasmatic optic tract
13. Lateral olfactory tract

ventricle, to reach the mamillary body of the hypothalamus. This caudally projecting column may be more evident on the intact right cerebral hemisphere. In the left cerebral hemisphere, pierce the septum and separate the corpus callosum from the column and body of the fornix.

The curved cavity exposed lateral to the septum pellucidum and ventral to the corpus callosum is the **lateral ventricle**. It communicates with the third ventricle of the diencephalon by the **interventricular foramen** (see Figs. 6-11, 6-13, 6-33), which is located caudal to the column of the fornix at the level of the rostral commissure. The caudodorsal wall of this foramen is the roof plate and choroid plexus of the third ventricle. This is usually pulled free and lost when the brain is removed.

Locate the caudal part of the lateral rhinal sulcus in the left temporal lobe. Cut through this sulcus into the lateral ventricle. The smooth,

curved bulge exposed in the wall of the ventricle is the caudal surface of the hippocampus as it courses in a dorsorostral curve.

To remove the hippocampus intact from the left lateral ventricle, cut the column of the fornix dorsal to the rostral commissure on the medial side. Grasp the fornix with the forceps and, with the blunt end of the scalpel, gently roll the hippocampus out of the lateral ventricle. Its attachment ventrally in the temporal horn may be cut to free the hippocampus completely.

Phylogenetically, the cerebral cortex can be divided into three regions: paleopallium, neopallium, and archipallium. The paleopallium consists of the cortex of the olfactory peduncle. This is separated laterally from the neopallium by the rhinal sulcus. The neopallium includes all of the gyri on the external surface of the cerebrum. The **hippocampus** belongs to the archipallium and is an internal gyrus of the telencephalon that has been rolled

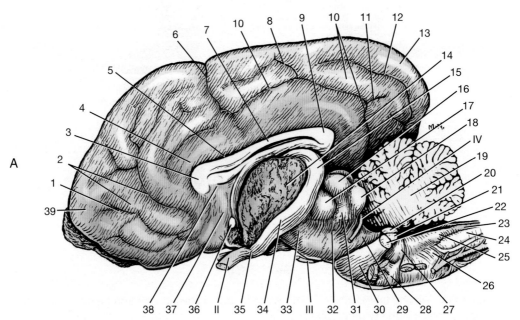

Fig. 6-34   A, Medial surface of right cerebral hemisphere and lateral surface of brain stem.
(**A** From Evans HE: *Miller's anatomy of the dog,* ed 3, Philadelphia, 1993, Saunders.)

1. Ectogenual sulcus
2. Genual sulcus and gyrus
3. Genu of corpus callosum
4. Cingulate gyrus
5. Callosal sulcus
6. Cruciate sulcus
7. Body of corpus callosum
8. Ramus of splenial sulcus
9. Splenium of corpus callosum
10. Splenial sulcus and gyrus
11. Caudal horizontal ramus of splenial sulcus
12. Suprasplenial sulcus
13. Occipital gyrus
14. Cut internal capsule between cerebral hemisphere and brain stem
15. Postchiasmatic optic tract at lateral geniculate nucleus
16. Rostral colliculus
17. Medial geniculate nucleus
18. Caudal colliculus
19. Arbor vitae cerebelli
20. Rostral cerebellar peduncle
21. Caudal cerebellar peduncle
22. Middle cerebellar peduncle
23. Fasciculus cuneatus
24. Spinal tract of trigeminal nerve
25. Lateral cuneate nucleus
26. Superficial arcuate fibers
27. Cochlear nuclei
28. Trapezoid body
29. Lateral lemniscus
30. Transverse fibers of pons
31. Brachium of caudal colliculus
32. Transverse crural tract
33. Crus cerebri
34. Postchiasmatic optic tract
35. Optic chiasm
36. Rostral commissure
37. Paraterminal gyrus
38. Septum pellucidum
39. Frontal gyrus
   II. Prechiasmatic optic tract
   III. Oculomotor nerve
   IV. Trochlear nerve

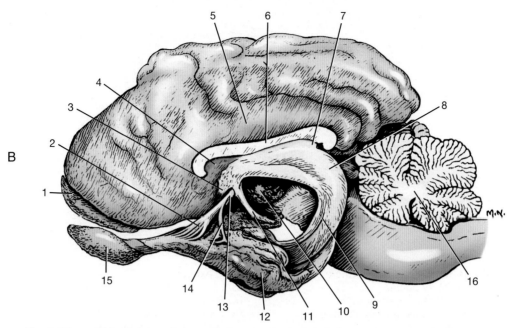

Fig. 6-34, cont'd   B, Lateral view of a brain with the left half removed except for most of the left rhinencephalon.

1. Right olfactory bulb
2. Rostral part of the rostral commissure
3. Precommissural fornix
4. Telencephalic septum
5. Medial surface of right cerebral hemisphere
6. Corpus callosum
7. Dorsal commissure of fornix
8. Alveus of hippocampus

9. Fimbria of hippocampus
10. Interthalamic adhesion
11. Column of fornix
12. Piriform lobe (from dorsal side)
13. Rostral commissure
14. Caudal part of rostral commissure
15. Left olfactory bulb
16. Cerebellar medulla

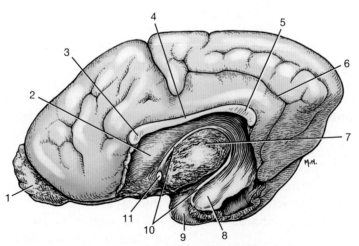

Fig. 6-35   Medial view of a right cerebral hemisphere with medial structures removed to show lateral ventricle. The rostral horn of the ventricle is bounded laterally by the caudate nucleus (2). The distal part of the temporal horn is bounded laterally by the amygdala (8); elsewhere, the ventricle is bounded by white matter.

1. Olfactory bulb
2. Caudate nucleus
3. Genu of corpus callosum
4. Body of corpus callosum
5. Splenium of corpus callosum
6. Splenial sulcus

7. Internal capsule
8. Amygdaloid body
9. Piriform lobe
10. Stria terminalis
11. Rostral commissure

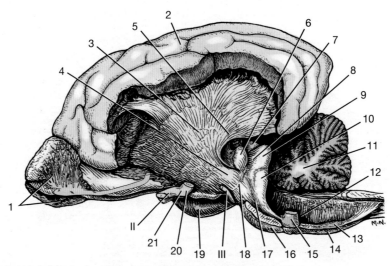

Fig. 6-36 Lateral view of the brain, internal capsule exposed.

1. Olfactory bulbs
2. Left cerebral hemisphere
3. Internal capsule (lateral view)
4. Crus cerebri
5. Acoustic radiation
6. Medial geniculate nucleus
7. Rostral colliculus
8. Brachium of caudal colliculus
9. Caudal colliculus
10. Lateral lemniscus
11. Cerebellum—arbor vitae
12. Location of dorsal nucleus of trapezoid body
13. Location of olivary nucleus
14. Pyramid
15. Trapezoid body
16. Transverse fibers of pons
17. Pyramidal and corticopontine tracts (longitudinal fibers of pons)
18. Transverse crural tract
19. Piriform lobe
20. Optic tract (cut to show internal capsule)
21. Optic chiasm
    II. Prechiasmatic optic tract
    III. Oculomotor nerve

into the lateral ventricle by the lateral expansion of the neopallium. Notice that the hippocampus begins ventrally in the temporal lobe and curves, first caudodorsally and then rostrodorsally, over the diencephalon to reach its caudodorsal aspect. At that point the hippocampus ends, and a **hippocampal commissure** connects the hippocampus of each cerebral hemisphere. The fibers of the hippocampus continue rostrally as the body and column of the fornix. Notice the crus of the fornix on its lateral surface. Place the previously removed hippocampus over the exposed left diencephalon to see its normal relationship with that structure. They are normally separated by arachnoid trabeculae and the subarachnoid space.

Attached to the lateral free edge of the crus of the fornix is a network of blood vessels covered by meninges and ependyma. This is the **choroid plexus of the lateral ventricle**. Its anatomical structure is the same as that of the choroid plexus of the third and fourth ventricles. The surface of the choroid plexus that faces the lumen of the ventricle is the ependymal layer derived from

the embryonic neural tube. This layer of ependyma is attached on one side to the free edge of the fornix. To complete the wall of the lumen of the lateral ventricle, it must be attached on its other side. This attachment is to a small tract, the **stria terminalis,** located in the groove between the thalamus and the caudate nucleus (Figs. 6-10, 6-35). The stria terminalis is a small tract that connects the amygdala with the septal nuclei. This layer of ependyma from the stria terminalis to the fornix forms part of the medial wall of the lateral ventricle. Branches of the middle and caudal cerebral arteries covered by pia push this layer of ependyma into the lumen of the lateral ventricle. The result is the formation of a choroid plexus that is continuous with the choroid plexus of the third ventricle at the interventricular foramen (Fig. 6-1).

Examine the **rostral commissure** (Figs. 6-11, 6-33 through 6-35). On each side this commissure connects rostrally to the olfactory peduncles and caudally to the piriform lobes.

In each cerebral hemisphere the neuronal cell bodies are located either on the surface in the

cerebral cortex or deep to the surface in a **basal nucleus**. Examine the floor of the lateral ventricle of the removed left hemisphere. The bulge that enlarges rostrally is the **caudate nucleus**. This is one of the subcortical basal nuclei of the telencephalon, a part of the corpus striatum. Its rostral extremity is the head. Caudal to this the body rapidly narrows into a small tail, which courses over the internal capsule fibers in the floor of the ventricle. With the blunt end of a scalpel, free the caudate nucleus from the medial side of the internal capsule.

Dorsolateral to the caudate nucleus, the internal capsule forms the lateral angle of the lateral ventricle. At the dorsolateral angle of the lateral ventricle, the fibers of the internal capsule meet those of the corpus callosum. Arising from this interdigitation of fibers, the **corona radiata** radiates in all directions to reach the gray matter of the cerebral cortex. A longitudinal section of the cerebral hemisphere in the dorsal plane at the level of this interdigitation reveals a mass of white matter in the center of the hemisphere. This mass is referred to as the **centrum semiovale**.

Remove the pia and arachnoid from the surface of the right cerebral hemisphere. Expose the corona radiata by removing the gray matter, the cerebral cortex, with the scalpel handle. Begin this removal of gray matter on the medial side of the hemisphere. The cingulate gyrus is located dorsal to the corpus callosum. Remove the gray matter of the cingulate gyrus to expose its fibers, which form the **cingulum**. Many of the fibers in the cingulum are long association fibers that course longitudinally from one end of the hemisphere to the other. Demonstrate this by freeing some fibers rostral to the genu of the corpus callosum and by stripping them caudally. Remove the cingulum and demonstrate the transverse course of the fibers of the corpus callosum by stripping these from their cut edge toward the hemisphere.

Remove the gray matter from the gyri on the lateral surface of the rostral half of the cerebral hemisphere. Examine the white matter of the gyri. Short association fibers, the arcuate fibers, course between adjacent gyri.

The **internal capsule** is situated lateral to the caudate nucleus. Expose the lateral surface of the internal capsule (see Fig. 6-36).

When you have completed the dissection of the right cerebral hemisphere, all that remains are the corpus callosum, the internal capsule, and part of the corona radiata.

Remove the corpus callosum of the right cerebral hemisphere to expose the lateral ventricle, with the caudate nucleus on the floor rostrally and the hippocampus on the floor caudally. The internal capsule forms the lateral wall (see Figs. 6-12, 6-14, 6-33, 6-36).

Make a median section of the brain stem from the optic chiasm through the medulla (see Fig. 6-11). Observe the interthalamic adhesion and note the smooth surface of the third ventricle surrounding it. The ventricle is bounded dorsally by the roof plate between each stria habenularis. It connects rostrally with each lateral ventricle through the interventricular foramen, which is caudal to the column of the fornix and dorsal to the rostral commissure. Caudally, it is continuous with the mesencephalic aqueduct. Rostroventral to the interventricular foramen, the ventricle is bounded by the **lamina terminalis,** the most rostral extent of the embryonic neural tube on the median plane. (From this point each cerebral hemisphere develops laterally.) The third ventricle extends into the infundibulum of the pituitary gland as the **infundibular recess** (see Figs. 6-11, 6-13).

Follow the ventricular system caudally from the third ventricle into the mesencephalic aqueduct and into the fourth ventricle. Note that the roof of the fourth ventricle consists of the rostral medullary velum, the cerebellum, and the caudal medullary velum. The choroid plexus of the fourth ventricle is formed in the caudal medullary velum. The fourth ventricle continues into the central canal of the spinal cord at the obex.

Functional and structural correlates of the nervous system are listed in Table 6-1.

SPINAL CORD

If a prepared dissection of the spinal cord is not available, do a complete laminectomy by removing all of the vertebral arches and the attached muscles from your specimen to expose the spinal cord. Observe the spinal cord with its dural covering. Between the dura of the spinal cord and the periosteum of the vertebrae is the **epidural space,** which contains loose connective tissue, fat, and blood vessels.

The spinal cord is divided into segments (Fig. 6-37). A group of dorsal and ventral rootlets

Table **6-1**	Functional and Structural Correlates of the Nervous System
Neuroanatomical Structure	**Function**
Frontal lobe	Behavior
Frontoparietal lobe (sensorimotor cortex)	Upper motor neuron (central motor system) Conscious perception of somatic, visceral, and proprioceptive sensations
Temporal lobe	Behavior, hearing, balance
Occipital lobe	Vision
Olfactory bulb, peduncle, tract, piriform lobe	Olfaction—smell
Pons—transverse fibers	Pathway from cerebrum to cerebellum
Middle cerebellar peduncle	Pathway from pontine nuclei to cerebellum
Rostral cerebellar peduncle	Pathway from cerebellum to brain stem and cerebrum
Caudal cerebellar peduncle	Pathway from spinal cord and medulla with vestibular proprioceptive systems to cerebellum
Mamillary bodies	Limbic system (behavior)
Crus cerebri	Pathway from cerebrum to brain stem and spinal cord—upper motor neuron, and from cerebrum to cerebellum via pons
Internal capsule	Pathway between cerebrum and brain stem—upper motor neuron and thalamocortical projections—sensory and motor, and from cerebrum to cerebellum via pons
Hypothalamus	Visceral functions Autonomic nervous system Limbic system Pituitary control
Lateral geniculate nucleus	Visual system (conscious perception)
Rostral colliculus	Visual system (reflexes)
Medial geniculate nucleus	Auditory system (conscious perception)
Caudal colliculus Brachium of caudal colliculus Lateral lemniscus Trapezoid body Acoustic stria Cochlear nuclei	Auditory system (reflexes and conscious perception)
Pyramid Corticospinal tracts	Upper motor neuron
Fasciculus gracilis Nucleus gracilis	Pelvic limb—conscious pathway of general proprioception
Fasciculus cuneatus Medial cuneate nucleus Lateral cuneate nucleus	Thoracic limb—general proprioception Conscious perception pathway Cerebellar pathway
Spinal tract of trigeminal nerve	Projection pathway of somatic afferent sensation from head
Septal nuclei	Limbic system
Fornix—hippocampus	Limbic system
Cingulum	Limbic system
Caudate nucleus	Upper motor neuron
Lentiform nucleus	Upper motor neuron
Stria habenularis	Limbic system
Habenular nucleus	Limbic system

leave each spinal cord segment on each side and combine, respectively, to form the **spinal nerve** at the level of the intervertebral foramen. Note the **spinal ganglia** in the intervertebral foramina (Figs. 6-37 through 6-39).

There are 8 cervical spinal cord segments, 13 thoracic, 7 lumbar, 3 sacral, and about 5 caudal.

The first cervical spinal nerves leave the vertebral canal through the lateral vertebral foramen in the arch of the atlas. The second cervical spinal nerves leave caudal to the atlas. The cervical spinal nerves of segments 3 through 7 leave the vertebral canal through the intervertebral foramina cranial to the vertebra of the same number. The

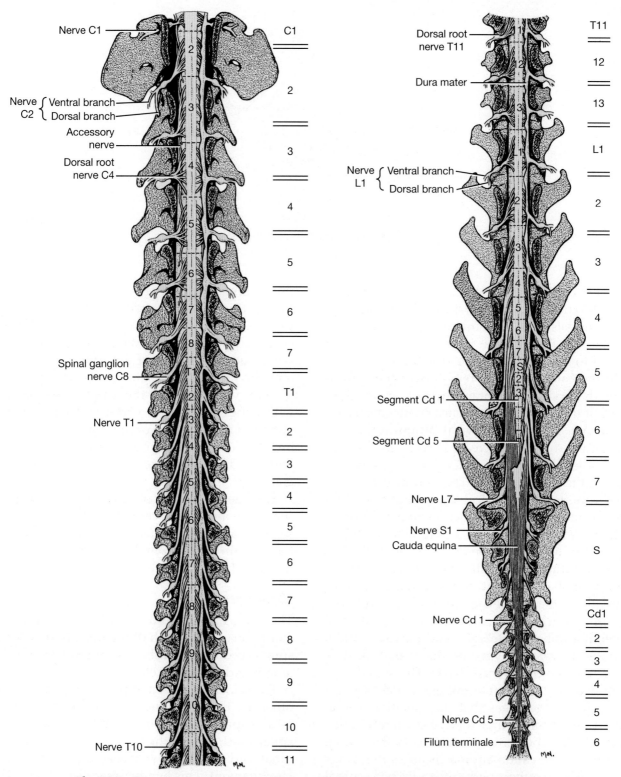

Fig. 6-37 Dorsal roots of spinal nerves and spinal cord segments. Dorsal view, vertebral arches removed. Dura removed on left side of both figures. (Figures on the right represent levels of vertebral bodies. On the right side the nerves are covered with epineurium so they are not yellow.)

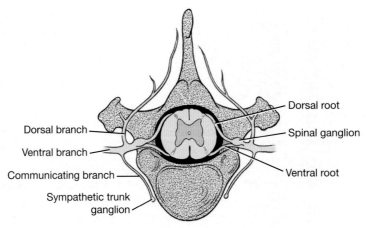

Fig. 6-38   Diagram of spinal nerve.

spinal nerves of the eighth cervical segment pass caudal to the seventh (last) cervical vertebra. The spinal nerves of all the remaining spinal cord segments pass through the intervertebral foramina caudal to the vertebra of the same number.

In the caudal cervical region over the fifth to seventh cervical vertebrae, there is an enlargement of the spinal cord that nearly fills the vertebral canal. This is the **cervical intumescence**. Its presence is due to an increase in white matter and cell bodies that are associated with the innervation of the thoracic limb. This intumescence occurs from the sixth cervical segment of the spinal cord through the first thoracic segment. Another enlargement occurs in the midlumbar vertebral region for the innervation of the pelvic limb. The **lumbar intumescence** that begins at about the fourth lumbar segment and gradually narrows caudally as the spinal cord comes to an end near the intervertebral space between the sixth and seventh lumbar vertebrae. The narrow caudal end of the parenchyma of the spinal cord is known as the **conus medullaris**. The spinal cord terminates in the **filum terminale,** which is a narrow cord of meninges that may include a long extension of the neural tube and central canal. This attaches the conus medullaris to the caudal vertebrae. The **cauda equina** includes the conus medullaris together with the adjacent caudal lumbar, sacral, and caudal roots that extend caudally in the vertebral canal.

Observe the relationship of the spinal cord segments to the corresponding vertebrae. The only spinal cord segments that are found entirely within their corresponding vertebrae are the last two thoracic and the first two (or occasionally three) lumbar segments. All other spinal cord segments reside in the vertebral canal cranial to the vertebra of the same number (see Fig. 6-37). This is most pronounced in the caudal lumbar and sacrocaudal segments of the spinal cord. In general, the three sacral segments lie within the fifth lumbar vertebra and the caudal segments lie within the sixth lumbar vertebra. There is a breed variation in the length of the spinal cord. In small breeds it extends about one vertebra farther caudally, and in large breeds one vertebra farther cranially.

The nerve roots of the first 10 thoracic segments and those caudal to the third lumbar segment are long because of the distance between their origin at the spinal cord and their passage through the intervertebral foramen (see Fig. 6-37).

Meninges

The thick, fibrous dura may be cut longitudinally along the entire length of the dorsal aspect of the spinal cord to reveal the dorsal rootlets and their length at different levels.

The thin arachnoid and pia are apposed to each other in the embalmed specimen and remain on the spinal cord. On the lateral surface of the spinal cord, the pia thickens and forms a longitudinal cord of connective tissue called the **denticulate ligament**. This ligament segmentally attaches to the arachnoid and dura laterally, midway between the roots of adjacent spinal cord segments (see Fig. 6-39).

Vessels

There is a longitudinal **ventral spinal artery** and one or two dorsal spinal arteries on the spinal

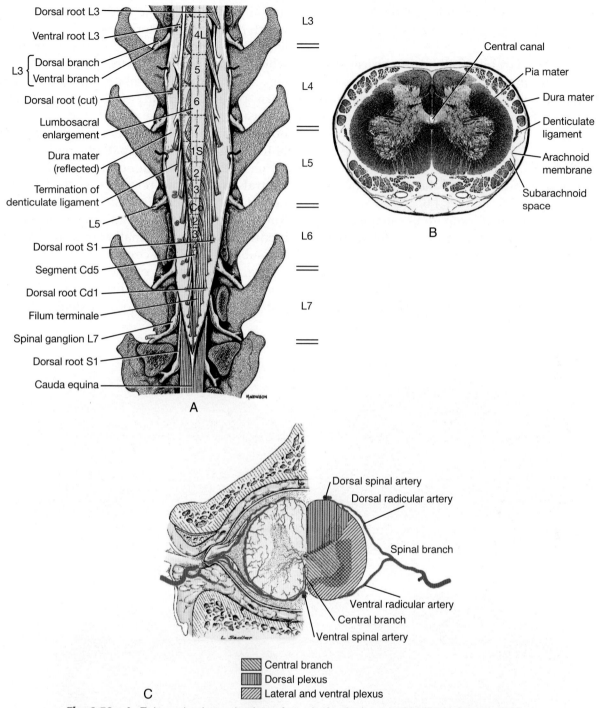

Dorsal root L3
Ventral root L3
L3 { Dorsal branch
      Ventral branch
Dorsal root (cut)
Lumbosacral enlargement
Dura mater (reflected)
Termination of denticulate ligament
L5
Dorsal root S1
Segment Cd5
Dorsal root Cd1
Filum terminale
Spinal ganglion L7
Dorsal root S1
Cauda equina

A

L3
L4
L5
L6
L7

Central canal
Pia mater
Dura mater
Denticulate ligament
Arachnoid membrane
Subarachnoid space

B

Dorsal spinal artery
Dorsal radicular artery
Spinal branch
Ventral radicular artery
Central branch
Ventral spinal artery

Central branch
Dorsal plexus
Lateral and ventral plexus

C

Fig. 6-39 A, Enlarged schematic view of terminal spinal cord with dura reflected. **B,** Enlarged transverse section of seventh lumbar segment. **C,** Arterial vasculature of the canine spinal cord. (Parts **A** and **B** courtesy Dr. Thomas Fletcher. Part **C** from Evans HE, de Lahunta A: *Miller's anatomy of the dog,* ed 4, St Louis, 2013, Saunders.)

cord. They are formed by **spinal branches** of the paired vertebral arteries in the cervical region, intercostal arteries in the thoracic region, and lumbar arteries in the lumbar region. The ventral spinal artery is continuous cranially with the basilar artery at the foramen magnum.

There are ventral internal vertebral venous plexuses on the floor of the vertebral canal in the epidural space (see Fig. 6-4). These were seen previously in the atlanto-occipital region to be continuous cranially with the basilar sinus, a branch of the sigmoid sinus. Anastomoses occur

---

[writing]

between the plexus of each side and the branches of the vertebral and azygos veins and caudal vena cava.

Although this is a bilaterally symmetrical segmental system, there is often considerable variation in the size of various segmental vessels, including an occasional absence of one or more vessels.

Transverse Sections

Study transverse sections of the spinal cord at segments C4, C8, T4, T12, L2, L6, and S1 under a dissecting microscope. Compare the shape of the gray matter of these segments and relate it to their areas of innervation (Fig. 6-40).

The gray matter of the spinal cord in transverse section is in the shape of a butterfly or the letter H. It consists primarily of neuronal cell bodies. The dorsal extremity on each side is the **dorsal horn**, which receives the entering dorsal (sensory) rootlets. The ventral extremity is the **ventral horn**, which sends axons out via the ventral (motor) rootlets. In the thoracolumbar region, the **lateral horn** projects laterally from the gray matter midway between the dorsal and ventral gray horns. This lateral horn contains the cell bodies of the preganglionic sympathetic neurons. In the center of the gray matter of the spinal cord is the **central canal**. This remnant of the embryonic neural tube is continuous rostrally with the fourth ventricle. At the caudal end of the conus medullaris, there is a small communication with the subarachnoid space.

The white matter of the spinal cord can be divided into three pairs of funiculi. Dorsally, a shallow, longitudinal groove extends the entire

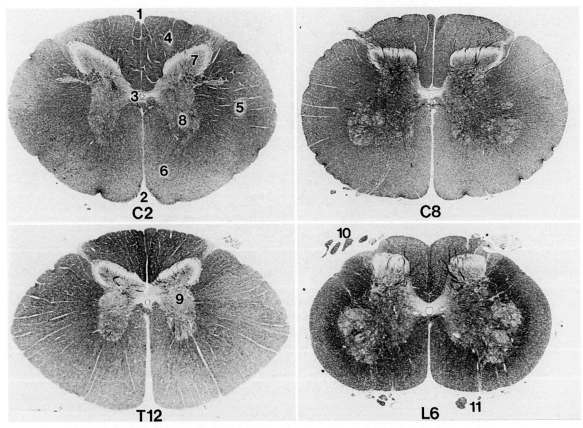

Fig. 6-40   Transverse section of spinal cord: second cervical segment (C2), eighth cervical segment (C8), twelfth thoracic segment (T12), and sixth lumbar segment (L6).

1. Dorsal median sulcus
2. Ventral median fissure
3. Central canal
4. Dorsal funiculus
5. Lateral funiculus
6. Ventral funiculus
7. Dorsal gray horn
8. Ventral gray horn
9. Lateral gray horn
10. Dorsal rootlets
11. Ventral rootlets

length of the spinal cord. This is the **dorsal median sulcus**. The longitudinal furrow along which the dorsal rootlets enter the spinal cord is the **dorsolateral sulcus**. Between these two sulci is the **dorsal funiculus** of the spinal cord.

Between the dorsolateral sulcus and the line of exit of the ventral rootlets, the **ventrolateral sulcus,** is located the **lateral funiculus**. The **ventral funiculus** is the white matter between the line of exit of the ventral rootlets and the longitudinal groove on the ventral side of the spinal cord, the **ventral median fissure**. In some species the funiculi have been subdivided topographically into specific cranially and caudally projecting tracts. Such anatomical information in domestic animals is still incomplete.

Bibliography

Adams, D.R. 2003. Canine Anatomy: A Systemic Study, 4th ed., Ames, Iowa State Press.

Anderson, W.D. & Anderson, B.G. 1994. Atlas of Canine Anatomy, Philadelphia, Lea & Febiger.

Auton, J.M.V. et al. 2000. Atlas de Anatomia perro y gato Clinica, AG Novograf, SA.

Barone, R. 2000. Anatomie Comparée des Mammifères Domestiques, 7 vols, Paris, Vigor Frères.fa.

Boyd, J.S. et al. 1991. A Color Atlas of Clinical Anatomy of the Dog and Cat, London, Wolf Pub. Ltd.

Budras K.-D. et al. 2002. Anatomy of the Dog, 4th ed., Hannover, Germany, Schlutersche GmbH & Co.

Constantinescu, G.M. 2002. Clinical Anatomy for Small Animal Practitioners, Ames, Iowa State Press.

Coulson, A. & Lewis, N. 2002. Interpretive Radiographic Anatomy of the Dog & Cat, Oxford, Blackwell Sci.

deLahunta, A., Glass, E. & Kent, M. 2015. Veterinary Neuroanatomy and Clinical Neurology, 4th ed., St. Louis, Elsevier.

deLahunta, A. & Habel, R.E. 1986. Applied Veterinary Anatomy, Philadelphia, Saunders.

Dyce K., Sack, W. & Wensing, C. 2002. Textbook of Veterinary Anatomy, 3rd ed., Philadelphia, Saunders.

Evans, HE. 1974. Prenatal Development of the Dog, Ithaca, NY, Twenty fourth Gaines Veterinary Symposium.

Evans, H.E. and de Lahunta, A. 2013. Miller's Anatomy of the Dog, 4th ed., St. Louis, Elsevier.

Evans, H. & deLahunta, A. 2010. Guide to the Dissection of the Dog, 7th ed., Philadelphia, Saunders (also published in Spanish, Japanese, Portuguese, Korean, and Chinese).

Feeney, D., Fletcher, T. & Hardy, B. 1991. Atlas of Correlative Imaging Anatomy of the Normal Dog, Philadelphia, Saunders.

Frewein, J. & Vollmerhaus, B. 1994. Anatomie von Hund und Katze, Berlin, Blackwell.

Konig, H. & Liebich, H-G. 2004. Veterinary Anatomy of Domestic Mammals, Schattauer, GmbH, Stuttgart.

Maggs, D. et al. 2008. Slater's Fundamentals of Veterinary Ophthalmology, 4th ed., Philadelphia, Saunders, Elsevier.

Noden, D.M. & deLahunta, A. 1985. The Embryology of Domestic Animals: Developmental Mechanisms and Malformations, Baltimore, Williams & Wilkins.

Nomina Anatomica Veterinaria (NAV) [electronic resource]. 2005, World Assoc. of Veterinary Anatomists, 5th ed., Knoxville, TN, International Committee on Gross Anatomical Nomenclature.

Pasquini, S. & Pasquini, C. 2009. Dog and Cat Dissection Guide: A Regional Approach, Pilot Point, Tex, Sudz Publishing.

Popesko, P. 1977. Atlas of Topographical Anatomy of the Domestic Animals, 2nd ed., Philadelphia, Saunders.

Ruberte, J. et al. 1995-1996. Atlas de Anatomia del Perro y del Gato, 3 vols, Univ. Autonoma de Barcelona.

Schaller, O. 1992. Illustrated Veterinary Anatomical Nomenclature, Stuttgart, Enke Verlag.

Schebitz, H. & Wilkins, H. 1986. Atlas of Radiographic Anatomy of the Dog and Cat, 4th ed., Berlin, Verlag Paul Parey.

Singer, M. 1962. The Brain of the Dog in Section, Philadelphia, Saunders.

Terminologia Anatomica (TA). 1998. Federative Comm. on Anatomical Terminology, Stuttgart, Thieme.

Index

Page numbers followed by *f* indicate figures; *t*, tables; *b*, boxes.